MRI From Picture to Proton

MRI *from Picture to Proton* presents the basics of MR practice and theory as the practitioner first meets them. The subject is approached intuitively: starting from the images, equipment and scanning protocols, rather than pages of dry physics theory. The reader is brought face-to-face with issues pertinent to practice immediately, filling in the theoretical background as their scanning experience grows. Key ideas are introduced in an intuitive manner which is faithful to the underlying physics but avoids the need for difficult or distracting mathematics. Additional explanations for the more technically inquisitive are given in optional secondary text boxes. Informal in style, informed in content, written by experienced teachers, MRI from Picture to Proton is an essential text for the student of MR whatever their background: medical, technical or scientific.

Donald W. McRobbie is Head of Radiological and MR Physics in the Radiological Sciences Unit, the Hammersmith Hospitals NHS Trust and Senior Lecturer in Imaging at Imperial College London.

Elizabeth A. Moore is MR Clinical Scientist for Philips Medical Systems UK.

Martin J. Graves is Consultant Clinical Scientist in the Department of Radiology at the University of Cambridge Hospitals NHS Foundation Trust.

Martin R. Prince is Professor of Radiology at Columbia College of Physicians and Surgeons and at Weill Medical College of Cornell University as well as Chief of MRI at New York Hospital.

D1579730

MRI From Picture to Proton

Second edition

Donald W. McRobbie

Elizabeth A. Moore

Martin J. Graves and

Martin R. Prince

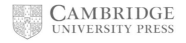
CAMBRIDGE
UNIVERSITY PRESS

CAMBRIDGE UNIVERSITY PRESS
Cambridge, New York, Melbourne, Madrid, Cape Town, Singapore, São Paulo, Delhi

Cambridge University Press
The Edinburgh Building, Cambridge CB2 8RU, UK

Pulished in the United States of America by Cambridge University Press, New York

www.cambridge.org
Information on this title: www.cambridge.org/9780521865272

First published 2003
Reprinted 2004
Second edition 2007
Reprinted 2008

Printed in the United Kingdom at the University Press, Cambridge

A catalogue record for this publication is available from the British Library

ISBN 978-0-521-86527-2 hardback
ISBN 978-0-521-68384-5 paperback

Cover illustrations: courtesy of Siemens Medical Solutions

To Fiona, Laura and Andrew
DWMcR

To all the people who kept asking me when this book would be written
EAM

To Philippa, Sophie, Katie and Chloe
MJG

To my brilliant colleagues, fellows, residents and technologists who have taught me the art of MRI
MRP

Contents

Acknowledgements   xi

1   MR: What's the attraction?   1
    1.1   It's not rocket science, but I like it   1
    1.2   A brief history of medical imaging   2
    1.3   How to use this book   4
    Further reading   7

Part A   The basic stuff

2   Early daze: your first week in MR   11
    2.1   Introduction   11
    2.2   Welcome to the MR unit   11
    2.3   Safety first   15
    2.4   The patient's journey   18
    2.5   Basic clinical protocols   19
    2.6   A week in the life of an MRI radiographer   27
    Further reading   29

3   Seeing is believing: introduction to image contrast   30
    3.1   Introduction   30
    3.2   Some basic stuff   31
    3.3 T_1-weighted images   32
    3.4 T_2-weighted images   33
    3.5   PD-weighted images   35
    3.6   GE T_1-weighted images   36
    3.7   GE $T_2{}^*$-weighted images   38
    3.8   GE PD-weighted images   40
    3.9   STIR images   40
    3.10   FLAIR images   41
    3.11   Contrast agents   42

Contents

3.12 Angiographic images 44
Further reading 46

4 The devil's in the detail: pixels, matrices and slices 47
4.1 Introduction 47
4.2 Digital and analogue images 47
4.3 Matrices, pixels and an introduction to resolution 51
4.4 Slices and orientations 57
4.5 Displaying images 57
4.6 What do the pixels represent? 58
4.7 From 2D to 3D 61
Further reading 64

5 What you set is what you get: basic image optimization 65
5.1 Introduction 65
5.2 Looking on the bright side: what are we trying to optimize? 65
5.3 Trading places: resolution, SNR and scan time 69
5.4 Ever the optimist: practical steps to optimization 74
Further reading 78

6 Improving your image: how to avoid artefacts 79
6.1 Introduction 79
6.2 Keep still please: gross patient motion 79
6.3 Physiological motion 80
6.4 Motion artefacts from flow 86
6.5 Lose the fat! 89
6.6 Partial volume artefact and cross-talk 96
6.7 Phase sampling artefacts 98
6.8 Susceptibility and metal artefacts 101
6.9 Equipment artefacts 103
6.10 What's causing this artefact? 107
Further reading 107

7 Spaced out: spatial encoding 108
7.1 Introduction 108
7.2 Anatomy of a pulse sequence 108
7.3 From Larmor to Fourier via gradients 109
7.4 Something to get excited about: the image slice 113
7.5 In-plane localization 117
7.6 Consequences of Fourier imaging 129
7.7 Speeding it up 133
7.8 3D FT 135
Further reading 136

8 Getting in tune: resonance and relaxation 137
8.1 Introduction 137
8.2 Spinning nuclei 137
8.3 Measuring the magnetic moment 141
8.4 Creating echoes 144
8.5 Relaxation times 148
8.6 Relaxation time mechanisms 153
8.7 Measuring relaxation times *in vivo* 161
8.8 Contrast agent theory 162
Further reading 166

9 Let's talk technical: MR equipment 167
9.1 Introduction 167
9.2 Magnets 167
9.3 Gradients 173
9.4 RF system 175
9.5 Computer systems 188
9.6 Open MRI systems 188
9.7 Siting and installation 189
Further reading 191

10 But is it safe? Bio-effects 192
10.1 Introduction 192
10.2 RF effects 192
10.3 Gradient effects 194
10.4 Static field effects 197
Further reading 200

Part B The specialist stuff

11 Ghosts in the machine: quality control 203
11.1 Introduction 203
11.2 The quality cycle 204
11.3 Signal parameters 204
11.4 Geometric parameters 211

11.5 Relaxation parameters 216
11.6 Artefacts 217
11.7 Spectroscopic QA 218
Further reading 219

12 Acronyms anonymous: a guide to the pulse sequence jungle 220
12.1 Introduction 220
12.2 Getting above the trees: a sequences overview 220
12.3 RARING to go: SE-based techniques 222
12.4 Spoiled for choice: GE 235
12.5 Ultra-fast GE imaging 248
12.6 Pulse sequence conversion chart 255
Further reading 257

13 Go with the flow: MR angiography 258
13.1 Introduction 258
13.2 Effect of flow in conventional imaging techniques 258
13.3 TOF MRA 263
13.4 PC angiography 265
13.5 CE MRA 271
13.6 Novel contrast agents 279
Further reading 281

14 A heart to heart discussion: cardiac MRI 282
14.1 Introduction 282
14.2 Artefact challenges 282
14.3 Morphological imaging 285
14.4 Functional imaging 288
14.5 Cine phase-contrast velocity mapping 298
14.6 Myocardial perfusion imaging 300
14.7 Myocardial viability 303
14.8 Coronary artery imaging 304
Further reading 305

15 It's not just squiggles: *in vivo* spectroscopy 306
15.1 Introduction 306
15.2 Some basic chemistry 307
15.3 Single-voxel spectroscopy 310
15.4 Processing of single-voxel spectra 316
15.5 Chemical shift imaging 318
15.6 ^{31}P spectroscopy 319

15.7 Other nuclei 321
15.8 Hyperpolarized gases 322
Further reading 324

16 To BOLDly go: new frontiers 325
16.1 Introduction 325
16.2 EPI acquisition methods 325
16.3 Diffusion imaging 329
16.4 Perfusion imaging 335
16.5 Brain activation mapping using 341 the BOLD effect 340
Further reading 345

17 The parallel universe: parallel imaging and novel acquisition techniques 346
17.1 Introduction 346
17.2 Groundwork 346
17.3 Making SENSE: parallel imaging in image space 348
17.4 SMASH hits: parallel imaging in k-space 351
17.5 k-t BLAST 357
17.6 Clinical benefits of parallel imaging 359
17.7 Image quality in parallel imaging 360
17.8 Non-Cartesian acquisition schemes 364
17.9 Epilogue: the final frontier 371
Further reading 373

Appendix: maths revision 375
A.1 Vectors 375
A.2 Sine and cosine waves 376
A.3 Exponentials 377
A.4 Complex numbers 377
A.5 Simple Fourier analysis 378
A.6 Some useful constants 379

Index 381

Colour plates between pages 324 and 325.

Acknowledgements

We thank the following for assistance in providing images for this book (in alphabetical order): Mitchell Albert, Caroline Andrews, Janet De Wilde, Jo Hajnal, Andrew Heath, Franklyn Howe, Derek Jones, Steve Keevil, Debiao Li, David MacManus, Erin McKinstry, James F. M. Meaney, Annie Papadaki, Simon Pittard, Rebecca Quest, Erica Scurr, Annette Schmidt, Stefan Schoenberg, Julie Shepherd, Catriona Todd, Dennis Walkingshaw, Barry Whitnall, Ian Young, and Honglei Zhang.

The permission of the Department of Radiology, University of Cambridge and Addenbrooke's NHS Trust to reproduce certain figures and images is gratefully acknowledged.

Other images were kindly provided by the Hammersmith Hospitals NHS Trust and Chelsea and Westminster Hospital London, and by the Lysholm Department of Radiology, National Hospital for Neurology & Neurosurgery, London.

We also thank Erin McKinstry of the Department of Radiology, Brigham and Women's Hospital and Harvard Medical School, Boston, MA, for helpful comments on hyperpolarized gas imaging and Jeff Hayden of the American College of Radiology for guidance regarding the ACR Accreditation Program.

Our mystery radiographer is thanked for providing access to her diary.

Figures and material relating to the ACR Accreditation Program are reprinted with permission of the American College of Radiology, Reston, VA. No other representation of this material is authorized without express, written permission from the American College of Radiology.

The subject matter of this book may be covered by one or more patents. This book and the information contained therein and conveyed thereby should not be construed as either explicitly or implicitly granting any license; and no liability for patent infringement arising out of the use of the information is assumed.

We would like to thank Sarah Price for invaluable editorial fine tuning and the team at Cambridge University Press, especially Peter Silver, Lucille Murby and Jane Williams. Thanks also to Greg Brown for suggesting the title.

MR: What's the attraction?

1.1 It's not rocket science, but I like it

How would you impress a stranger you meet at a party with your intelligence? You might claim to be a brain surgeon or a rocket scientist. Well **M**agnetic **R**esonance (MR) is not rocket science, it's better. MR involves an amazing combination of advanced science and engineering, including the use of superconductivity, cryogenics, quantum physics, digital and computer technology – and all within the radiology department of your local hospital. MR imaging has evolved from unpromising beginnings in the 1970s to become nowadays the imaging method of choice for a large proportion of radiological examinations and the 'jewel in the crown' of medical technology. A modern MRI scanner is shown in figure 1.1.

So what is it? It is an imaging method based principally upon sensitivity to the presence and properties of water, which makes up 70% to 90% of most tissues. The properties and amount of water in tissue can alter dramatically with disease and injury which makes MR very sensitive as a diagnostic technique. MR detects subtle changes in the magnetism of the nucleus, the tiny entity that lies at the heart of the atom. This is probing deeper than X-rays, which interact with the clouds or shells of the electrons that orbit the nucleus. MR is a truly powerful modality. At its most advanced, MR can be used not just to image anatomy and pathology but to investigate organ function, to probe in vivo chemistry and even to visualize the brain thinking.

In the early days, the scanners were the domain of the physicists and engineers who invented and built them, and the technique was called NMR imaging (NMR stands for nuclear magnetic resonance). The cynics may say that the technique really took off clinically when the 'N-word' was dropped. This was sensible as the term 'nuclear', although scientifically accurate, implied a connection with nuclear energy and, in the last of the cold war years, resonated in the public's mind with the spectre of nuclear weapons.

Because of the diversity of sciences and technologies that gave birth to and continue to nurture MR, it is an extremely hard subject to learn. A lifetime is not enough to become expert in every aspect. Clinicians, technologists and scientists all struggle with the study of the

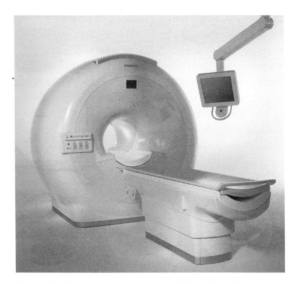

Figure 1.1 Modern superconducting MR system. Courtesy of Philips Medical Systems.

subject. The result is sometimes an obscurity of under-standing or a dilution of scientific truth resulting in mis-conceptions. This is why we have chosen to write this book. Our aim is to introduce you to MR as a tool – rather like learning to drive a car. Once you are confident on the road, we can then start to learn how the engine works.

1.2 A brief history of medical imaging

Radiology began after the accidental discovery of 'X-rays' by Roentgen in 1895. At about the same time (1896) Becquerel and the Curies were discovering radioactivity and radium and making possible the future development of nuclear medicine. Within a couple of years most of the basic techniques of radiog-raphy were established, e.g. the use of fluorescent screens (Pupin 1896), contrast media (Lindenthal 1896), even the principle of angiography. Early fluoroscopy entailed direct viewing from a fluorescent plate, i.e. putting your head in the main beam, a prac-tice frowned upon today! Unfortunately radiation pro-tection followed slightly too late for the pioneers of radiology. The next real technical breakthrough was the development of the image intensifier in the 1950s, but the basis of conventional radiography remained the same until the recent IT and digital revolutions. Computed Tomography (CT) was a huge breakthrough earning Hounsfield and Cormack the Nobel Prize for medicine and physiology in 1979. X-ray CT was unique in producing tomographic images or slices of the living human body for the first time and with a higher contrast than achievable by conventional planar techniques. The combination of a moving X-ray gantry and the computing power necessary to reconstruct from pro-jections made CT possible.

In nuclear medicine a similar evolution was occur-ring, from the development of the gamma camera by Anger in 1958 to tomographic imaging in the form of Single Photon Emission Computed Tomography (SPECT) and Positron Emission Tomography (PET) which is ongoing today. PET's clinical use is increasing, particularly in detecting metastases in oncology. Its ability to image minute concentrations of metabolites is unique and makes it a powerful research tool in the aetiology of disease and the effects of drugs.

Ultrasound was developed in the 1950s following the development of SONAR in World War II and was unique in involving no ionizing radiation and offering the pos-sibility of safe, noninvasive imaging. Its ability to image in real time and its sensitivity to flow, through the Doppler effect, have been key factors in its widespread role in obstetrics, cardiology, abdominal and vascular disease, real-time biopsy guidance and minimally inva-sive surgery.

As early as 1959, J. R. Singer at the University of California, Berkeley, proposed that NMR could be used as a noninvasive tool to measure in vivo blood flow. In 1971 Raymond Damadian discovered that certain mouse tumours displayed elevated relaxation times compared with normal tissues in vitro. This opened the door for a complete new way of imaging the human body where the potential contrast between tissues and disease was many times greater than that offered by X-ray technology and ultrasound (figure 1.2). At the same time developments in cryogenics, or the study of very low temperatures, made the development of whole-body superconducting magnets possible. Damadian and his colleagues at the State University of New York, starved of mainstream research funding, went so far as to design and build their own superconducting magnet operating in their Brooklyn laboratory and the first human body image by NMR is attributed to them. There is some dispute about who actually is the founder of modern Magnetic Resonance Imaging (MRI), but one thing is certain, Damadian coined the first MR acronym, namely FONAR (Field fOcussed Nuclear mAgnetic Resonance). This set a trend, and you can see the development of the acronym family tree in chapter 12!

In 1973, in an article in *Nature*, Paul Lauterbur pro-posed using magnetic field gradients to distinguish between NMR signals originating from different loca-tions combining this with a form of reconstruction from projections (as used in CT). The use of gradients still forms the basis of all modern MRI as recognised by the Nobel Committee in 2003. This is the basis of all modern MRI. Unfortunately Lauterbur's brilliant invention was not accompanied by a brilliant acronym; he coined the

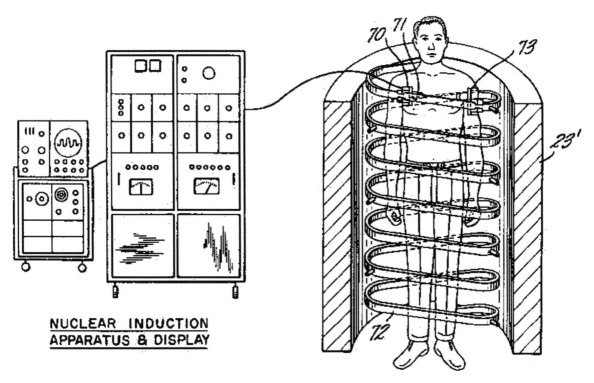

NUCLEAR INDUCTION
APPARATUS & DISPLAY

Figure 1.2 Raymond Damadian's "Apparatus and method for detecting cancer in tissue". US patent 3789832 filed 17 March 1972, issued 5 February 1974. Image from the US Patent and Trademark Office.

obscure term 'zeugmatography', meaning imaging from a joining together (of the main field and the gradients). In contemporary MR terms Lauterbur can be said to have invented frequency encoding. Whilst the term 'zeugmatography' sunk without trace, fortunately the technique it described has gone from strength to strength.

Selective excitation, or the sensitization of tomographic image slices, was invented at the University of Nottingham, England in 1974 by Sir Peter Mansfield's group, a contribution also recognised by the 2003 Nobel Committee, whilst in 1975 Richard Ernst's group in Zurich invented two-dimensional Fourier transform imaging (2D FT). The first practical 2D FT imaging method, dubbed 'spin warp', was developed by Edelstein and Hutchison at the University of Aberdeen, Scotland in 1980. Many other researchers contributed to the early development of MR, and in this short introduction it is impossible to do justice to them all

(see Further reading). And what of the commercial development? EMI, the creators of X-ray CT through Sir Godfrey Hounsfield, were involved from very early on. Clow and Young produced the first published human head image in 1978 (figure 1.3). EMI sold their research interest to Picker International, which became Marconi and is now part of Philips. The 'Neptune' 0.15T superconducting system installed at the Hammersmith Hospital, London, was the first commercial clinical system. Elsewhere in Europe, Philips Medical Systems also dedicated substantial early investment (figure 1.4). General Electric introduced high field (1.5T) systems in around 1984. The technique developed rapidly through the late 1980s to become the method of choice for non-trauma neurological scanning. By 1996 there were in excess of 10 000 scanners worldwide.

Due to problems of low signal and high sensitivity to motion, body MR did not really take off until the 1990s.

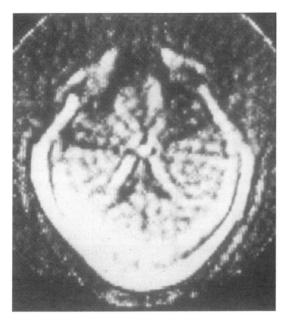

Figure 1.3 First ever human head image using MRI at 0.1 T from EMI Central Research Laboratories. For this image CT type "back projection" was used. Courtesy of Ian Young.

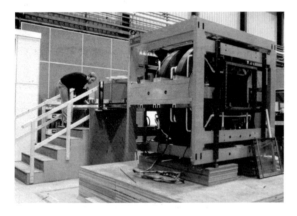

Figure 1.4 0.15T resistive magnet used by Philips in the early development of MRI. Courtesy of Philips Medical Systems.

The key factors were the development of fast imaging techniques, particularly gradient echo, and phased array coil technology. The 1990s also saw the coming of age of earlier developments, namely cardiac MRI and Echo **P**lanar **I**maging (EPI). EPI, which is the fastest and

The early history of NMR

'Nuclear induction', as it was first described, was discovered in 1945, soon after the close of World War II, by Bloch and independently by Purcell and Pound. It is said that the development of radio communications in the war effort, to which Purcell had contributed scientifically, was one of the factors underpinning this important scientific discovery. Another important factor, as in the development of atomic physics, was the expulsion or fleeing of European physicists from the Nazi regime, an exodus that included Bloch and Bloembergen. What did these MR pioneers discover? That you can detect a signal (a voltage in a coil) when you place a sample in a magnetic field and irradiate it with radiofrequency (RF) energy of a certain frequency, the resonant or Larmor frequency. The signal is produced by the interaction of the sample nuclei with the magnetic field. The spin echo was 'stumbled upon' by Hahn in 1949. He discovered that you could get a repeat of the NMR signal at a delayed time by adding a second burst of RF energy. That's all you need to know for now. So what were NMR researchers doing between the forties and the seventies – that's a long time in cultural and scientific terms. The answer: they were doing chemistry, including Lauterbur, a professor of chemistry at the same institution as Damadian, albeit on different campuses. NMR developed into a laboratory spectroscopic technique capable of examining the molecular structure of compounds, until Damadian's ground-breaking discovery in 1971.

one of the most cutting edge methods, was actually one of the first imaging methods to be proposed, by Sir Peter Mansfield. EPI is now extensively used in neurological imaging through functional MRI (fMRI) and diffusion imaging.

1.3 How to use this book

Everyone starts MRI with the same basic problem: it's like nothing else they've learnt in the past. All that knowledge you have about radioactive isotopes and

The spin doctors: Nobel Laureates' roll-call (figure 1.5)

In 1952 Edward Purcell (Harvard) and Felix Bloch (Stanford) jointly received the Nobel Prize for physics 'for their development of new methods for nuclear magnetic precision measurements and discoveries in connection there-with'. Of Purcell's discovery, the Boston Herald reported that 'it wouldn't revolutionize industry or help the house-wife'. Purcell himself stated that 'we are dealing not merely with a new tool but a new subject which I have simply called nuclear magnetism. If you will think of the history of ordinary magnetism, the electronic kind, you will remember that it has been rich in difficult and provocative problems and full of surprises.' It seems that the Boston Herald misjudged the importance of NMR!

Bloch, a Swiss-born Jew and friend of quantum physicist Werner Heisenberg, quit his post in Leipzig in 1933 in disgust at the Nazi's expulsion of German Jews (as a Swiss citizen, Bloch himself was exempt). Bloch's subsequent career at Stanford was crammed with major contributions to physics and he has been called 'the father of solid state physics'.

Nicolaas Bloembergen, a Dutch citizen, was forced to hide from the Nazis for the duration of the War, reputedly living on boiled tulip bulbs, until becoming Purcell's first graduate student at Harvard two months after the discovery of NMR. With Purcell and Robert Pound he developed the theory of NMR relaxation, known now by their initials BPP. In 1981 he won a Nobel Prize for his work in laser spectroscopy. In 1991 Richard Ernst joined the MRI Nobel Laureates 'for his contributions to the development of the methodology of high resolution nuclear magnetic resonance spectroscopy'. You could say Richard Ernst achieved the same trick twice: by his novel applications of 2D FT in both spectroscopy and imaging.

The 2003 Nobel Prize for Physiology or Medicine was awarded to Professor Paul Lauterbur and Sir Peter Mansfield for 'for their discoveries concerning magnetic resonance imaging'. Peter Mansfield left school at 15 with no qualifications, aiming to become a printer. His scientific curiosity was sparked by the V1 and V2 flying bombs and rockets that fell on London in 1944, when he was 11. After working as a scientific assistant at the Jet Propulsion Laboratory and a spell in the army, he went back to college to complete his education, eventually becoming Professor of Physics at the University of Nottingham. He was knighted in 1993.

Paul Lauterbur is said to have been inspired to use field gradients to produce an image whilst eating a hamburger. His seminal paper 'Image Formation by Induced Local Interactions. Examples Employing Nuclear Magnetic Resonance' (*Nature* **242**, March 16, 1973) was originally rejected. 30 years later, Nature placed this work in a book of the 21 most influential scientific papers of the 20th century.

Other Nobel Laureates associated with NMR include Norman Ramsey (1989), a spectroscopy pioneer who developed the theory of the chemical shift, Isidor Rabi (1944), Ramsey's PhD mentor, 'for his resonance method for recording the magnetic properties of atomic nuclei' and Kurt Wüthrich (2002) for his development of NMR spectroscopy for determination of the three-dimensional structure of biological macromolecules in solution.

film-screen combinations is useless to you now. Where do you start? Most MRI books start at the beginning (a very good place to start, according to the song), and introduce protons, net magnetization, precession and the Larmor equation all in the first three pages. We think there is another way, starting at the end with the images that are produced, which is much more useful if you're already working in the MR unit. After all, you don't expect to understand how the internal combustion engine works before you learn to drive.

The book is divided into two parts. In part A you will find everything you need to know about the basics of MRI, but presented in reverse order. We start with things you can touch and look at: the equipment you find in an MR unit and what the images look like, using terms like 'T_1-weighted' simply as labels. Later on we talk about how the images are produced and finally we cover the underlying physics. By that stage you will be able to link these rather difficult concepts back to things which matter – the images.

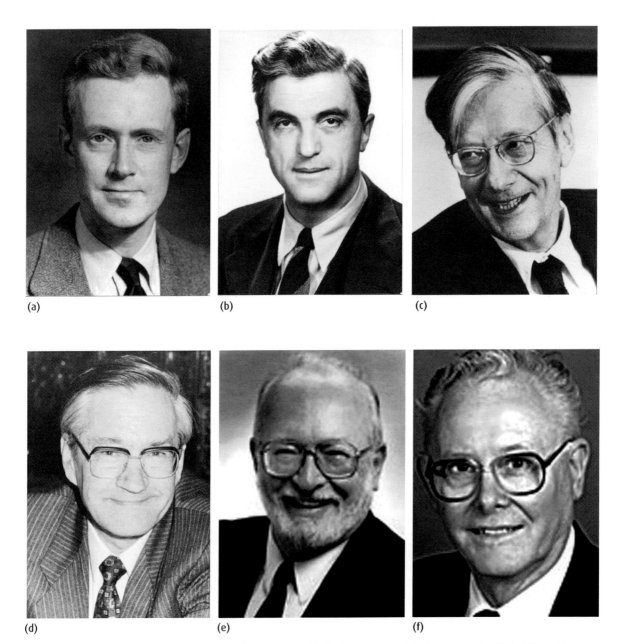

Figure 1.5 Nobel prize-winners in NMR: (a) Purcell 1912–1997, (b) Bloch 1901–1999, (c) Bloembergen b. 1920, (d) Ernst b. 1933, (e) Lauterbur b. 1929 and (f) Mansfield b. 1933. Courtesy of the Nobel Museum.

Part B contains more advanced topics, such as cardiac MR and spectroscopy, in no particular order. You don't have to work right through part A before you read these chapters, we just couldn't fit them neatly into the reverse order!

In all the chapters you will find the most basic information in the main text. Advanced boxes, shaded in blue, deal with various topics in more detail and are placed at appropriate places through the text. If you're completely new to MR, we suggest you read straight through skipping all the advanced boxes. When you need to understand something a bit better, re-read the chapter this time taking in the blue boxes. The topics can seem to jump around a bit by splitting them up this way, but we think it is a good compromise, which allows us to include enough information for everyone, whether you are a new radiographer hoping to make a good impression in your new job, a radiologist trying to get the best images for making diagnoses or a physicist studying for a postgraduate degree.

FURTHER READING

Christie DA and Tansey EM (eds) (1996) *Making the Human Body Transparent: The Impact of Nuclear Magnetic Resonance and Magnetic Resonance Imaging.* London: Wellcome Institute for the History of Medicine. Available from: http://www.wellcome.ac.uk/en/images/witness_vol2_pdf_1 905.pdf [accessed 24th October 2001]

Mattson J and Simon M (1996) *The Pioneers of NMR and Magnetic Resonance in Medicine: The Story of MRI.* Jericho, NY: Dean Books Co (ISBN: 0961924314)

Thomas AM, Isherwood I and Wells PNT (eds) (1995) *Invisible Light: 100 Years of Medical Radiology.* Oxford: Blackwell Science (ISBN: 0865426279)

Part A

The basic stuff

Early daze: your first week in MR

2.1 Introduction

In any first week of a new job or in a new environment, it takes a little time to become orientated and to find your way around. This chapter aims to ease those initial experiences so that you will feel more like a seasoned campaigner than a raw recruit. The following are your essential instructions:

- Magnet safety, especially from ferro-magnetic projectiles, is paramount to the safe operation of any MR unit; the MR examination room is probably the most dangerous environment in the imaging department.
- Aside from the magnet itself, the coils are the main items of equipment that you will have to learn to handle (don't break them!), and learn how to position patients comfortably and effectively with them.
- Good patient cooperation is essential for safe and effective scanning: you will need good people skills.
- Typically the most common MR examinations are brain, spine and musculoskeletal but we also look at some others in section 2.5.
- Enjoy the experience!

2.2 Welcome to the MR unit

The MR suite will probably be arranged differently from the remainder of the imaging department. It is likely to have its own dedicated reception, administration, waiting and patient handling areas. Security will be high on the staff's agenda and the suite may have its own lockable doors. In general accommodation may comprise:

- facilities for patient management: reception, waiting areas, changing facilities, toilets, anaesthesia and recovery area, counselling room;
- MR system: the MRI scanner room (magnet room), control room, computer/technical room and film printing area;
- facilities for staff: reception/office, administration office, reporting rooms;
- dedicated storage areas: trolley bay, general store, resuscitation trolley bay, cleaner's store.

An example of a typical MRI suite layout is given in figure 2.1.

The MR system itself is actually distributed between three of the rooms in the suite: the magnet room which houses the *magnet* and *coils*, an air-conditioned technical (computer) room which is full of supporting electronics and electrical plant, and the control room which houses the MR console. You will spend most time in the control room where you operate the MR scanner by entering patient details, selecting and modifying the scan acquisition parameters, viewing and post-processing images, selecting images for hard copy on a remote laser imager and archiving images. There may be an adjacent reporting room and one or more independent image viewing and post-processing workstations.

Other accommodation may be required for MR-specific patient handling accessories, such as nonferromagnetic trolleys and wheelchairs, a dedicated preparation room for inducing general anaesthesia, and recovery bays. Even the cleaners' equipment for general household chores about the suite should be specifically designated for MR. The MR unit is, in all likelihood, a miniature department in its own right. The

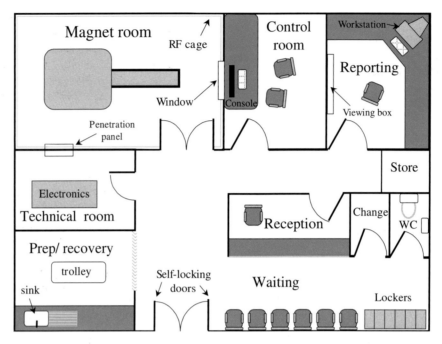

Figure 2.1 Typical MR suite layout.

magnet room, in addition to housing the magnet, will have storage for all the coils, physiological monitoring accessories and may have piped medical gases.

The preoccupation with security and the 'separateness' of the MR suite is principally to prevent anyone introducing ferromagnetic items into the vicinity of the magnet, where the outcome could be disastrous. On your first day you will be asked to complete a staff safety questionnaire and should undergo a thorough safety induction. (Once you are MR trained you will find yourself doing strange things such as taking off your watch and emptying your pockets when you go into a CT room!)

The MR system itself consists of:

- a magnet that produces a strong, constant magnetic field;
- radiofrequency transmit and receive coils, which excite and detect the MR signal;
- magnetic field gradients, which localize the MR signals;
- a computer system for scanner control, image display and archiving;
- patient couch, comfort and positioning aids;
- physiological monitoring equipment.

2.2.1 The magnet

The magnet is the heart of the MR system. The principal types of magnet used in MRI are:

- *superconducting magnets* – used in mid and high-field systems (0.5 T and higher);
- *permanent magnets* – capable of sustaining fields up to about 0.3 T;
- *resistive and electromagnets* – capable of fields up to about 0.6 T.

A modern 1.5 T superconducting magnet was shown in figure 1.1. The main field may point horizontally or vertically depending on whether the magnet is 'closed' or 'open' bore (the bore is the opening where the patient goes). Closed bores are more common in diagnostic systems. For superconducting and permanent magnets the magnetic field is always present. Resistive magnets are electrically powered and can have their field switched off. Superconducting magnets require liquid helium to be used as a *cryogenic* cooling fluid. A sudden loss of superconductivity results in a magnet *quench* where the windings heat up, the field collapses in less

The size of an MR system is expressed in terms of its operating magnetic field strength. The unit of magnetic flux density or induction is the *tesla (T)*. You may also come across the *gauss (G)* as a measure of field strength. One tesla equals 10 000 gauss, i.e. 1 G equals 0.1 mT (milli tesla). The Earth's magnetic field is approximately 0.05 mT (0.5 G).

A higher magnetic field produces stronger MR signals, with the signal-to-noise ratio (SNR) theoretically increasing linearly with the field, i.e. you get twice as much SNR at 1 T compared with 0.5 T. In practice the gains in SNR from field strength are often partially offset by other factors, discussed elsewhere in this text. At mid and low field strengths, it is easy to make the magnet design more open to reduce claustrophobia. The majority of systems in clinical use are 1.5 T. Higher field strengths are sometimes used clinically but are more commonly used in research.

The *homogeneity* of a magnet describes the quality or uniformity of its field. Poor homogeneity can result in image degradation and artefacts. When scanning patients, homogeneity may be degraded by so-called *susceptibility* problems (small differences between the magnetic properties of adjoining tissues, or tissue–air boundaries). The quality of the magnetic field within the scanner may also be adversely affected by neighbouring ferromagnetic structures or objects. Ferromagnetic articles in or on a patient, in addition to posing a serious hazard (see section 2.3), are disastrous for image quality.

than one minute and large amounts of helium boil off as gas. Accidental quenches are a rare occurrence in modern systems. In an emergency a quench can be initiated deliberately. In normal operation, small amounts of helium 'boil off' and are released into the atmosphere outside. The helium level is normally maintained by the manufacturer's service personnel.

2.2.2 Radiofrequency coils

The MR *signals* that provide the diagnostic information are produced within the patient's tissue in response to radiofrequency (RF) pulses. These are generated by a *transmitter coil* which surrounds the whole or a part of the body. A *body coil* is usually built into the construction of the magnet. For imaging the head or extremities, smaller transmitter coils are sometimes used.

The MR signals produced in the body are detected using a *receiver coil*. The MR signals are very weak and are sensitive to electrical interference. Special shielding is built into the magnet room (known as a Faraday cage) to minimize interference from radiofrequency sources outside the MR room. It is important to keep the magnet room door closed during scanning to complete the Faraday cage.

All MR systems have a head coil and integral body coil. Other coils you may encounter include the spine coil, neck coil, knee coil, wrist coil, shoulder coil, breast coil, endo-cavitary coils (e.g. prostate or endovaginal coil), peripheral vascular coil, flexible coils and **T**emporo-**M**andibular **J**oint (TMJ) coils. Some coils are called 'arrays'. This generally means they will produce better images than a nonarray version of the same sort of coil. Array coils have multiple elements and you may have to select which of them you wish to scan with. You can actually use any coil to obtain an image provided it encompasses the anatomical region of interest, but specialist coils, which fit closer and are smaller, usually do a better job. You must store coils carefully. They are the one part of the MR system most prone to failure due principally to excessive or careless handling. Be careful when connecting or disconnecting the coils: all the MR signals have to go through the coil connectors, so treat them with due respect. Examples of coils are shown in figure 2.2.

2.2.3 Gradients

The localization of the MR signals in the body to produce images is achieved by generating short-term spatial variations in magnetic field strength across the patient. These are commonly referred to as the *gradients*. The use of stronger gradients permits smaller anatomical features to be seen in the images, and enables faster scanning. The gradient fields are produced by three sets of *gradient coils*, one for each direction, through which large electrical currents are applied repeatedly in a carefully controlled *pulse sequence*. The

(a)

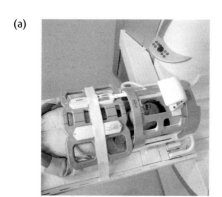

(b)

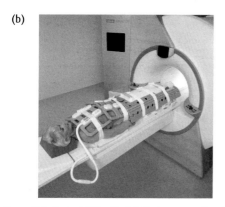

(c)

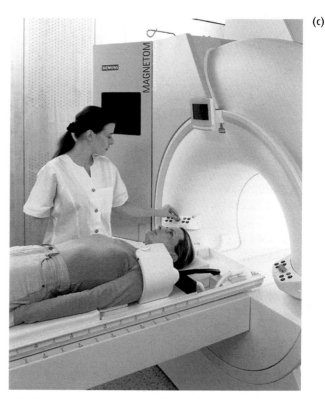

Figure 2.2 Typical MR coils. (a) Body array coil and head coil, (b) peripheral angiography coil and (c) flexible coil. Courtesy of Siemens Medical Solutions.

gradient coils are built in to the bore of the magnet. The gradient coils generate a loud tapping, clicking or high pitched beeping sound during scanning, like a loud-speaker. The cumulative effect of all three gradients can be so loud that ear protection is required. Generally the acoustic noise level is worse for high field strength systems with high power gradients.

2.2.4 Computer system and console

The MR system is controlled via the operator's console situated in the control room. An independent workstation may also permit other post-processing functions to be carried out without interfering with the operation of the scanner. Computer networking will allow the scanner and workstation to send and receive data from the hospital networks, **P**icture **A**rchiving and **C**ommunications **S**ystem (PACS) and teleradiology systems.

2.2.5 Patient handling system

The patient couch (sometimes called 'table') is integral to the magnet system to allow for patient positioning. For motor-driven couch systems emergency stop buttons are provided. Patient positioning accuracy is achieved using light alignment markers, e.g. with halogen lights or lasers. An intercom is provided between the operator's console and the bore of the magnet for communication with the patient. A hand-held alarm or 'panic button' is also provided. Closed circuit TV may be used for additional visual monitoring of the patient. Equipment for physiological measurement – peripheral pulse, ECG (electrocardiograph) and respiration – is often provided as part of the MR system. The physiological signals may be used to control the timing of the scan (*gating* or *triggering*) to prevent motion (e.g. from breathing) spoiling the images, but they are unsuitable for monitoring the patient's condition. MR-compatible anaesthetic and physiological monitoring systems should be used when the patient is being scanned under a general anaesthetic or sedation. Other patient handling accessories include nonferromagnetic wheelchairs, trolleys and drip stands.

2.3 Safety first

MRI is a relatively safe imaging technique in that it does not involve ionizing radiation and there are no clearly demonstrated biological effects (see chapter 10). However, the MRI system and its environment are potentially very hazardous to both patients and staff working in the MRI unit if metal objects get pulled into the magnet bore.

2.3.1 Beware: strong magnetic field

The primary hazard associated with the static magnetic field is that of ferromagnetic attraction. When a ferromagnetic object, e.g. one containing iron or steel, is brought close to the magnet, it will experience a force. If sufficiently close, this can turn the object into a dangerous projectile. Items such as scissors could become deadly in such a scenario; even a coin could inflict serious damage or injury. The bigger the object the stronger the forces involved and there has recently been a death caused by an oxygen cylinder being accidentally taken too close to the magnet. This attractive force requires the field to be changing over position, as in the fringe field.

Even in the absence of a field change any ferromagnetic object will twist with a force considerably greater than its mass in an attempt to align its long axis with the static magnetic field lines of force. This twisting force is called torque (see 'Force fields').

It is obvious therefore that this ability to twist objects and to turn them into high-velocity projectiles is a major risk to both staff and patients within an MRI unit. In modern MRI systems the stray field may decrease very rapidly with distance: an object that does not appear to demonstrate ferromagnetic properties as you approach the magnet may suddenly be torn from your grasp or pocket as you take one further step closer.

Force fields

The translational force (F) on a volume V with magnetic susceptibility χ is proportional to the product of the static field (B) and its spatial gradient:

$$F \propto \chi V B \cdot \frac{dB}{dr}$$

where dB/dr is the rate of change of B with position (r). F gets stronger the closer you are to the opening of the magnet bore. The torque (T) is proportional to the square of the static field

$$T \propto \chi^2 V B^2$$

Thus ferromagnetic objects will experience a torque even in a uniform field.

Table 2.1 Limit of fringe field for various objects affected by the scanner. Values are typical for a 1.5 T MR system

Fringe field (mT)	Item	Minimum distance (m)	
		On axis	Radially
3	Magnetic media	2.8	2.0
1	Computer hard disks	3.4	2.2
	Shielded colour monitors		
	X-ray tubes		
0.5	Pacemakers	4.0	2.5
0.1	Colour monitors	5.6	3.0
	Image intensifiers		
	CT scanners		
0.05	Photomultiplier tubes	6.8	3.7
	Linear accelerators		
	Gamma cameras		

2.3.2 Fringe field

The magnetic field extends beyond the physical covers of the scanner. This is referred to as the *fringe field*. The strength of the fringe field decreases rapidly with distance and has implications for safety and for the proper functioning of nearby sensitive electronic equipment (see table 2.1). To ensure safety a *controlled area* is defined within the vicinity of the magnet, and there should be a diagram in the local safety rules. Access of persons and equipment to the controlled area is restricted. A typical fringe field is illustrated in figure 2.3. A more detailed plot is shown in chapter 9.

2.3.3 Do not enter!

Implanted ferromagnetic items such as vascular aneurysm clips may also experience these forces and torques. There has been at least one reported death of a patient scanned with a ferromagnetic aneurysm clip that moved, rupturing the blood vessel, as they were moved into the magnet. Similar hazards arise with patients who may have metallic foreign bodies located in high-risk areas such as the eye. Alternatively the function of implanted medical devices such as pacemakers or cochlear implants may be severely impaired by the static magnetic field and persons with pacemakers are normally excluded from the 0.5-mT fringe field. This book is not intended to give comprehensive advice on the MR compatibility or otherwise of medical devices, since this is covered in great detail in specialized books and on the Internet. However, it is imperative that any person responsible for their own safety or the safety of patients undergoing an MRI investigation is aware of the risks associated with taking metallic objects into the vicinity of an MRI magnet.

The same rules apply to any pieces of medical equipment that may also need to be taken into the room; for example, a pulse oximeter for monitoring a sedated patient. Devices such as these must be MR compatible. Even though the device may be labelled as MR compatible it may have a maximum operating proximity to the magnet and care must be taken that the device is not moved any closer.

2.3.4 I hear you knocking: acoustic noise

The MR scanner is very noisy during operation. In some MR imaging sequences the noise level can exceed safety guidelines and it is recommended that all patients and any other person that may be in the room during scanning are given ear-plugs to reduce the noise level. Some newer magnets use vacuum isolaton of the gradients to reduce the gradient switching noise to a lower level,

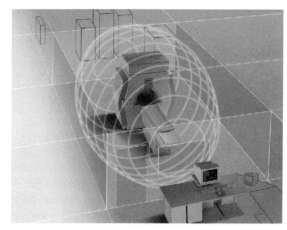

Figure 2.3 Extent of the 0.5 mT fringe field around a 1.5 T system. Courtesy of Philips Medical Systems.

however we recommend you use ear-plugs with all patients.

2.3.5 Bio-effects

Biological effects of field exposures are examined in chapter 10. As staff you will be primarily exposed to only the fringe static field. There are no known hazardous bio-effects for this.

Your patients will be exposed to the main static field, the gradient fields and RF fields. In extreme cases, the gradients can induce peripheral nerve stimulation. This may be alarming or annoying, but it is not harmful. If it occurs the scan should be stopped.

The main effect of RF is the heating of tissue. The scanner does not let you exceed certain values of RF exposure (or **S**pecific **A**bsorption **R**ate 'SAR'). Sometimes you may need to alter the scan parameters to keep within the permitted values. Care is required when physiological monitoring is used in the scanner. Contact with cryogens – the ultra cold liquids that maintain superconducting magnets – will usually be restricted to fully trained MR engineering staff (see 'Burning issues and cold sores').

Adverse reactions to common MR contrast agents, injected into the patient to provide better diagnostic information, are rare. However, whenever contrast agents are used, there should be an MR compatible crash

Burning issues and cold sores

There is a small risk of patients receiving burns through the coupling of RF energy into wires or cables, such as those used for ECG triggering, that are touching the patient. Care must be exercised in ensuring that cables are not formed into loops, that dry flame-retardant pads are placed between cables and the patient and that any unnecessary cables are removed from the patient prior to imaging. All cables should also be inspected every time before use to ensure that there is no damage to the insulation. Furthermore, only ECG cables specifically deemed MR compatible should be used.

Potential hazards of working with cryogens (liquid helium and nitrogen) include asphyxiation in oxygen-deficient atmospheres, cold burns, frostbite and hypothermia. Additionally there is the possibility of inducing asthma in susceptible persons if cold gas is inhaled. Resist the temptation to touch the feed pipes just after a helium fill to see how cold they get!

International standards

The international standard for the safety of MR equipment intended for medical diagnosis is the International Electrotechnical Commission (IEC) 60601-2-33. IEC 60601-1 is the general standard for the safety of medical electrical equipment. An important aspect of the IEC standard is the establishment of three operating modes:

- Normal mode – requires only routine monitoring of the patient;
- First-level controlled mode – requires medical supervision and a medical assessment of the risk versus benefit for the patient having the scan;
- Second-level controlled mode – requires an approved human studies protocol. Security measures, e.g. a lock or password, must be provided to prevent unauthorized operation in this mode.

cart nearby equipped with the necessary medications to treat any complications and for resuscitating patients. In addition, there should be medical personnel nearby who know how to recognize and treat these rare complications. Restrictions on the use of contrast agents may apply during pregnancy and to nursing mothers.

2.3.6 Practical guidelines

Everyone entering the magnet room should be carefully screened, using a checklist and/or detailed questioning, to ensure that they do not have any contraindications to MRI either internally or about their person. This includes the patient's relative(s), friend(s) or nurse who may enter the MR scanner room to assist the patient. The key to MR safety in this respect is to be acutely vigilant at all times. Metallic objects taken into the bore of a magnet may at worse cause serious injury or death and at best may produce unwanted artefacts on the images. Patient and staff safety is of paramount importance in running an MRI system. The MRI unit should have clearly written policies and procedures for checking that patients and staff have no contraindications.

MRI examinations require particular caution in the following cases:

- Patients with implanted surgical clips or other ferromagnetic material;
- Patients who have engaged in occupations or activities that may have caused the accidental lodging of ferromagnetic materials, e.g. metal-workers, or anyone who may have embedded metal fragments from military duties;
- Neonates and infants, for whom data establishing safety are lacking;
- Patients with tattoos, including permanent eye-liner;
- Patients with compromised thermoregulatory systems, e.g. neonates, low-birth-weight infants, certain cancer patients;
- Patients with metallic implants which may cause artefacts in the images due to distortion of the static magnetic field;
- Patients with prosthetic heart valves;
- Pregnant patients: although no MRI effects on embryos or fetuses are known and fetal MRI is routinely performed, most sites avoid scanning during the first trimester. The unknown risk to the fetus must be weighed against the alternative diagnostic tests, which may involve ionizing radiation.

2.4 The patient's journey

In this section we walk with you through the journey made by the patient on their visit to the MR unit.

2.4.1 Before the examination

Patient cooperation is essential for obtaining high quality images, and their initial chat with MR staff can make all the difference. All patients require counselling to explain the nature of the examination and must complete a questionnaire to assess their suitability and safety for being scanned. This should take place in an appropriate quiet and private place. During this interview you should also ensure that the correct examination is being performed on the correct region of anatomy. For example, it is always essential to ask which knee is symptomatic because a clerk may accidentally mix up 'right' and 'left' on the request form. It can also be useful to mark the specific site of any symptoms with an MRI marker (vitamin E or cod liver oil capsules make good markers). This is important when there is a 'lump' being imaged, especially the ones which are there one minute and gone the next!

Patients need to remove all metallic objects, jewellery, watches and credit cards, which can be stored in lockers. Lockers should have nonmagnetic brass or plastic keys which will be safe in the magnet. Local policy will determine whether patients should undress and wear a gown for the examination. Generally it is preferable to wear an MR compatible gown because clothing often has embedded metal, e.g. underwired bras, zippers, buttons/fasteners. Nonambulatory patients will be transferred to nonferromagnetic, MR-compatible trolleys or wheelchairs prior to being taken into the MRI examination room. Some MR systems incorporate removable patient couch systems or table-tops to allow for efficient and comfortable moving of bed-bound patients.

The patient will usually be weighed before entering the scanner. This is required for RF safety purposes (see chapter 10). You will quickly become expert at estimating patient weight, so in instances when weighing the patient is impractical you don't need to worry too much.

2.4.2 During the examination

Choose the coil which is able to completely cover the region of interest with the highest SNR and homogeneity. The patient can then be positioned on the scanner couch and made comfortable. Maximizing patient comfort and relieving anxiety is essential to the success of the examination. 'Landmarking' on the region of interest allows the scanner to place this anatomy at the very centre of the magnet (the *isocentre*). This is the 'sweet spot' with the best magnetic field homogeneity, thereby ensuring highest image quality. After landmarking the initial scan position using the laser light guides, the couch is moved into the centre of the magnet.

While the patient moves into the scanner watch carefully for any sign that the patient may be claustrophobic or may not fit into the bore of the scanner. Especially for large patients, the arms may need to be repositioned to fit comfortably into the magnet. When the fit is too tight with the arms by the side, it may be possible to get the patient into the scanner with one or both arms overhead. If you place the arms overhead though, make sure to scan very quickly and to give the patient opportunities to come out of the magnet to rest the arms by the side to avoid rotator cuff impingement. Scanning may also be initiated from the buttons along the side or on the front of the magnet.

Once the patient is comfortably inside the magnet, MRI staff then leave the scanner room closing the door to completely seal the Faraday cage around the scanner. The first series of pictures is typically a scout or positioning scan. These are quick, low-resolution, large field-of-view images which are then used to plan the longer, higher resolution diagnostic scans which home in on the region of interest. The positioning of slices and saturation bands is usually prescribed graphically using these scout scans (figure 2.4). The diagnostic scans or sequences can often be queued to run automatically leaving you free to do other tasks on the console such as filming or archiving.

All patients need to be observed during the examination either through the observation window from the control room or by closed-circuit TV. An intercom enables two-way audible communication between the patient in the magnet and the control room. At some point during the examination, the administration of a

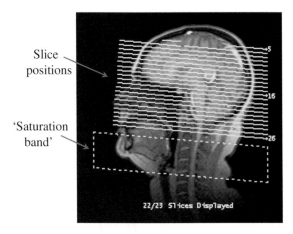

Slice
positions

'Saturation
band'

22/23 Slices Displayed

Figure 2.4 Quick localizer or scout scan for planning. Slice positions are shown as lines. A regional saturation band is also shown.

MR *contrast agent*, usually a gadolinium compound, to the patient may be required. Since gadolinium alters the image contrast, gadolinium-enhanced imaging is always performed at the end of the examination. Local policy may determine who can give this injection. Whether the injection is done by technologist or nurse, responsibility for the patient will rest with the consultant radiologist.

During an MRI examination, patients may be fully conscious (this is the norm), naturally asleep (e.g. for infants), sedated or anaesthetized. In the latter instances they may require life support and physiological monitoring, e.g. ECG and pulse oximetry.

It may be necessary for a patient to be moved quickly from the scanner room – either for an emergency procedure, such as resuscitation, or because of a situation related to equipment failure, for example in the event of a magnet quench. Local safety rules will detail the evacuation procedures for various emergencies. As a general rule, when a patient needs resuscitating or other emergency treatment, the number one priority is to get the patient out of the scanner room as quickly as possible. This is because arriving emergency personnel, who may not understand the dangers of the strong magnetic field, can unintentionally make matters worse by bringing MR-incompatible ferromagnetic equipment into the scanner room such as stethoscopes, laryngoscopes, oxygen tanks or even metal crash carts (no pun intended).

2.4.3 After the MRI examination

Patients are escorted from the magnet room and will need to retrieve their personal possessions. They will often want to see their images and ask questions about their medical condition. The radiologist may review the images with the patient but as a general rule they are recommended to get this information from their primary physician who ordered the study since the results of the MR need to be incorporated into the full clinical picture in order to provide the best patient counselling. If the patient had an adverse event such as allergic reaction to a contrast injection, contrast extravasation or became hysterical from claustrophobia, it may be prudent to watch the patient until they return to their baseline condition.

2.5 Basic clinical protocols

Although there are many ways to perform any particular MRI examination depending upon the patient's medical issues or the philosophy of the radiologist interpreting the images, some general approaches have emerged for most examinations. In this section we briefly review typical strategies for these commonly performed exams that tend to have some consensus.

2.5.1 Brain

MRI of the brain is the most commonly performed examination at most institutions which reflects the enormous amount of information that MR provides about this complex organ. The most basic examination consists of a sagittal T_1-weighted, axial proton density and axial T_2-weighted images. An improvement in T_2-weighted images known as FLAIR (**FL**uid **A**ttenuated **I**nversion **R**ecovery) has become popular for being able to visualize the periventricular tissues without interference from bright cerebrospinal fluid (CSF). Diffusion imaging is also popular because of its exquisite sensitivity to ischaemic injuries, which allow cellular fluids to diffuse through cell membranes. For some specific conditions, it may be useful to obtain additional images at higher resolution through a specific region of interest, such as the brainstem, or specific cranial nerves such as the cochlear nerve or optic nerve. Sagittal T_2-weighted images are useful for optimal definition of the characteristic T_2 bright changes of multiple sclerosis.

Postgadolinium T_1-weighted images typically acquired in axial and coronal planes give the greatest sensitivity for detecting pathological processes that break down the normal blood–brain barrier. Tumours, infection and inflammation all break down the blood–brain barrier and light up vividly on postgadolinium T_1-weighted images. Accordingly, gadolinium is particularly useful when these are suspected. For patients with cancer, postgadolinium imaging is essential for the optimal detection and characterization of metastatic disease. It is also helpful to determine the extent of primary tumour growth and the precise boundary between normal and neoplastic tissue.

2.5.2 Spine

Imaging the spine is another important application of MRI because of the high prevalence of back pain. MRI readily detects herniated discs, discitis and tumours which may be the underlying cause of pain. To maximize the SNR in spine imaging the patient is positioned with the portion of spine to be imaged directly on top of a surface coil or coil array. Typically the spine coil array is divided into cervical, thoracic and lumbar regions, with multiple elements covering the entire spine. One can then select the particular elements appropriate for each patient or even image the entire spine all at once.

It is essential to image the spine with a sagittal T_1-weighted sequence in order to evaluate the bone marrow and for a high SNR assessment of the anatomy. Sagittal T_2-weighted imaging is essential to assess the hydration of the intervertebral discs and to help characterize any pathology. Finally axial images through each disc are important to better assess the extent of any disc herniations and to look for compression of nerve roots. These axial images may be individually obliqued to align perfectly with the plane of each intervertebral disc.

In patients who have a spine tumour, other spinal cord pathology or a history of previous surgery on the spine, it is useful to acquire T_1-weighted images postgadolinium.

2.5.3 Breast

The possibility of injury to patients from the silicone material within breast implants has led to the initial widespread use of MRI for detecting breast implant rupture and leakage of the silicon into the surrounding tissues. This exam is performed with a special surface coil utilizing two elements, one for each breast. The patient lies prone on top of the coil so the breasts suspend down into each element (figure 2.5(a)). The prone position minimizes the effect of respiratory motion on the breasts. T_1-weighted, T_2-weighted and **S**hort **TI I**nversion **R**ecovery (STIR) images are obtained with at least one of those sequences in each cardinal plane (axial, coronal and sagittal). It may also be useful to perform a three-point Dixon image (see box 'Dixon method for fat/water separation', section 6.5.2) to separately image the water, fat and silicon peaks, or to perform a silicon image with fat saturation to optimally assess for leakage of silicon into the surrounding tissues.

More recently, recognition of the limitations of conventional X-ray mammography, especially in younger women with dense breasts, has led to the use of MRI for evaluating women suspected of having breast cancer. On dynamic gadolinium-enhanced MR imaging, breast cancer enhances rapidly in the first 90–180 s and then washes-out over the next several minutes while normal breast parenchymal tissue enhances more slowly. To detect this differential enhancement between cancer and normal breast tissue, a 3D gradient-echo sequence with fat saturation is acquired in either the sagittal plane (for a single breast at high resolution, figure 2.5(b)) or in the axial plane (for both breasts at lower resolution). Eight to ten repetitions of the 3D sequence are repeated every 60 to 90 s. The gadolinium injection is performed by rapid bolus just as the second 3D acquisition begins. A workstation is used to interrogate the enhancement kinetics and borders to determine if enhancing lesions have benign or malignant features. When suspicious lesions are identified, breast MR may be used to guide biopsy of the lesion or marking the lesion to make it easy for the breast surgeon to locate and remove.

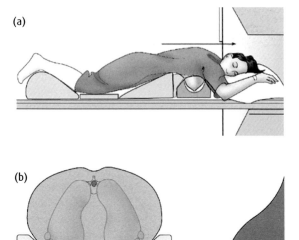

Figure 2.5 (a) Patient position for breast imaging. (b) Slice positioning for high resolution sagittal breast images.

2.5.4 Cardiac

Cardiac imaging is becoming more useful, albeit more complicated because of the increasing capabilities of MRI for evaluating cardiac morphology, as well as cardiac wall motion and contraction, myocardial perfusion and myocardial viability. Coronary MR angiography is also gaining acceptance for assessing coronary anomalies. For all cardiac applications, it is crucial to synchronize data acquisition with the ECG in order to freeze cardiac motion on the images. ECG gating is discussed in greater detail in chapter 14. The most basic cardiac examination evaluates cardiac morphology using axial spin-echo (black blood, see section 2.5.10) images followed by cine imaging to assess cardiac function including wall motion and valvular competence. Cine images are performed in planes oriented to the shape of the heart including 2-chamber, 4-chamber and short axis views (see figures in chapter 14). Typically cine imaging is performed with steady state techniques which maximize blood signal and contrast with respect to myocardium.

Myocardial perfusion is assessed using fast ECG gated T_1-weighted images obtained repeatedly over 1 minute during and after rapid bolus injection of gadolinium contrast. For maximum sensitivity, perfusion imaging may be obtained while infusing dobutamine or adenosine via an IV in the other arm to stress the heart. Myocardial infarcts are dark during the fast pass, but later take up the gadolinium and are identified on breath-hold T_1-weighted images 10 to 20 minutes post gadolinium using an inversion pulse to null signal from normal myocardium.

Flow in the aorta, main pulmonary artery, across the mitral and tricuspid valves or through cardiac defects such as atrial septal defect, ventricular septal defect or patent ductus arteriosus can be assessed with cine phase contrast images. Phase contrast image data has higher SNR post gadolinium so these flow measurements can be obtained after perfusion imaging during the 10-20 minute wait for optimum post-Gd infarct imaging.

If a cardiac mass is identified, it can be further characterized with ECG gated breath hold T_2 weighted images and by obtaining pre and post-gadolinium T_1-weighted images with fat saturation. When there is congenital heart disease, contrast-enhanced MR angiography (CE-MRA) of the pulmonary arteries and aorta is used to assess for coarctation, pulmonary artery stenoses and pulmonary venous anomalies. Anomalous coronary arteries may be detected by imaging the origins with thin black blood images and bright blood cine images obliqued to the plane of the aortic root.

2.5.5 Liver

MRI of the liver is commonly performed to look for hepatocellular carcinoma in patients with cirrhosis, to screen for metastases in patients with cancer, to characterize hepatic lesions identified on other imaging studies such as ultrasound or CT, to look for biliary obstruction and to assess iron accumulation in patients with blood dyscrasia or hemochromatosis. A comprehensive approach starts with steady state T_2 imaging (balanced FFE, trueFISP, single-shot fast spin echo), typically in the coronal plane (see

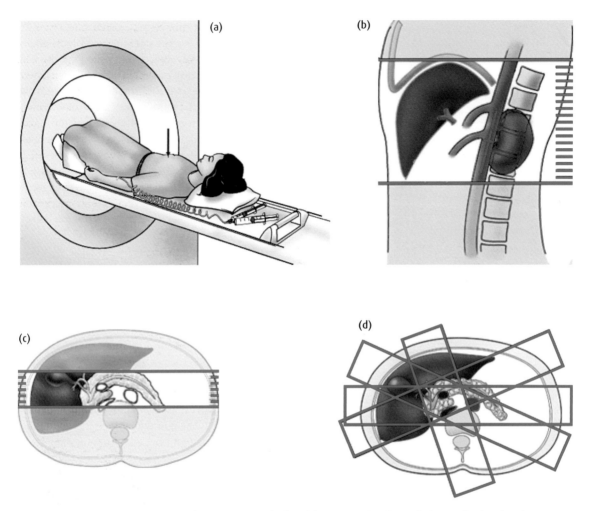

(a)　　　　(b)

(c)

(d)

Figure 2.6 Liver MR. (a) Patient prepped for intravenous (i.v.) gadolinium. Landmark: just below xyphoid at the rib cage margin. (b) Positioning of axial slices for liver imaging. (c) Thin slab MR Cholangiopancreatography (MRCP) with imaging volume from posterior to the common bile duct (CBD) as it passes through the head of the pancreas to anterior to the parta hepatis. (d) Thick slab MRCP acquired at various angles.

figure 2.6) to evaluate the biliary system and to serve as a localizer for subsequent axial acquisitions. This is often known as MR cholangiopancreatography (MRCP). Axial T_2-weighted images can detect focal neoplastic lesions. T_2 can be acquired with or without fat saturation. If fat saturation or breath-holding is not utilized then respiratory triggering or at least an anterior saturation pulse is necessary to minimize artefact from the movement of anterior subcuta-neous fat during breathing. Spoiled gradient-echo T_1-weighted images can be performed in-phase and out-of-phase in order to assess for any fatty lesions and to evaluate the liver on T_1-weighted images. Finally dynamic gadolinium enhanced spoiled gradient-echo imaging with fat saturation is performed, pre-gadolinium, during the arterial phase of the gadolinium injection, at 30 s, 1 min, 3 min and 5 min. This helps to identify malignant lesions, which may only be seen during the arterial phase of the gadolinium bolus and also helps to characterize lesions by showing their homogeneity and time course of enhancement.

2.5.6 Pelvis

Imaging the male pelvis is controversial because a large multi-centre study in the late 1990s showed that MRI of the prostate gland, even with an endo-rectal prostate coil, did not accurately diagnose and stage prostate cancer. Recently, however, prostate MRI and spec-troscopy has improved and is becoming popular again in many centres for the more limited task of identifying gross invasion of prostate cancer beyond the capsule, into seminal vesicles or lymph nodes. T_1-weighted images are obtained in the axial plane to look for lymph nodes and hemorrhage related to prostate biopsies. T_2-weighted images are obtained in axial coronal and sagittal planes to identify tumour which is dark on these images compared with the normally bright peripheral zone and seminal vesicles.

For the female pelvis, MRI provides a comprehensive assessment of the uterus and ovaries with much more

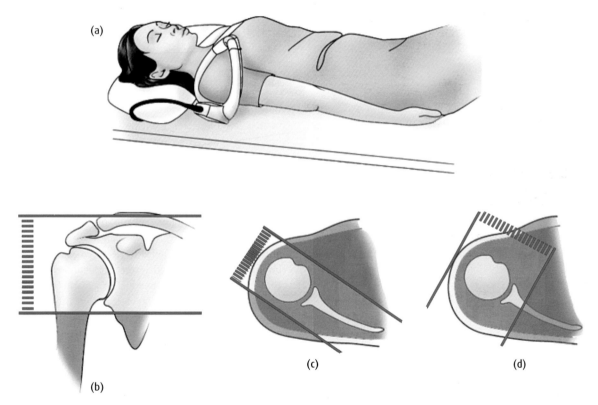

Figure 2.7 (a) Shoulder MRI. Positioning: supine with arm at side and palm facing up. It is useful to tuck the hand under the hip to help keep the shoulder motionless. It is important to shift the patient to one side of the magnet so the shoulder being imaged is closer to the centre 'sweet spot' of the magnet. This is especially helpful for fat saturation. A vitamin E capsule may be placed at the site of any mass or symptoms. A wide strap over the shoulder can help reduce shoulder motion during breathing. Landmark: mid-coil. (b) Axial slices from the top of the acromion to below the gleno-humeral joint, (c) coronal oblique parallel to the supraspinatus tendon and gleno-humeral joint and (d) sagittal parallel to glenoid and perpendicular to coronal.

detail than ultrasound. As a result MRI of the female pelvis has become the trouble-shooting technique for evaluating patients in whom ultrasound is inadequate. Pelvic MRI is also useful preoperatively and pre-embolization of the fibroid uterus. Use a pelvic or torso array coil to maximize SNR. T_2-weighted imaging is performed in all three planes to assess the ovaries, uterus, endometrium, free fluid in the pelvis and any pathology. If the uterus has an unusual angle, then the coronal T_2-weighted image can be angled such that it is coronal to the uterine fundus to better assess for uterine anomalies. T_1-weighted imaging is performed in at least one plane, typically axial, to assess for adenopathy and again with fat saturation to look for endometriosis or haemorrhagic cysts, which are bright on these images. The fat saturation images can also demonstrate fat in dermoid tumours.

2.5.7 Shoulder

The frequency of injury to the rotator cuff as well as impingement syndrome and the ability of MRI to diagnose soft-tissue injuries including tendonosis and frank tears of the rotator cuff has made this a popular exam, which has largely replaced the more invasive shoulder arthrogram. It is performed with a dedicated shoulder coil for maximum SNR. Axial proton density imaging is performed first and used as a guide to position coronal proton density and T_2-weighted images, with fat saturation aligned with the supraspinatus muscle and tendon. Finally a sagittal oblique T_2-weighted image is performed perpendicular to the coronal obliques as in figure 2.7.

2.5.8 Hip

The availability of MRI for evaluating the hips has enabled the accurate diagnosis of two important conditions that are not seen well by conventional X-rays. One is osteonecrosis of the femoral head and the other is occult femoral neck fractures and insufficiency fractures of the pelvis, which occur in older patients with osteoporosis. The standard exam includes axial and coronal T_1-weighting to assess the bone marrow and then axial and coronal STIR or T_2-weighting with fat saturation to look for the oedema characteristically associated with these conditions. It is important to always image both hips because

these conditions are often bilateral even if symptoms are present on just one side. Also be sure to extend high enough up into the pelvis to include the sacro-iliac joints since a sacro-iliac insufficiency fracture can present with pain that is similar to an occult hip fracture. For a more comprehensive assessment of a particular hip joint, a combination of surface coils can be placed over the symptomatic joint to obtain a higher SNR for more detail of just the one hip. For example, it may be possible to combine the shoulder coil with a small circular coil or flexible coil. Then high-resolution proton density imaging is performed in all three planes (figure 2.8).

2.5.9 Knee

Although knee injuries are common, the incidence of actual fractures is rare. Since X-rays of the painful knee only show fractures or large effusions, they are often not very helpful. The ability of MRI to evaluate the soft tissues, tendon, ligaments and menisci has revolutionized management of knee pathology. The relatively small size of the critical structures around the knee joint requires high-resolution, high-SNR imaging that is only possible with specialized coils optimized to encompass just the knee. It is also important to image with the pulse sequence that yields the highest SNR and a lot of slices; this means using proton density sequences. Proton density is performed at high resolution in axial and coronal planes as well as in a sagittal oblique plane aligned with the expected course of the anterior cruciate ligament. In order to assess for bone contusion and to see effusions better, it is useful to perform a T_2-weighted image with fat saturation or STIR in coronal or sagittal planes (figure 2.9).

2.5.10 Thoracic aorta

With conventional spin-echo imaging, the flow of the blood during gradient activity and between the initial 90° RF pulse and the subsequent 180° refocusing pulse causes loss of signal, creating a flow void effect sometimes referred to as black blood imaging. This allows spin-echo MRI to evaluate large vascular structures with high blood flow, such as the thoracic aorta. The black blood effect is good for evaluating the aortic wall

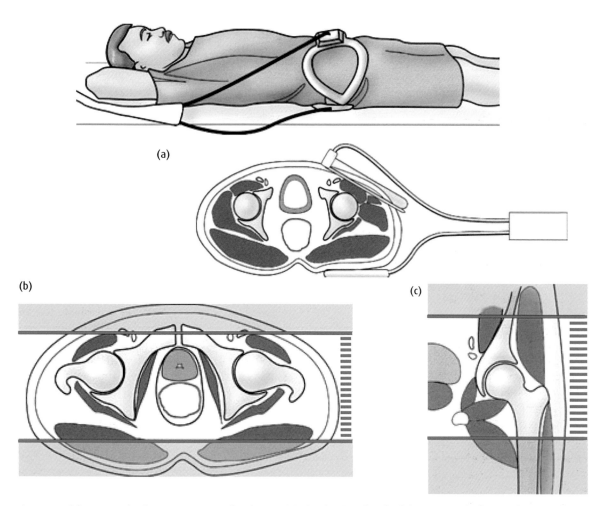

Figure 2.8 (a) Suggested coil arrangements and patient positioning (supine, feet first) for imaging the hip. Landmark: pubic symphysis. (b) Positioning for coronal slices, (c) axial slices.

and the relationship of the aorta to other structures. Recently simple spin echo imaging has been largely replaced with an ECG gated breath hold sequence that utilizes inversion pulses to more effectively null blood signal. Bright blood, cine gradient echo or steady state images provide greater lumenal detail and a sense of the blood flow especially where coarctation or valvular disease creates jets of spin dephasing.

Because of the complex anatomy of the thoracic aorta, its complete evaluation requires 3D imaging. 3D CE-MRA is a fast technique that resolves most issues.

For a more comprehensive evaluation axial black blood images plus cine images in coronal and sagittal planes are obtained prior to 3D CE-MRA. Ideally the sagittal acquisition is angled into the right anterior oblique (RAO) position to show the ascending aorta, arch and descending aorta on a single image. The coronal cine images are most useful for the aortic root. When vasculitis is suspected, triple IR and axial T_1-weighted images with gradient-moment-nulling and fat-saturation are useful to look for mural thickening and perivascular inflammation.

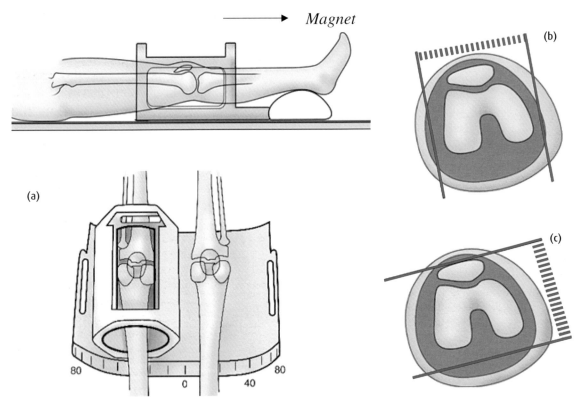

Figure 2.9 (a) Knee imaging in an extremity coil. The foot is externally rotated by about 10–15° to stretch the anterior cruciate ligament. Packing cushions around the knee helps to keep it motion free. A small cushion under the ankle helps to keep the leg straight. Landmark: inferior region of patella. Patient positioning: supine, feet first. (b) Sagittal scans oblique to the intercondylar notch. (c) Coronal oblique scans, perpendicular to sagittal.

2.5.11 Carotid and intracerebral arteries

Because flow to the brain is fast even while the patient is resting, time of flight images generally show the intracerebral vessels well. The circle of Willis and intracerebral arteries are well seen on 3D time-of-flight MRA. To reduce in-plane saturation of the blood signal, the 3D data may be acquired as **M**ultiple **O**verlapping **T**hin **S**lab **A**cquisitions (MOTSA) or a variation thereon. Outside the brain, blood flow is slower because most organs and muscles are at rest in a patient lying comfortably on the couch. With slower flow spin saturation becomes more problematic. Accordingly, carotid arteries are typically imaged with 3D CE-MRA in a coronal acquisition covering from aortic arch to the circle of Willis. Gadolinium eliminates the spin saturation to allow imaging of even tortuous vessels at high resolution. Ideally 2D projectional MR fluoroscopy is used to watch for the arrival of gadolinium. When Gd is seen arriving in the aortic arch, 3D CE-MRA of carotids is initiated with k-space ordered so that the central portion that dominates image contrast is acquired near the beginning of the scan. More recently plaque imaging has been performed with 2D black blood and bright blood techniques using specialized high SNR coils localized to the carotid bifurcation.

2.5.12 Renal arteries

Regulation of blood pressure by the renin – angiotensin system, which ensures adequate perfusion of each kidney even in the setting of renal artery stenosis, leads to a suspicion of renal artery stenosis in every severely hypertensive patient. This is an important diagnosis to make because treating essential hypertension prolongs life but using medication to lower blood pressure in the setting of renal vascular hypertension will eventually destroy the kidney. When the hypertension is caused by severe renal artery stenosis the correct treatment is balloon angioplasty or stent. However, a mild renal artery stenosis is unlikely to be haemodynamically significant and should be left alone. Thus the renal MR angiography exam must not only identify renal artery stenosis but also determine if the stenosis is haemodynamically significant. The exam is performed with 3D CE-MRA in the coronal plane during breath-holding followed by 3D phase contrast MR angiography to look for the characteristic spin dephasing that identifies the turbulent jet-like flow in haemodynamically significant stenoses. It is also useful to perform a 5 to 10-min delayed coronal 3D gradient-echo image to assess the excretory phase since asymmetry in excretion can also help with determining if a stenosis is haemodynamically significant.

2.5.13 Peripheral MRA

When the legs become tired and painful with walking and recover immediately with rest, peripheral vascular disease is suspected. Since an arterial stenosis or occlusion anywhere from aorta down to the ankle can be the cause, it is necessary to perform MR angiography over this entire distance. To image such an extensive region of anatomy quickly and with a single bolus injection of gadolinium, a technique known as bolus chase MR angiography is used. Blood pressure cuffs are wrapped around the thighs to slow down venous enhancement but they are left deflated until just before the MRA scan. The patient is immobilized on the table and if the peripheral vascular coil doesn't have suitable feet shaping, the feet are bound together with a soft strap to minimize motion.

Fast 2D time-of-flight localizer images are used to prescribe 3 coronal volumes over the abdomen-pelvis, thighs and calves. The thigh blood pressure cuffs are inflated to 60 mmHg, then a mask image is acquired at each station to use for subtraction. 3D CE-MRA is performed with a large dose (typically 30 to 45 ml) of gadolinium and fluoro-triggering to ensure optimal bolus timing at the first station (abdomen-pelvis). While the bolus is still in the arteries, the table advances to the thighs for another 3D CE-MRA coronal volume and finally the calves for the last 3D CE-MRA volume. If k-space is ordered centrically for the final calf station, data can be acquired for at least 1 min to obtain extremely high resolution which is useful for resolving fine details in the smaller calf arteries.

Some centres start the peripheral MRA examination with a time-resolved MRA of the calf and feet in order to determine how fast the blood flows to the legs and how quickly venous enhancement occurs. This information can then be used to fine tune how much scanning time is spent on each station of the bolus chase examination in order to optimally share the bolus between the three stations.

2.6 A week in the life of an MRI radiographer

A scarily all-true but slightly tongue-in-cheek description of the typical working pattern in a UK MRI unit, with apologies to other better known diarists.

MONDAY

Quality Assurance Tests	Done
Patient Alarm	Checked
Cryogen Level	83%
Chocolate	0 (This is diet week – even though the MRI scales are at least 5 kilos out.)
Alcohol	0 (Liver guilt.)

Why is it that when it rains everything grinds to a halt? Train signals fail, buses disappear, train drivers lose the ability to rise from their beds and MRI patients turn up late!

Not a good start for a Monday morning – we're already 30 minutes behind schedule – first patient had trouble parking – 'and wasn't it about time we improved our parking facilities'?

And why is it that when the day starts badly and you desperately want to catch up, all the patients arrive, especially the ones that didn't confirm . . . and the further behind you are the earlier they arrive (must be the rain) . . . and then comment that they hope not to be waiting too long . . . mmm.

Try to catch up with my reading (hey I take my continuing professional development seriously). If I could only remember where I put that article on 'mag lag'.

(Editor's note: There is no such thing as 'mag lag' so there's no need to worry about it. You can read all about the bio-effects of magnets later in this book in chapter . . . damn . . . can't remember which chapter it was . . . I'm sure it's in the book somewhere . . .)

TUESDAY

Quality Assurance Tests	Done
Patient Alarm	Checked
Cryogen Level	82.9%
Chocolate	0 (It's nice to know I can do without.)
Alcohol	1 Gin & Tonic (I decided that Monday is a difficult day on which to start a voyage of self sacrifice. In order to be effective I need to break myself in gently.)

First patient (thin, rather-too-attractive model type) feels sure my scales are wrong. 'Yes, I know, they do over estimate rather – I have new ones on order . . .'

Next was the one who said 'Are you going to scan my whole body while you're at it? That's what they're doing in the States now – I saw it on the Internet.'

In the afternoon the intensive care unit phoned: could I come up to do a scan as the patient was far too unwell to

come down. I asked if they wanted the mobile radiographer to come up to do a chest X-ray, but sure enough – they wanted MRI. I suggested they might like to pay us a visit in the very near future, as it was highly unlikely I could fit the scanner in the lift or haul it up the stairs.

WEDNESDAY

Quality Assurance Tests	Done
Patient Alarm	Checked
Cryogen Level	82.8%
Chocolate	0 (Jaffa cakes don't count do they?)
Alcohol	2 (My other half is entirely to blame: I could not stand by and watch a perfectly good Merlot be swilled down an unappreciative gullet.)

Hurrah – new scales have arrived.

Had to start the list early today to accommodate the intensive care patient from yesterday. New anaesthetist (George Clooney look-a-like) gives me a hard time about filling out a safety checklist – he's got that 'know it all' look about him that always spells trouble. Sure enough, half an hour later 'George' yells 'does it matter if I've had my credit cards in my back pocket?' 'Oh dear, George' I say . . . and he says 'my name's Nigel' . . .

THURSDAY

Quality Assurance Tests	Light bulbs need attention. Will have to write out a requisition and remember to get it triple-signed. How many hospital staff does it take to change a light bulb?
Patient Alarm	Checked
Cryogen Level	82.7%
Chocolate	0 (Bad news, the new scales measure just the same as the old ones – what

are the chances of there being a duff batch. If the dreadful truth must be faced then it's no more chocs for me.)

Alcohol   0 (Mine's a diet coke.)

Today was the day I met a medium for the first time. 'A medium what?', I hear you ask. NO! The other sort of medium – the ones that have special powers.

    Anyway, this chap came along with the patient to help guide us to the source of her pain, and to make sure that we did the scan properly. We thought it best to mark the site of pain with an oil marker, as the clinical information on the request form was so vague. After sticking a whole box of cod liver oil tablets onto a mound of quivering flesh I began to suspect that the problem may not be purely physical.

FRIDAY

Quality Assurance Tests	What's the point! (Note to reader – see chapter 11)
Patient Alarm	Does it matter? (Note to reader, yes it does)
Cryogen Level	0 for all I care.
Chocolate	3 Snickers and M&Ms (what diet?)
Alcohol	4 Gin & Tonics, 6 Bloody Marys

Had a problem with the network going down. Phoned IT department's 'helpdesk' to have the following conversation:

Me: 'We have a problem with the network and our MR scanner'.
Helpdesk girl: 'OK, can you bring it down to the workshop'.
Me (oh dear, not that can-you-bring-your-scanner-here one again!): 'No it is an MRI scanner. It doesn't move.'
Helpdesk girl: 'Well, is the green light on the front of it lit up?'
Me (losing patience): 'No it's not a flatbed scanner. It's an Emm Are Eye scanner.'

Helpdesk girl: 'How do you spell M.R.I?'
Roll on the weekend – and then back on X-ray duty!

And finally some questions we may never know the answers to . . .

- Why do patients only turn up early when you're running late?
- Why do patients want both knees to be scanned when you've only been asked to do one?
- Why do people ask for the 'Mister' Unit?
- Why do weighing scales in MRI never lie?
- Why don't all doctors look like George Clooney?
- Do magnetic fields stimulate a craving for chocolate and alcohol?
- Where is that mag lag article?

See also: Chapter 10: But is it safe? Bio-effects

FURTHER READING

International Electrotechnical Commission (2002) *Medical Electrical Equipment* – Part 2-33: *Particular Requirements for the Safety of Magnetic Resonance Equipment for Medical Diagnosis Edition: 2.0.* IEC 60601-2-33. Available direct from IEC at http://www.iec.ch/webstore/ [accessed 23rd October 2004]

Medical Devices Agency (2002) *Guidelines for Magnetic Resonance Diagnostic Equipment in Clinical Use with Particular Reference to Safety.* 2nd edn. London: Medical Devices Agency.

National Radiological Protection Board (1991) *Principles for the Protection of Patients and Volunteers During Clinical Magnetic Resonance Procedures.* Documents of the NRPB Vol 2 No 1 (ISBN: 0859513394). Available direct from NRPB at http://www.nrpb.org.uk/ [accessed 1st November 2001]

Shellock FG (2003) *Reference manual for Magnetic Resonance Safety 2003.* Salt Lake City: Amirsys Inc (ISBN: 1931884048)

International Commission on Non-Ionizing Radiation Protection (2004) *Medical Magnetic Resonance (MR) Procedures: Protection of Patients.* Health Physics 87:197-216

http://www.mrisafety.com [accessed 23rd October 2004] The Institute for Magnetic Resonance Safety, Education and Research.

Seeing is believing: introduction to image contrast

3.1 Introduction

Now that you have a basic idea of what MR images can show, we need to look a little more closely at the different types of contrast that are produced. We will use a very simple classification of the body tissues, which will be good enough to describe the basic appearances:

- fluids – cerebrospinal fluid (CSF), synovial fluid, oedema;
- water-based tissues – muscle, brain, cartilage, kidney;
- fat-based tissues – fat, bone marrow.

Fat-based tissues have some special MR properties, which can cause artefacts. Fluids are separated from other water-based tissues because they contain very few cells and so have quite different appearances on images. (Flowing fluids are rather complicated and their appearance depends on many factors including their speed; they will be dealt with in detail in chapter 13.) Pathological tissues frequently have either oedema or a proliferating blood supply, so their appearance can be a mixture of water-based tissues and fluids.

The various tissues have different signal intensities, or brightness, on MR images. The differences are described as the image contrast, and allow us to see the boundaries between tissues. For example, if a tumour is bright and brain tissue is mid-grey, we can detect the extent of the tumour (figure 3.1(a)). MRI allows us to produce a wide range of contrasts by using different imaging techniques (known as pulse sequences) and by controlling the timing of the sequences. So it is also possible to make the tumour

dark and brain tissue brighter (figure 3.1(b)). Note that this is quite separate from changing the window and level: that can make the whole image darker or brighter on the screen or film, but the tumour will always be darker than the brain tissue. Compare this with Computerized Tomography (CT) images. CT contrast depends only on the attenuation of X-rays by the tissues (measured in Hounsfield units). We can produce 'soft tissue' or 'bony' windows by changing the reconstruction algorithm, but bone will always be the brightest tissue and grey matter will always be darker than white matter.

In this chapter we will:

- learn the basic terminology: T_1, T_2, proton density, and so on (you've probably noticed that MRI has an entirely new language, most of which seems to start with the letter 'T'!);
- describe the main types of image contrast (T_1-weighted, T_2-weighted, PD-weighted and T_2^*-weighted);
- show how to achieve different contrasts with the basic pulse sequences, spin echo and gradient echo, by changing the TR and TE times and changing the flip angle (gradient echo only);
- show how STIR and FLAIR work for suppressing fat or CSF respectively leaving a T_2-weighted appearance in the remaining tissues;
- show how special contrast agents can improve image contrast by enhancing signal intensity in tumours;
- introduce MR angiography techniques to show flowing blood with suppression of the background static tissues.

(a) (b)

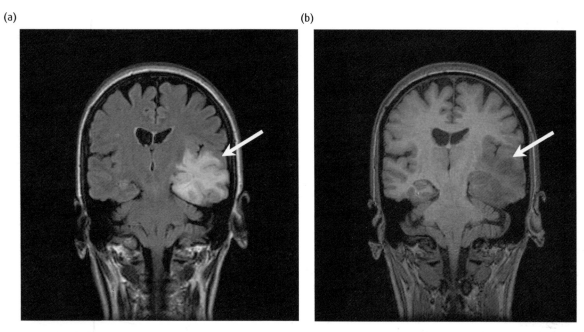

Figure 3.1 (a) Coronal image of the brain showing a tumour (arrow). In this image the tumour is bright against the darker grey of the normal brain tissue. (b) The same slice with a different pulse sequence, this time showing the tumour darker than the surrounding brain.

3.2 Some basic stuff

In this section we will introduce some important terminology and give a simple explanation of the processes involved in MR for those who like to know 'why'. You can skip this for now and come back to it later if you don't want to go into the details just yet.

All MR images are produced using a *pulse sequence*, which is stored in the scanner computer. The sequence contains *radiofrequency (RF) pulses* and *gradient pulses* which have carefully controlled durations and timings. The gradient pulses make the characteristic 'knocking' noise when the imager is acquiring a scan. There are many different types of sequences, but they all have timing values called TR, and TE, which can be modified. Usually you (the operator) set TR and TE in order to get the required image contrast.

MRI uses the natural properties of hydrogen which, as part of water or lipids, makes up 75–80% of the human body. The most important properties are the

proton density (often abbreviated to PD), and two characteristic times called *spin-lattice relaxation time* and *spin-spin relaxation time*, denoted T_1 and T_2 respectively. Proton density is related to the number of hydrogen atoms in a particular volume; fluids such as CSF and blood have higher PD than tendon and bone. Relaxation times describe how long the tissue takes to get back to equilibrium after an RF pulse. T_1 and T_2 depend on the different tissues (full explanations of the mechanisms are given in chapter 8). Fluids have long T_1s (e.g.1500–2000 ms), water-based tissues are usually mid-range (e.g. 400–1200 ms), and fat-based tissues generally have short T_1s (e.g. 100–150 ms). T_2 is always shorter than T_1 for a given tissue. Fluids have the longest T_2 (700–1200 ms), while water-based tissues tend to have longer T_2s than fat-based tissue (40–200 ms and 10–100 ms respectively).

In general images have contrast which depends on either PD, T_1 or T_2. In PD images, high PDs give high signal intensities which in turn have bright pixels on the

Table 3.1 Choice of TR and TE for conventional spin echo sequences

TR	TE	
	Short (less than 40 ms)	Long (more than 75 ms)
Short (less than 750 ms)	T_1-weighted	Not useful
Long (more than 1500 ms)	PD-weighted	T_2-weighted

Table 3.2 Choice of TR, TE and α for gradient-echo sequences

Flip angle α	TE	
	Short (less than 15 ms)	Long (more than 30 ms)
Small (less than 40°)	PD-weighted	T_2-weighted
Large (more than 50°)	T_1-weighted	Not useful

Notes:
TR is always short (less than 750 ms) compared with SE sequences. (N.B. Longer TRs require larger flip angles to show T_1 weighting; at short TRs even 45° flip angles may have T_1 weighting.)

image. In T_2-weighted images, tissues with long T_2 give the highest signal intensities, producing a bright appearance. T_1-weighted images are completely different; long T_1 tissues give the weakest signal, i.e. bright pixels on T_1 are associated with short T_1s.

There are two principle types of pulse sequence, called *spin echo* and *gradient echo*, abbreviated *SE* and *GE*. SE sequences use two RF pulses to create the echo which measures the signal intensity. SE can produce T_1-, T_2-, or PD-weighted images depending on the choice of TR and TE as shown in the table 3.1. SE sequences generally produce the best quality images but they take a relatively long time – several minutes rather than seconds. GE sequences use a single RF pulse followed by a gradient pulse to create the echo, which also measures the signal intensity. GE sequences can produce images with T_1-, T_2- or

PD-weighting (see table 3.2) and generally have much shorter TRs than SE, so they have shorter scan times. However, they are influenced by the quality of the main magnetic field (called the *inhomogeneity*) as well as by timing parameters. This affects the apparent spin-spin relaxation time which becomes shorter. The combined T_2 and magnetic field inhomogeneity is known as T_2^* (pronounced 'tee two star'), so GE sequences really depend on T_2^* not just T_2. However, with modern magnets GE T_2^*-weighted images have very similar contrast to SE T_2-weighted images, and so we often just refer to 'gradient-echo T_2s'.

3.3 T_1-weighted images

T_1-weighted images can be produced using either the SE or the GE sequence. For now we will just consider SE images, leaving GE images until later. We need to use a short TR and a short TE to enhance the T_1 differences between tissues. T_1-weighted images usually have excellent contrast: fluids are very dark (unless they are flowing into the imaging volume), water-based tissues are mid-grey and fat-based tissues are very bright. They are often known as 'anatomy scans', as they show most clearly the boundaries between different tissues (figure 3.2).

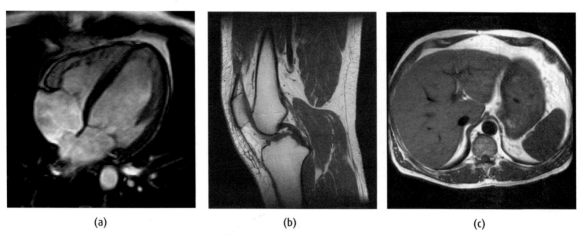

(a)   (b)   (c)

Figure 3.2 T$_1$-weighted images of normal anatomy. (a) Oblique '4-chamber' view of the heart, (b) sagittal knee, (c) axial liver.

How does the sequence timing affect T$_1$ contrast?

T$_1$ is the relaxation time for the recovery of magnetization along the z axis and we use a short TR to get T$_1$-weighted images. Let's see what happens if we acquire several spin-echo (SE) images with different TRs but the same TE (figure 3.3(a)). If we measure the signal intensity of various tissues we find that they all increase as TR is increased, as shown in figure 3.3 (b). Notice that at the longest TR there is very little signal difference between grey and white matter, but at shorter TRs the contrast is improved. These curves are the T$_1$ relaxation curves for the tissues and show that at short TRs we get T$_1$-weighted images – i.e. the contrast depends mostly on the T$_1$ differences between the tissues.

You will probably have noticed by now that long-T$_1$ tissues such as fluids are dark on T$_1$-weighted images while short-T$_1$ tissues are bright. So we can predict that pathology which has oedema or a lot of capillaries will be darker than the surrounding normal tissue, while fatty lesions will have higher signal intensities (figure 3.4). In fact, anything which changes the T$_1$ of a tissue will change its appearance on T$_1$ images.

3.4 T$_2$-weighted images

T$_2$-weighted contrast can also be produced by SE or GE sequences, but GE images are affected by the magnetic field inhomogeneity, and we will leave discussion of this until later. SE T$_2$ images require long TR and long TE, so they take longer to acquire than T$_1$-weighted images (the scan time depends directly on the TR). On these scans fluids have the highest intensity, and water- and fat-based tissues are mid-grey. T$_2$ images are often thought of as 'pathology' scans because collections of abnormal fluid are bright against the darker normal tissue. So for example the meniscal tear in the knee shows up well because the synovial fluid in the tear is brighter than the cartilage (figure 3.5).

Notice that the relationship between T$_2$-weighted image appearance and the actual T$_2$ value is different from the case of T$_1$ weighting. On T$_2$ images long T$_2$s are brighter than short T$_2$s, whereas on T$_1$-weighted images long T$_1$s are darker than short T$_1$s. This can be confusing and difficult to remember at first, but you will quickly get used to it. For the next few days, try to take a little extra time when you look at images and think carefully about the relationship between the tissue relaxation times and the image contrast.

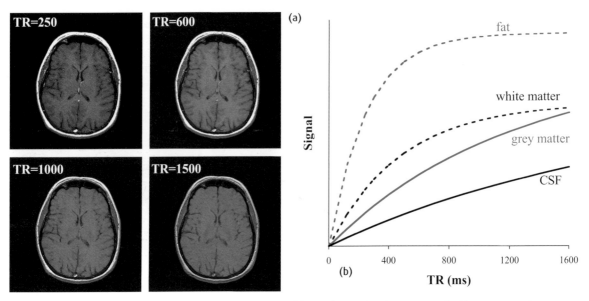

Figure 3.3 (a) SE brain images with TE = 10 ms and various TR. (b) Signal intensity of CSF, grey and white matter, and subcutaneous fat plotted against TR.

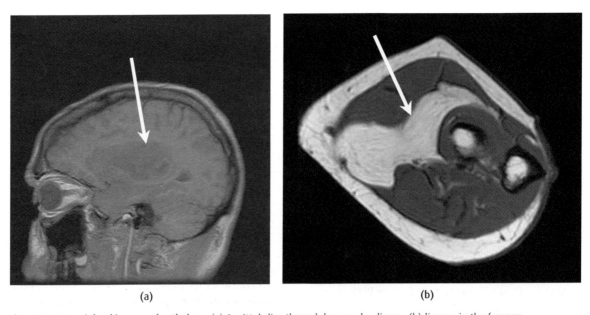

Figure 3.4 T_1-weighted images of pathology. (a) Sagittal slice through low-grade glioma, (b) lipoma in the forearm.

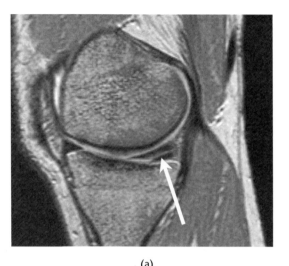

(a)

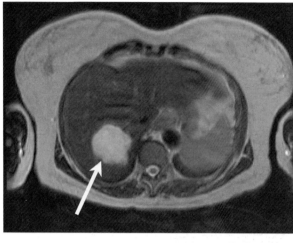

(b)

Figure 3.5 T_2-weighted pathology images. (a) Sagittal image of meniscal tear (arrow) and (b) axial liver scan showing haemangioma.

How does the sequence timing affect T_2 contrast?

Suppose we acquire several images at different TEs, keeping the TR long to allow full T_1 relaxation (figure 3.6 (a)), and again we measure the signal intensity of various tissues. Plotting the intensity against TE (figure 3.6 (b)) we find that they all decrease with increasing TE, but fluids stay bright for longest. We have made a rough measure of the T_2 decay curves. At short TE there is little contrast between grey matter, white matter and CSF, while longer TEs improve the T_2 weighting of the images.

Figure 3.6 shows how important it is to choose the right timing parameters. If TE is mid-range, we lose much of the T_2 contrast, but it is not quite short enough to produce a 'true' PD image. The same is true of changing TR: at intermediate values, images have contrast which is neither one thing nor the other. There is quite a wide range of acceptable values for TR and TE to produce T_1, T_2 or PD images, but the exact figures will depend on the scanner's field strength and manufacturer, and the tissues being imaged.

3.5 PD-weighted images

Bearing in mind that the proton densities (i.e. water content) for most tissues are rather similar, you might wonder why we bother to produce PD-weighted images since they will have less contrast than either T_1 or T_2 images. The reason is partly historical: when MRI was first used clinically, GE images had very poor quality so only SE images tended to be used. As we've just found out, T_2-weighted SE images require a long TR and they therefore take a long time to acquire. However, it is possible to create another echo at a shorter TE. This produces an image at the same slice location and within the same scan time, but with PD weighting instead of T_2 weighting. So PD images were 'free' if you wanted a T_2 image, and the 'dual echo' sequence is still popular even though these days we can do a fast spin echo (FSE) T_2 scan in a very short time.

Of course we have been making some very sweeping statements about contrast, and PD scans do have some useful clinical applications; for example, in the knee you can distinguish articular cartilage from the cortical bone and menisci (figure 3.7).

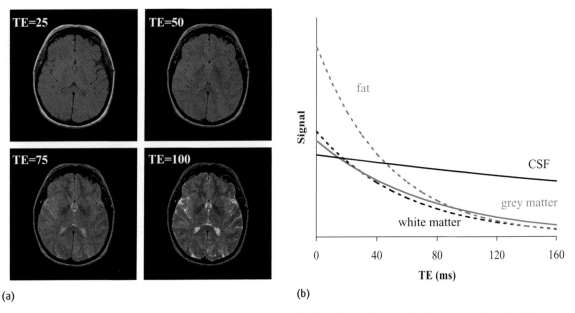

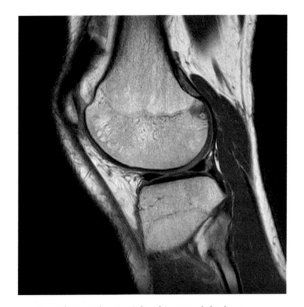

(a)   (b)

Figure 3.6 (a) SE brain images with TR = 1500 ms and various TE. (b) Signal intensity for brain tissues plotted against TE.

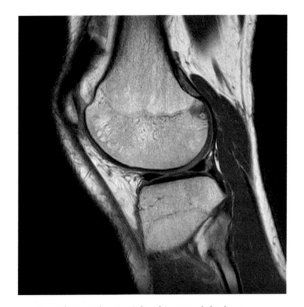

Figure 3.7 Sagittal PD-weighted image of the knee.

Timing parameters for PD-weighted images
From the T_1 and T_2 decay curves we have produced, we can also work out the best timing for a PD-weighted image. We need to allow full T_1 relaxation, so TR must be long (figure 3.3 (b)), and we want to avoid T_2 weighting so TE must be short (figure 3.6 (b)). The curves also tell us that we won't have a lot of contrast between grey and white matter, but CSF will still be slightly darker and fat rather bright.

3.6 Gradient-echo T_1-weighted images

As you know by now, gradient-echo (GE) sequences can produce T_1-, T_2*- or PD-weighted images. However, there are lots of different gradient sequences with different names – how do you know which one to choose? There are important differences between these sequences, so we eventually have to learn which is which (see chapter 12). To start with though, for basic GE T_1 images you should use the following sequences depending on your scanner: FLASH (Siemens), SPGR (General Electric), T1-FFE (Philips), RF-FAST (Marconi, formerly Picker). For other manufacturers, consult your applications specialist.

Although the sequence choice is important, the choice of flip angle, α, is much more important for getting T_1-weighted images. GE sequences generally use small flip angles (less than 90°) and very short TRs, e.g. around 150 ms. Looking back at figure 3.3 (b), we would expect to have very little signal-to-noise ratio (SNR) with such short repetition times. However, if we use a 30° RF pulse instead of a 90° pulse, we can avoid this signal loss. Immediately after a 30° pulse, the z magnetization is not zero but left at approximately 86% of the equilibrium value M_0 (see figure 3.8). This means the T_1 recovery is already nearly complete, and full relaxation can be achieved in a very short time (typically less than 500 ms). So even with a short TR, using $\alpha = 30°$ will not have T_1 weighting.

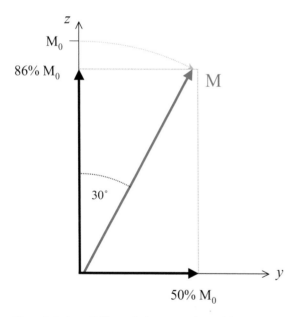

Figure 3.8 A small flip angle leaves a substantial magnetization along the z axis, e.g. after a 30° flip angle, the z magnetization $\approx 86\% M_0$ and in the x-y plane we have $50\% M_0$.

Alternatively, using $\alpha = 50°$ or higher reduces the z magnetization immediately after the RF pulse a lot more, and we can create better T_1 weighting. (The exact choice of α depends on which GE sequence you are using; check with your applications specialist.) You can see the effect of changing α on the signal intensities of brain tissues in figure 3.9. Notice that intermediate values of α give contrast that is not good for either T_1 or PD.

We can summarize by saying that TR has much less effect on the image contrast, and we can just use α to

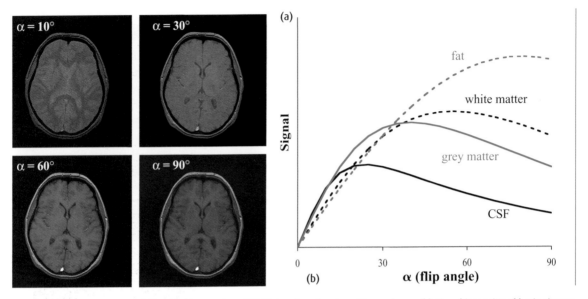

Figure 3.9 (a) GE images with fixed TR (150 ms) and TE (4.6 ms) and various flip angles α. (b) Signal intensity of brain tissues plotted against α.

control the T_1 weighting of the scans. For GE T_1-weighted scans we need a relatively large α of at least 50°, and a short TE; TR can be either as short as possible for rapid scanning or just long enough to get the required number of slices. Note that even if you don't use one of the sequences mentioned above, you can still get a T_1 GE image with these parameters.

GE T_1 images are very quick to acquire and can have excellent SNR and resolution. They are often used for 3D volume scanning, where the scan times with SE would be hours, and for breath-hold chest or abdomen imaging.

3.7 Gradient-echo T_2*-weighted images

Remember that GE images should be called T_2* weighted not T_2 weighted? This is because of the effects of an imperfect magnetic field: a perfectly uniform magnetic field simply can't be produced, and even if it could the patient would make it imperfect due to *susceptibility* effects. Air pockets (sinuses or intestines), dense bone (skull base), and iron-rich blood breakdown products (met-haemoglobin or haemosiderin) all change the main magnetic field in their immediate

vicinity, so tissues around such inhomogeneities will experience different magnetic fields.

These inhomogeneities affect the relaxation of tissues after an RF pulse, speeding up the apparent spin-spin relaxation T_2*. An SE sequence can correct for this effect but GE sequences can't, and so GE images depend on the apparent spin-spin relaxation time T_2*.

For any particular tissue T_2* is closely related to T_2, so the basic contrast in T_2*-weighted images is the same as in SE T_2-weighted scans (fluids are bright, other tissues are mid-grey).

T_2, the spin-spin relaxation time, is a fundamental property of the tissue which describes how fast the transverse magnetization decays. Spin-spin relaxation T_2 would occur even in a perfectly homogeneous magnetic field. However, if there are different magnetic field strengths in different regions of the body, either due to susceptibility effects or inhomogeneities in the main magnetic field, transverse relaxation is speeded up (but spin-lattice relaxation is not affected). In a GE sequence, we see the combined effect of T_2 and magnetic field inhomogeneities. We can call this relaxation the 'apparent' relaxation time and give it the shorthand notation T_2*.

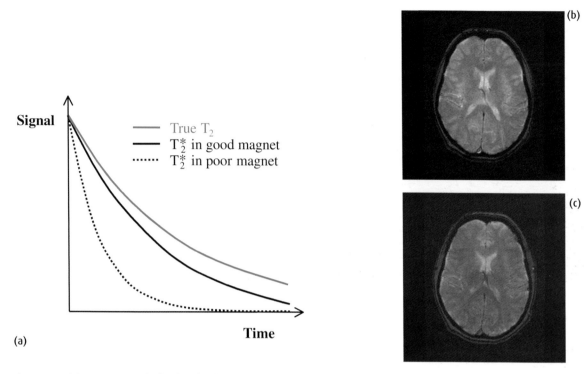

(a)

(b)

(c)

Figure 3.10 (a) Comparison of T$_2$* with T$_2$ for the same tissue in different magnet homogeneities. (b) T$_2$* image of the head produced in a modern well shimmed magnet. (c) The same image with deliberately reduced homogeneity. Notice the overall loss of signal and the loss of grey–white matter contrast. TE was 40 ms in (b) and (c).

Magnetic properties of tissues

Magnetic susceptibility is a natural property of all tissues and is given the symbol χ (pronounced 'ki' to rhyme with 'sky'). It is a measure of how magnetized the tissue becomes when it is placed in a strong magnetic field, which depends on the arrangement of electrons in the tissue. There are four descriptions of different magnetic susceptibilities.

- *Diamagnetic* materials have a very weak susceptibility which actually produces an internal field in the opposite direction to the applied field. Most body tissues are diamagnetic, while air and dense bone have almost zero susceptibility.
- *Paramagnetic* materials have a stronger susceptibility and produce a field in the same direction as the main field; examples include gadolinium (used as an MR contrast agent), deoxy-haemoglobin and met-haemoglobin.
- *Superparamagnetic* is a term used to describe materials intermediate between paramagnetic and ferromagnetic. Examples include iron oxide particles (used as MR contrast agents), ferritin and haemosiderin.
- *Ferromagnetic* materials become strongly magnetized and experience a large force when placed in an external field. Metal alloys containing iron, nickel and cobalt are often ferromagnetic.

Although the magnetic susceptibility of tissues is small, the differences between the tissues and air are big enough to set up local magnetic field gradients. So hydrogen atoms on either side of the boundary will be in different magnetic fields and will relax more quickly as they interact with each other.

To produce basic GE T_2^* images, use the following sequence depending on your scanner: FISP (Siemens), GRE (General Electric, also called GRASS on earlier scanners), T2-FFE (Philips), CE-FAST (Marconi). For other manufacturers consult your applications specialist. Whichever sequence you use, you need to keep α small to avoid T_1 weighting, and TR can be short for rapid scanning or long enough for multiple slices. The TE is increased to achieve T_2^* weighting. T_2^* images are particularly useful in musculoskeletal imaging or to detect haemorrhage.

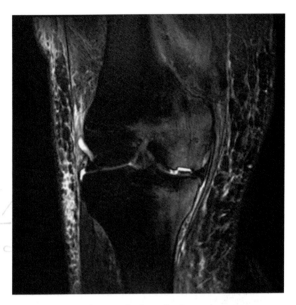

Figure 3.11 STIR image of a bone bruise

How good is yours?

T_2^* depends on the quality of your scanner's magnet. In the ideal case of a nearly uniform field, T_2^* is almost identical to T_2 (figure 3.10 (a)), which means that GE T_2^* images will look very similar to SE T_2 scans. Conversely the same tissues in a poor magnet will have much shorter T_2^*s which will be almost the same for all tissues. GE T_2^*-weighted images acquired with the same timing parameters will have less contrast and reduced SNR, especially around areas with susceptibility differences (figure 3.10 (b)). In the early days of MRI it was difficult to produce a homogeneous field and GE images often had a very low SNR and produced poor T_2^* contrast. Modern scanners are much better and we find that GE T_2^* images have very similar contrast to SE T_2-weighted scans.

Try it for yourself 2: contrast on gradient echo images

Using your oil and water bottles again, try changing TR, TE and α to see the effect on contrast. You need to use different GE sequences to show T_1 or T_2^* contrast: refer back to the last two sections. As before, there are pitfalls to avoid:

- Short TRs and long TEs don't allow many slices: check first how many you can get.
- Keep all the other scanning parameters the same.
- Keep the same receiver gains for all the scans within a set (e.g. for several different TEs). Measure the signal intensity within regions on the images, and then plot curves.

3.8 Gradient-echo PD-weighted images

You can probably work out for yourself how to get a gradient echo PD image. You need to use the same type of sequence as you did for a GE T_1-weighted image, setting the TR to be as short as possible (for a 3D scan) or long enough to get the required number of slices. Since we don't want any T_2 decay the echo time must be short, and α must be small to avoid creating T_1 contrast.

3.9 STIR images

You will often hear people ask for STIR images, especially for musculoskeletal imaging (figure 3.11). STIR images have very low signal from fat but still have high signal from fluids, i.e. they can be thought of as a 'fat-suppressed pathology' imaging technique. STIR uses a variation on the spin echo (SE) sequence called '*inversion recovery*' which has an extra 180° RF pulse separated by a new timing parameter (the inversion time TI) before the 90° pulse.

IR sequences can produce excellent T_1-weighted images (see chapter 12); however they are most often

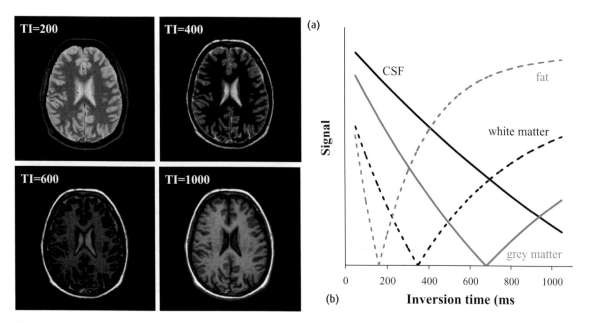

Figure 3.12 (a) Inversion recovery images at various TI with TR = 4000 ms and TE = 19 ms. (b) Inversion recovery curves showing magnitude signals (as most commonly used in scanners) with only positive values. The curve for fat indicates the appropriate TI for a STIR image.

used for tissue suppressed images, since by selecting the TI carefully the signal from any particular tissue can be nulled. The appropriate TI depends on the T_1 of the tissue and should be about 70% of the T_1. For example, fat has a T_1 of 220 ms at 1.5 T, so if we set TI to 150 ms, the signal from fat can be suppressed. At other field strengths TI should be different, e.g. 110 ms at 0.5 T. This short inversion time gives STIR its name: **S**hort **TI** **I**nversion **R**ecovery. However, bear in mind that STIR images will suppress all tissues with the same T_1 as fat, so they should not be used after gadolinium contrast injection when there may be T_1 changes in the pathology as well as in normal tissues.

At this short TI, other tissues have nonzero (mostly negative) z magnetization immediately before the 90° pulse and therefore they produce large signals. By acquiring images at various TIs we can measure the signals and plot the inversion recovery curves (figure 3.12). Now it is easy to see that fluids (with the longest T_1s) will have the highest signals on STIR images – just like T_2 'pathology' scans.

There are other methods for removing or reducing the signal from fat, and STIR may not be the best choice. See section 6.5 for a more detailed explanation and evaluation of the strengths and weaknesses of the techniques.

3.10 FLAIR images

The IR sequence makes another frequent appearance, this time with a different TI, to produce T_2-weighted images with a suppressed CSF signal. This sequence, known as FLAIR (**FL**uid **A**ttenuated **I**nversion **R**ecovery), is commonly used for neurological imaging where lesions may be close to the ventricles. For example, it is more sensitive than simple T_2-weighted images for multiple sclerosis lesions (figure 3.13 (a,b)). The principles are the same as for STIR, but this time we want to remove the signal from CSF which has a much longer T_1. Because of the long T_1, there is a wider range of TIs which will give reasonably good fluid

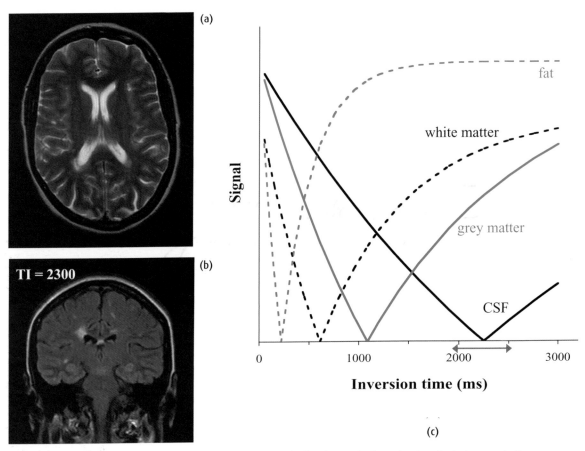

Figure 3.13 (a) SE T$_2$ and (b) FLAIR images in a patient with multiple sclerosis (MS). Notice that the lesions are better seen when the CSF signal is suppressed. (c) Inversion recovery curves showing the range of null point for CSF.

When to use STIR for fat suppression

STIR is a good fat-suppression technique for lower field systems (typically less than 1 T) where chemical-shift-based suppression doesn't work well because of the low field strength. It is also useful for images with large fields of view, when magnetic field inhomogeneities will cause patchy chemical-shift fat suppression. Fat-suppressed imaging of the orbits can be a difficult area due to susceptibility effects (see 'Magnetic properties of tissues') and STIR may be the best sequence for these scans, especially at low- or mid-field strengths.

suppression, typically between 1800 and 2500 ms depending on the magnet's field strength (figure 3.13 (c)). Again, all tissues with T$_1$s similar to CSF will be suppressed, and FLAIR is not recommended after gadolinium injection because of the rather unpredictable changes to T$_1$s.

3.11 Contrast agents

With all those different sequences and timing choices, why do we need to give patients artificial contrast agents? Surely it is possible to find the right technique

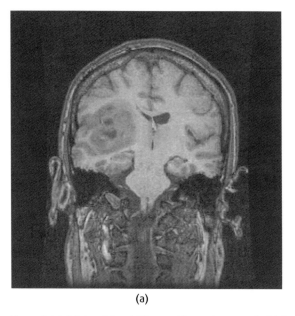
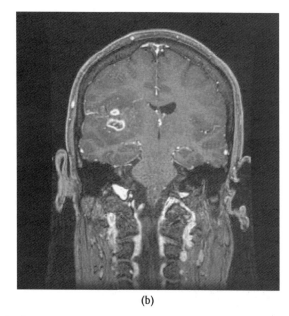

(a)   (b)

Figure 3.14 (a) Pre-Gd and (b) post-Gd SE T_1 images of a high-grade glioma.

to show the optimal contrast for each pathology? Well yes, it probably is possible, but not in the time available for a clinical MR scan! MR imaging is considered to be highly sensitive (that is, it shows up pathological conditions easily) but not very specific (i.e. several different pathologies have similar appearances). Contrast agents help to improve the specificity by producing an extra set of images with different contrast with only a short increase in the total patient scan time. Contrast agents can also increase SNR which improves image quality and allows higher resolution.

The most commonly used contrast agents are based on gadolinium, a metallic element with a strong paramagnetic susceptibility. When gadolinium is injected into the body, it is initially in the arteries but rapidly redistributes into the extracellular fluid spaces (11 min half-life), and is then gradually excreted via the kidneys with a 90 min half-life in patients with normal renal function. It is completely eliminated after 24 h. It has the effect of shortening T_1 in tissues where it accumulates, so on postcontrast T_1-weighted images these tissues will have enhanced signals. For example,

highly vascular tumours will become brighter and where the blood–brain barrier is disrupted gadolinium will leak into the region and enhance that area (figure 3.14). Gadolinium is also available in an oral preparation for gastro-intestinal applications, giving increased signal on T_1-weighted images of the bowel contents.

A more recent introduction but one which is gaining wide acceptance is the SPIO (**S**uper-**P**aramagnetic **I**ron **O**xide) group of contrast agents. These are available in a variety of formulations, for intravenous injection or oral administration. The effect of a SPIO agent is to reduce the T_2 of tissues in which it accumulates, causing lower signal intensities on T_2 or T_2^*-weighted images postcontrast. They are commonly used for liver and spleen imaging, where normal Kupffer cells take up the contrast agent. Thus the signal intensity of normal tissue is reduced, leaving pathological tissues with a relative enhancement postcontrast (figure 3.15). As oral agents, SPIOs dramatically reduce the signal within the bowel, leaving other abdominal and pelvic tissues relatively bright.

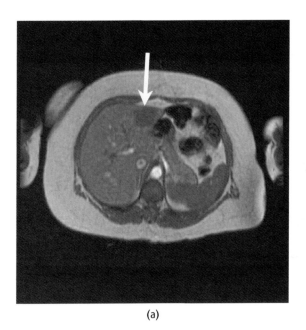

(a)   (b)

Figure 3.15 (a) Pre-SPIO and (b) post-SPIO T$_2$*-weighted images of a metastatic liver tumour.

Why doesn't gadolinium affect T$_2$?

The real answer is that gadolinium *does* affect T$_2$ as well as T$_1$, and similarly SPIOs have a T$_1$-shortening effect as well as reducing T$_2$ and T$_2$*. The precise effect of contrast agents depends on their concentration in the tissue concerned, and also on the imaging sequence being used. Remember that although images are described as T$_1$-weighted, T$_2$-weighted, etc., the signals have contributions from all the magnetic properties of the tissues concerned – T$_1$, T$_2$, PD, susceptibility, and so on. At high concentrations and in sequences with longer TEs, gadolinium may actually reduce the signal intensity of the tissue due to shortening of T$_2$.

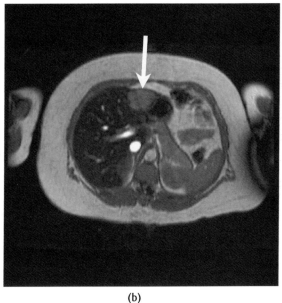

Blood flowing in vessel

Image slice

Figure 3.16 The time-of-flight or in-flow effect. The blood vessel is shown crossing through the imaging slice. When the sequence is repeated, the previously excited blood (coloured grey) has moved on and the bolus within the slice (coloured blue) has fully relaxed magnetization M$_0$.

3.12 Angiographic images

When we were describing T$_1$-weighted imaging, we mentioned that fast-moving fluids do not behave like other fluids. You may have noticed that the signal within vessels is very high on GE images and can also cause artefacts, which must be removed. How can a long-T$_1$ fluid give a high signal on T$_1$-weighted images? It is because the blood is flowing.

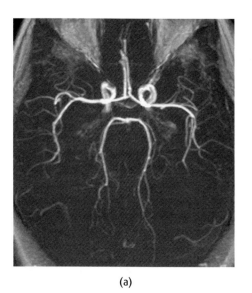

(a)

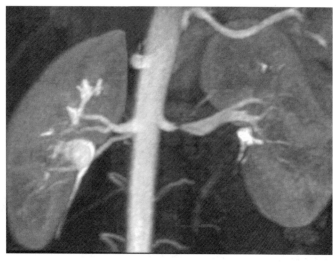

(b)

Figure 3.17 MR angiograms of (a) the Circle of Willis and (b) the renal arteries.

Consider a blood vessel passing through the imaging slice (figure 3.16). During the repetition time of the sequence, the little bolus of blood within the slice flows on and is replaced by a new bolus. This blood has not been tipped by the RF pulse, so when the next pulse is applied the blood has a stronger signal (refer back to 'How does the sequence timing affect T_1 contrast?'). Thus, it will give a high signal even though TR is short and the T_1 of blood is long. This process repeats itself during each TR, so each bolus of flowing blood always gives a high signal. It is known as the 'in-flow' or 'time-of-flight' effect.

We can exploit the high signal of flowing blood in MR angiography (MRA), using a variety of techniques to suppress almost all the signal in static tissues. The three most important sequences are 'time-of-flight MRA' (also known as 'in-flow MRA'), 'phase-contrast MRA', and 'contrast-enhanced MRA' which uses a very rapid imaging sequence during the injection of gadolinium. All three MRA sequences leave the blood vessels as the only high-signal structures against a dark background. Using a special kind of processing technique called 'Maximum Intensity Projection' (MIP), we can produce images which show the blood vessels (figure 3.17).

Warning: MRA is not as simple as it looks!
MRA seems to be an easy technique for producing angiographic images without subjecting the patient to a risky intra-arterial procedure or ionizing radiation. However, it is not without problems. For example, time-of-flight sequences may not distinguish freshly thrombosed clots from flowing blood (because the met-haemoglobin is starting to affect the MR signal), stenoses may be exaggerated in terms of length and severity, and very slow flowing blood may disappear altogether. All these pitfalls will be explained in detail in chapter 13, along with ways of avoiding them. In spite of these potential problems, MRA is a common and very useful imaging technique which you will undoubtedly use regularly.

See also:
- Details of T_1, T_2 and T_2^*, including the effects of gadolinium and SPIOs: chapter 8.
- Gradient-echo sequences: section 12.5.
- Fat-suppression techniques: section 6.5.
- MR angiography: chapter 13.

FURTHER READING

Hashemi RH and Bradley WG Jr (1997) *MRI The Basics.* Baltimore, MD: Lippincott, Williams & Wilkins (ISBN: 0683182404), chapters 7, 8 & 20.

Mitchell DG (1999) *MRI Principles.* London: WB Saunders Co. (ISBN: 0721667597), chapters 3 & 4.

Rinck PA (2005) *Magnetic Resonance in Medicine, 5th* edn. Oxford: Blackwell Science. (ISBN: 0632059869), chapter 10.

Smith H-J and Ranallo FN (1989) *A Non-mathematical Approach to Basic MRI.* Medical Physics Publishing Corp. (ISBN: 0944838022), chapters 10, 14, 15 & 21.

The devil's in the detail: pixels, matrices and slices

4.1 Introduction

MR images are not like photographs or plain X-radiographs; they are made up of thousands of tiny squares known as *pixels* (a contraction of 'picture elements') or *voxels* ('volume elements'). CT images are also made up of pixels, as are digital subtraction angiograms (DSA). The common link between MR, CT and DSA is that all these images are acquired digitally, by a computer, whereas plain X-radiographs or ordinary photographs are analogue processes.

Digital data have many advantages – they can be easily manipulated by computers, stored in a very small physical space and reproduced many times – but they also require some special understanding. In this chapter we show:

- that the analogue MR signal is digitized in order to create the image, and data can be misrepresented due to the digitization process;
- the organization of the image as pixels in a matrix with phase and frequency encoding directions;
- the relationship between the image matrix and the physical field of view, and how each pixel represents the MR signal from a small volume of tissue;
- the size of the voxel can be calculated from the FOV and matrix, which defines the resolution in MR images;
- that MR images can be acquired as either multi-slice two-dimensional scans, or as a three-dimensional volume, each of which has advantages and disadvantages.

Some of this may seem to be rather tedious and even trivial, but it is important to understand how the digital MR image is related to the human body it represents, and we need to deal carefully with these details.

4.2 Digital and analogue images

As we said in the introduction, MR images are digitally acquired and are made up of pixels (figure 4.1(a)). CT images are also digital. This means that each pixel is a number ('digital' refers to digits, i.e. numbers) which is stored in the computer memory or on a hard disk. The MR signal is a rapidly changing (analogue) electric voltage in the receiver coil, oscillating at high frequencies. It has to be converted to a digital signal which is stored temporarily in the computer before being reconstructed into the final image. Of course it is very important to make sure that the digital signal is an accurate representation of the analogue MR signal, by sampling it at a high enough rate. Once it is reconstructed the image can be converted back to an analogue physical image by printing it on photographic film or on paper. In comparison, conventional X-radiographs are acquired and stored as analogue images. The X-rays pass through the patient, being partially absorbed on the way, and then hit a fluorescent screen in a cassette, emitting light which is then detected by a sheet of film. The film has no pixels, just an even distribution of silver grains in the emulsion. The signal intensity on the final X-radiograph depends on the density of silver grains which have absorbed X-rays. After fixing the film, the intensity cannot change, and the X-radiograph becomes a permanent physical record of the patient's anatomy (figure 4.1(b)).

(a)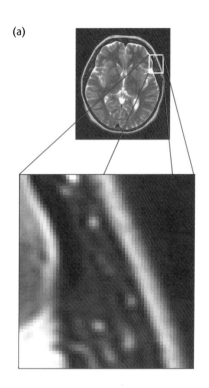

(b)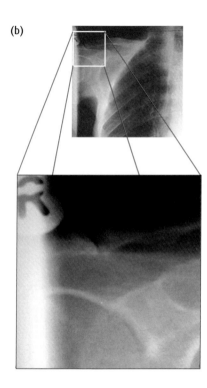

Figure 4.1 (a) A close-up of an MR image, showing the square pixels which make up the image. (b) When a conventional X-ray is magnified, you can see that the image doesn't have boxes like the MR image.

Digital versus analogue data

The *analogue* MR signal is described as *continuous* which means that it has a value (an electric voltage) at every point in time, no matter how closely you zoom in. So we can measure the signal every second, or every millisecond, or every microsecond: no matter how small the time interval, the signal always has a value (figure 4.2(a)). Because it is analogue, it also varies smoothly; whether we use a meter working in volts, millivolts or microvolts, there is a changing voltage.

When the signal is digitized (by an *analogue-to-digital converter*, or *ADC*), the changing voltage is represented as a series of numbers. The ADC makes a measurement of the voltage, calculates the appropriate number and stores the digital value in the computer. Although this happens very fast each conversion takes a certain length of time, so the ADC can only measure the signal at certain time intervals (figure 4.2(b)). The digital data are described as sampled because there are gaps between the measured values.

You may have wondered why we use values such as 256 and 512 for image matrices, instead of the more obvious 250 or 500. The reason is that computers store all their information in *binary* form using 0s and 1s. The computer can count up to 256 using 8 *bits* (a contraction of **B**inary dig**ITS**), or 512 using 9 bits. Due to the way binary arithmetic works, it is very efficient to do 256 calculations during reconstruction, rather than 250. In fact almost everything is easier for the computer if it is based on numbers that fit the pattern of 2 to the power n (2^n). The digitized signal is usually stored by 12 bits, giving a range of numbers from 0 to 4095, or more usefully -2048 to +2047. So the most negative and positive values of the MR signal will be converted to -2048 and +2047 respectively. All the values in between will be scaled to this range. However, the computer can only store whole numbers (*integers*), so the signal changes from being continuous to stepped or *discrete* data (figure 4.2(c)).

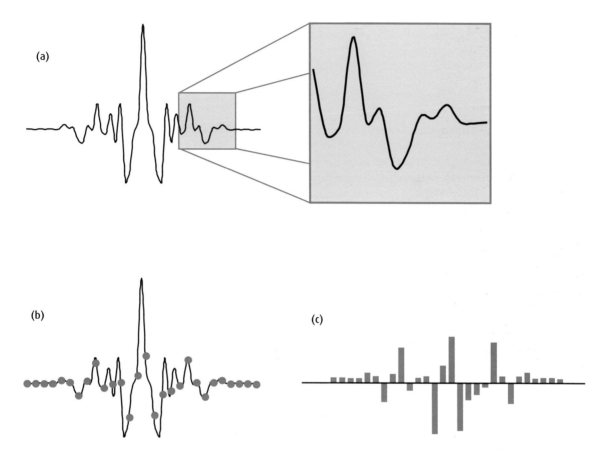

Figure 4.2 (a) The MR signal in the receiver coil is a continuously changing voltage; no matter how closely we zoom in, it still varies smoothly. (b) When it is digitized, there are gaps between sample points due to the analogue-to-digital converter's (ADC) performance. (c) Digital data are stored as integers, so the digitized MR signal has a stepped appearance.

The Nyquist theorem

An ADC can work at different speeds, defined as its *sampling rate* or *sampling frequency*, denoted f_s. If f_s is high, there is only a small gap between signal measurements, known as the *sample period*, T_s. T_s and f_s are related mathematically:

$$T_S = \frac{1}{f_s}$$

So if f_s is low there is a larger T_s and you can see that there is a chance that the digitized signal will lose some of the real MR signal (figure 4.3(a)). Mathematicians and engineers have done a lot of theoretical work on this problem, and have found a rule to characterize it, called the *Nyquist theorem* (Henry Nyquist was an engineer working for AT&T in the 1920s). According to Nyquist, the highest frequency signal that can be accurately digitized at a certain sampling frequency f_s is equal to half of the sampling frequency. This is known as the Nyquist frequency f_N, and we can write

Nyquist frequency $= \frac{1}{2} \times$ sampling frequency

or $f_N = \frac{1}{2} \cdot f_S$

Let's look carefully at various frequency signals all digitized at the same frequency f_s. First, a signal with frequency lower than f_N (figure 4.3(b)) is accurately digitized and the digital signal made by 'joining the dots' clearly has the same frequency as the original. What about a signal at exactly the Nyquist frequency (figure 4.3(c))? Now the digital samples occur at every peak and trough and again the digital signal represents the correct frequency. However, if the signal frequency is higher than f_N, you can see that the digital samples miss some of the peaks and troughs (figure 4.3(d)). When you connect up the digital samples (shown by the blue line), the frequency appears to be low instead of the correct high frequency. This is known as aliasing; we say that for any f_s, all frequencies higher than the Nyquist frequency f_N are aliased as low frequencies.

You can see a good visual example of aliasing by watching an old Western film: look at the spokes on the wagon wheels as they start to move. When the wheels are turning slowly the individual frames of the film are fast enough to show the motion accurately. As the wagon gets faster and the wheels turn more quickly, the spokes appear to slow down, stop still and then they seem to turn backwards! This is because the wheel has gone through more than one complete turn between each frame, i.e. the frequency of the spokes is higher than the sampling frequency of the film.

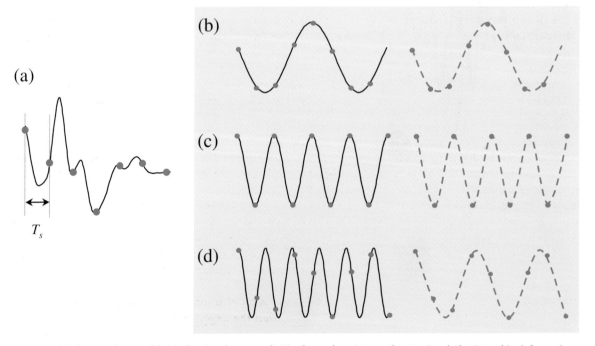

Figure 4.3 (a) The sample period (T_s) is the time between digitized sample points on the MR signal. If T_s is too big, information may be lost. (b) Digitization of a frequency lower than the sampling frequency, f_s. (c) Digitization of a signal at the Nyquist frequency f_N. (d) Signals at frequencies higher than f_N are aliased and the digital frequency appears to be low.

The receive bandwidth and oversampling

The MR signal is based at an RF frequency (which we will see later is fixed by the strength of the main magnetic field) but it contains many different frequencies that encode information about the location of various tissues (section 7.5). The base RF frequency is removed from the signal before it is digitized, leaving the *receive bandwidth* of the signal which is typically several kilohertz wide. Most of the signal-to-noise and contrast information is at very low frequencies, while the higher frequencies contain information about resolution in the image (see 'An easy introduction to k-space'). Electronic noise is distributed evenly across the whole bandwidth (figure 4.4). High receive bandwidths have a worse signal-to-noise ratio than low receive bandwidths because they include more noise. However, low receive bandwidths tend to cause chemical shift artefacts (see section 6.5); advice about choosing the right bandwidth for your images is given in chapter 5.

Earlier we learned that frequencies higher than f_N will be aliased and appear as low frequencies. In order to avoid this messing up the spatial information, we use a filter to remove all the MR signals with frequencies higher than f_N. This is known as a *low-pass filter* because it allows low-frequency signals to pass through, ideally without changing their appearance. Its cut-off frequency, defined by f_N, is set to match the receive bandwidth, and on certain MR systems you can control this parameter directly. In reality filters tend to attenuate signals close to the cut-off frequency, i.e. the signals have reduced intensity. If we look at the effect of the filter on all frequencies, we would see a sloping edge at the cut-off (figure 4.5(a)), known as 'filter roll-off'.

Does this matter? Well yes unfortunately it does. The MR signal contains all sorts of information about the tissues in the body, and its height is very important. The filter roll-off makes it look as if the number of protons fades away at the edges of the field of view – like a soft-focus filter on a photograph. That's not very useful for a diagnostic scan! To get round the problem, we use a technique called *oversampling*.

Frequency oversampling means that the ADC runs at double the required frequency. The Nyquist frequency is therefore doubled, and the filter cut-off frequency is also doubled. The filtered digital signal still has a roll-off edge, but we can now discard all the information above our original required frequency (figure 4.5(c)). The remaining signals are accurately represented and have no attenuation due to the filters. Most systems automatically use frequency oversampling, but on some scanners you can control whether it is on or off. Phase oversampling is similar in principle but it is always controlled by the operator because it has a direct effect on the scan time; it will be fully explained in section 6.7.

X-rays can also be detected digitally, for example in a DSA system, but MR and CT images cannot be detected as analogue images. This is because both MR and CT require many thousands of calculations to reconstruct an image from the received signals, which can only be performed by computers.

4.3 Matrices, pixels and an introduction to resolution

Let's start this section with a few simple definitions. The pixels in MR images are organized into rows and columns in a *matrix* (plural 'matrices'). Each pixel in the reconstructed image can be thought of as a location in the computer memory or hard disk, containing a number which controls the signal intensity. Although most images look square, the matrix doesn't have to be square, in other words it doesn't have to have equal numbers of rows and columns. You will have already come across some typical matrix sizes for MR; for example, 256×128, 256×192, 512×256 and 512×384, but there are many others in common use.

A lot of scanners quote the image matrix starting with the largest number, but this is not always the case. Check which way your scanner displays it. Most of the time the largest number refers to the frequency-encoding (FE) matrix and the smaller is the phase-encoding (PE) matrix (diffusion or perfusion images

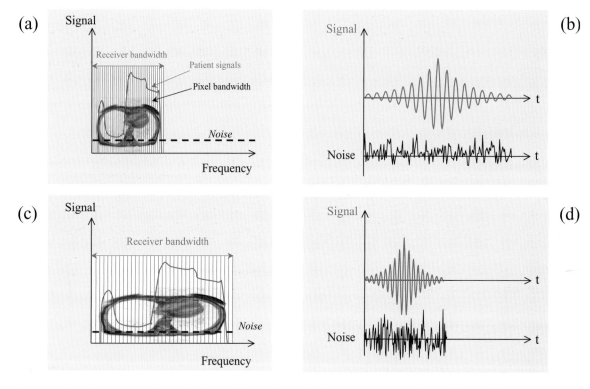

Figure 4.4 Signal and noise in the receive bandwidth. (a) The patient's signals in a narrow bandwidth and (b) the corresponding echo signal and noise. (c) and (d) as (a) but with a wider receive bandwidth; more noise gets into each pixel.

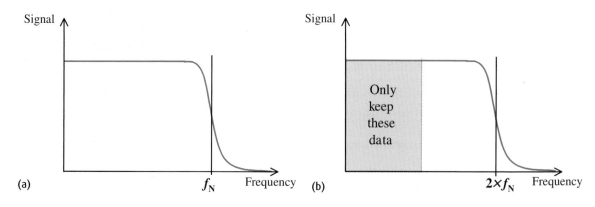

Figure 4.5 (a) The filter at the Nyquist frequency (f_N) has a sloping edge, which distorts the MR signal. (b) By frequency oversampling we can create a sharp cut-off at the original Nyquist frequency.

may be the exceptions). Don't worry for now what frequency and phase encoding actually mean, that will be covered in chapter 7. You will often hear people refer to the 'frequency-encode axis' and 'phase-encode axis': these are the two dimensions of the image. Bear in mind that the images have a third dimension too, the slice thickness. The matrix not only controls the final image size, it is also used for the raw data space, and defines how the scanner samples the signals. The raw data space is also known as k-space. Each time the sequence is repeated a full line of data in the frequency-encode direction is acquired (256 or 512 points). The phase-encode gradient is changed for each repetition and each line has a different position in the phase-encode direction. Thus as the sequence is acquired k-space is filled line by line. Once the matrix is full it is reconstructed into the final image using a clever piece of maths called a

Fourier transform. Notice that when you set the phase-encode matrix, you define how many times the sequence must be repeated and therefore how long the scan will take to acquire. The frequency-encode matrix doesn't have an effect on the scan time, which is why you usually just have to choose between 256 and 512.

Rather confusingly, the FE and PE directions are not always the same. For example, frequency encoding may be either the horizontal or the vertical axis of the displayed image, and it may be along any one of the three anatomical axes (superior-inferior SI, right-left RL or anterior-posterior AP) or even an oblique direction. There may be an annotation on the image for the FE direction; check your manufacturer's manual if you're not sure where it is. If it's not labelled you can usually recognize the PE axis by looking for motion artefacts as these always go across the PE direction.

An easy introduction to k-space

Many people get very worried about understanding k-space, but don't panic, it's really quite easy. You probably know that the raw data has to be processed or 'reconstructed' before you can see the final image. Simply, you can think of k-space as the 'raw data space' which is used to store the digitized MR signals during data acquisition (figure 4.6(a)). When k-space is full (at the end of the scan) the data can be reconstructed to produce the image (figure 4.6(b)) The clever bit is that k-space contains lots of information about the real space that it represents, although it's in a coded form. For now we will just look at the basic features of k-space.

When you set the frequency- (FE) and phase-encoding (PE) matrix, you are controlling the matrix size of the final image and also the size of k-space. If you choose 256 for frequency encoding, each MR echo will have 256 sample points, thus requiring 256 columns in the k-space matrix for temporary storage. When you set the PE matrix, you control how many echoes have to be acquired and thus how many rows are needed in k-space. So every digitized sample point has its own unique location in k-space, which you can imagine as rows and columns of little boxes waiting to be filled with a number.

Although both k-space and real space have the same matrix size, the pixels do not correspond directly with each other. That means that the information in the bottom left pixel in k-space does not contain the raw information for the bottom left pixel in the image. This is because the reconstruction processing uses a Fourier transform (which will be fully discussed in chapter 7). Instead, *data in the middle of k-space contain all the signal-to-noise and contrast information* for the image, and *data around the outside contain all the information about the image resolution* (edges and boundaries). You can see this if we take a set of raw data and reconstruct just the middle (figure 4.7(a)) or just the outside (figure 4.7(c)).

We can use this information in practical ways to design new pulse sequences or to re-order the data acquisition avoiding artefacts. k-space is linked mathematically to real space, and we will deal with this in section 7.5.

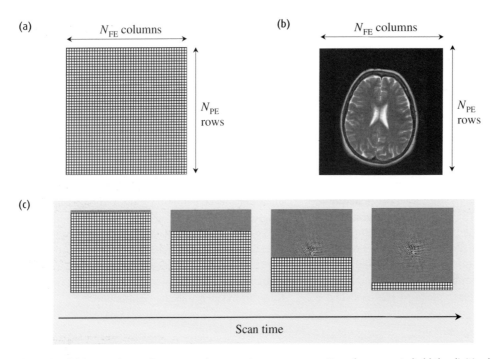

Figure 4.6 (a) k-space is raw data space. The computer reserves a section of memory to hold the digitised raw data during the scan, which has the same number of rows and columns as (b) the final image. (c) During a conventional SE or GE scan k-space is filled with raw data one line per TR.

Choosing anatomical axes for frequency and phase encoding

You will probably notice after working in MR for a while that the scanner automatically selects the directions for frequency and phase encoding depending on the orientation of the scan and the part of the body. Although it seems confusing at first, it is worthwhile learning what the system is doing.

The principle is to set up frequency encoding on the longest anatomical axis on the scan, in order to minimize the possibility of phase wrap-around artefacts by phase encoding the shortest axis (see section 6.7 for details of phase artefacts). To work it out for yourself, you need to imagine the final image and decide which axis has anatomy extending outside the field of view (FOV). For example, on a coronal head scan, the right-left direction is contained within the FOV, while the superior-inferior direction has anatomy below the bottom of the FOV (the rest of the body!). So the default frequency-encode direction for this scan is superior-inferior (figure 4.9(a)): if you put frequency encode along right-left, you will get artefacts (figure 4.9(b)). An axial body scan is less obvious, but the right-left direction is usually longer than the anterior-posterior direction, so right-left is the default frequency-encode direction (figure 4.9(c)).

It is sometimes useful to swap the frequency and phase-encode directions from this default, for example to avoid flow artefacts in the phase-encoding direction on sagittal spines. Techniques for swapping phase and frequency vary between the different manufacturers, but it is always important to know which is the default.

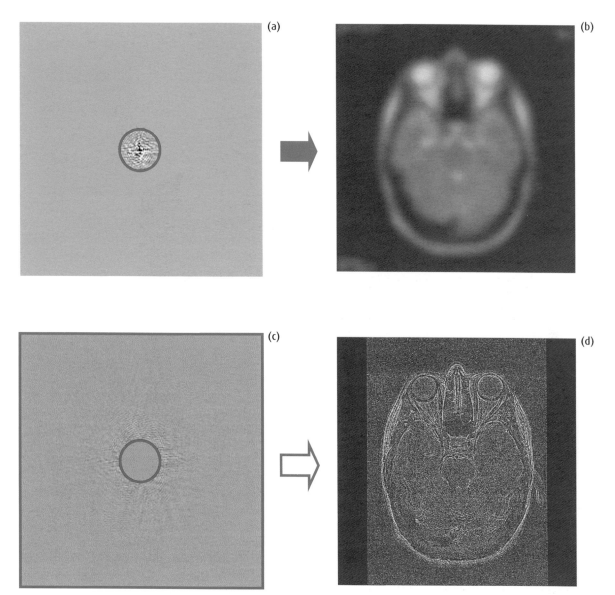

Figure 4.7 Signal and resolution information in k-space. (a) By reconstructing only the data from the middle of k-space we get all the signal and contrast information (b), but it is very blurred. (c) If we erase the middle of k-space and just reconstruct the outside data we can see where the tissue boundaries are (d), but the signal-to-noise ratio is very low and we have no contrast information. Clearly we need both parts of k-space to get a useful MR image!

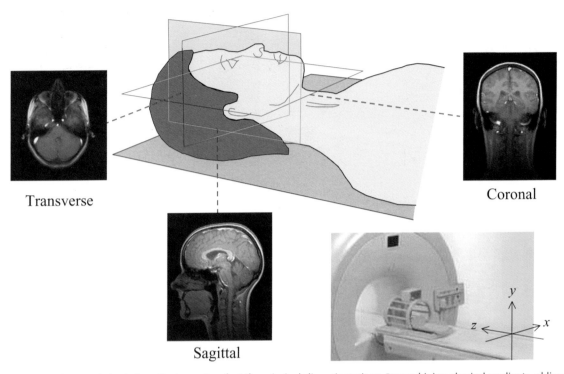

Figure 4.8 The use of physical gradient axes to select the principal slice orientations. By combining physical gradients, oblique and double oblique views are also possible.

When you set the frequency-encoding (FE) matrix, it makes no difference to the scan time (although it might affect the number of slices possible). The phase encoding (PE) matrix however has a direct effect on the scan time. Thus a PE matrix of 256 takes twice as long to acquire as a 128 PE matrix. To get the best possible resolution, we should ideally use a square matrix (256×256 or 512×512), but we have to strike a balance between resolution and scan time, so the phase matrix is often reduced. As a general rule you should not make the PE matrix less than half the FE matrix, because it makes the pixels too pencil-like. Chapter 5 has more information on optimizing parameters to get the best signal-to-noise ratio, resolution and scan time.

Obviously the size of the voxel is very important and it determines the image resolution. We can calculate the voxel size in all three dimensions from the field of view (FOV), matrix and slice thickness, all of which are parameters that you can control. We have to calculate the size in the frequency and phase-encode directions separately, because we usually have different matrix sizes in those directions. So,

$$\text{FE pixel size} = \frac{\text{FE field-of-view}}{\text{FE matrix}}$$

$$\text{PE pixel size} = \frac{\text{PE field-of-view}}{\text{PE matrix}}$$

Slice pixel size = slice thickness

The FOV is often square, which makes things a little simpler than they appear. For example, with a 32-cm FOV, a matrix of 256 (FE) $\times$ 192 (PE) and a slice thickness of 4.5 mm, we can define the voxel size as $1.25 \times 1.67 \times 4.5$ mm^3. Note that in this book we always use the order FE $\times$ PE $\times$ slice when quoting voxel sizes (or just FE $\times$ PE for pixel size); some manufacturers and textbooks use a different order.

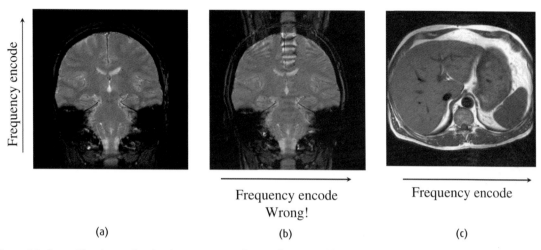

Figure 4.9 Coronal head scan showing frequency encoding on the SI axis (a) and the RL axis (b) – you can see what happens if it's wrong! (c) Axial body scan with frequency encoding on the RL axis.

4.4 Slices and orientations

We've introduced the idea of slice thickness as an important part of the voxel size. You already know that MR can produce slices in any direction – axial, coronal, sagittal, obliques and even double obliques. For comparison, CT produces only axial scans, although if you tilt the gantry you can get obliques. But to get coronals e.g. for sinuses, you have to position the patient prone with their head in a rather uncomfortable position and the gantry tilted to its maximum. Actually CT is catching up with MR now that multi-slice helical scanners are the norm; effectively they acquire an axial 3D block which is then reformatted into other orientations.

Getting back to MR, let's take a look at how the slice orientation is defined relative to the scanner. With a standard superconducting system, B_0 is along the bore, and we conventionally define this as the Z direction. This corresponds to the superior-inferior axis of the patient (the foot-head direction). By convention, the horizontal axis across the bore is known as X and the vertical axis as Y, corresponding to the right-left and anterior-posterior directions respectively. When we select an axial slice, we are creating images perpendicular to the Z direction. Sagittal images are perpendicular to the X direction, and coronal images are perpendicular to the Y

direction. Figure 4.8 shows the principle anatomical axes and corresponding images of the head.

4.5 Displaying images

So the pixels are just numbers that represent the MR signal intensity. They are not much good to us on the computer hard disk – we want to look at the images. When the computer displays an image on the screen, it is doing a *digital-to-analogue conversion* to change the pixel values to different intensities on the display screen. Display systems usually have 12- or 16-bit depth (4096 or 32 768 grey levels respectively). However, the human eye can only distinguish about 200 grey levels, so it makes more sense to compress the range of values in the image into relatively few grey levels. To achieve this a **Look-Up Table** (LUT) is used to link the pixel values to the screen brightness. The maximum pixel value in the image is found during the reconstruction process and is stored in the image *header* – the data tacked on to the front of the image file which holds all the information about the acquisition, including the patient's details. So it is quite straightforward to calculate an LUT to scale the pixel values to grey levels (figure 4.10(a)). In this example, the highest pixel value has the

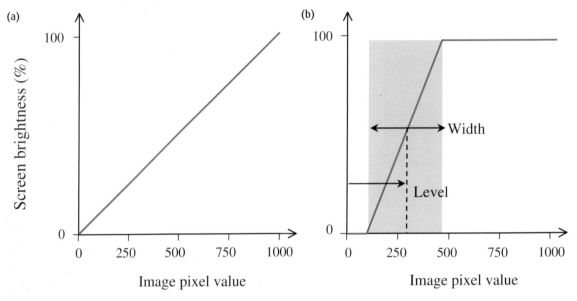

Figure 4.10 (a) A simple look-up table (LUT) scaling the pixel values (0–1000) to the screen brightness controls (0–100%). (b) Reducing the window width changes the LUT to make noise pixels very dark, and to bring out the detail in the mid-intensity pixels.

brightest screen intensity, zero-valued pixels are black, and everything in between is scaled accordingly.

While this is simple, it rarely shows the image in the sort of detail necessary for diagnostic imaging. Often there are only a few high-value pixels, so the whole image looks very dark. We can improve things if the LUT has a steeper slope, so that all pixel values above a certain level are displayed at maximum brightness. On the other hand it is also helpful to make the background noise as dark as possible, and this is done by setting all pixel values below the noise level to have minimum brightness (figure 4.10(b)). This type of modification to the LUT is known as setting the window width and level.

The *window width* is the range of pixel values which are displayed across the screen's brightness range, while the *level* is the central value of the window width. Reducing the window width increases the contrast of the displayed image, while moving the level up or down makes the whole image darker or brighter respectively (figure 4.11). Many MR systems use the mouse to change the window width and level, while others use trackballs or rotating dials. This aspect of changing the

displayed image is very similar to that used in CT and DSA. However, remember that you are only changing the displayed pixel intensities, not the values in the underlying MR image.

4.6 What do the pixels represent?

We have been talking about pixels and matrices in a rather abstract way. Let's see how they correspond to the physical reality of the patient being scanned. What does the number in each pixel actually mean? We know that it is calculated during image reconstruction, and we have already said that it represents the MR signal intensity. In fact it represents the signal from just a small volume of tissue within the patient's body, known as a *voxel* (a contraction of 'volume element'). You can imagine the front face of the voxel as the pixel which is displayed on the scanner (figure 4.12(a)). The third direction is determined by the slice thickness of the image.

So if we could chop up the patient into slices of the right width, cut each slice into the appropriate

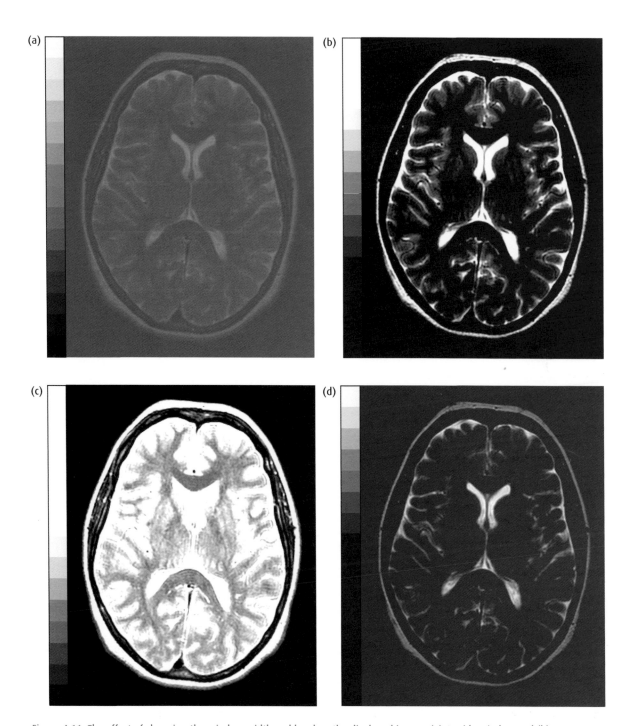

Figure 4.11 The effect of changing the window width and level on the displayed image. (a) A wide window and (b) a narrow window. (c) A low window level makes the image very bright, (d) a high level makes it much darker.

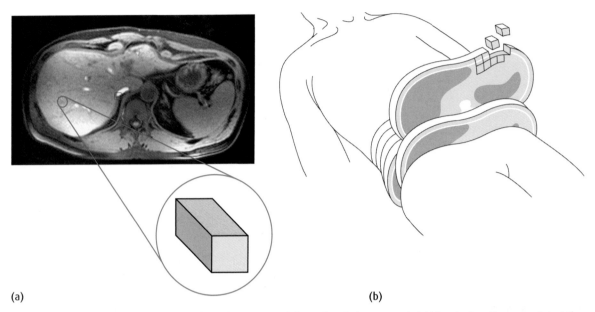

(a)

(b)

Figure 4.12 The relationship between pixels on the screen and the patient being scanned. (a) The pixel on the screen is just the front face of a three-dimensional voxel within the patient. (b) Chopping up the patient into voxels!

Partial volume effects

If we chopped up a patient into 5-mm slices and subdivided each slice into 256×256 pixels, would each voxel contain just one type of tissue? That would depend on which part of the body was being scanned and the relative size of the voxels. If we were imaging the thorax, we might expect most of the voxels to contain only lung, cardiac muscle or intercostal muscle. However, at the boundaries, where the lung is next to the mediastinum or rib cage, there will be some voxels which contain a mixture of tissues. If we imagine the same situation in the head, there will be many voxels that contain both grey and white matter, and around the cerebellum they would also include contributions from CSF. The signal from such mixed voxels will be the weighted sum of the signals from the various tissues.

Let's now take this imaginary situation to two extremes. First let's consider the effect of very small voxels, e.g. $0.25 \times 0.25 \times 3.00$ mm^3. In a head scan many of the voxels will contain just one tissue and the intensity is an accurate representation of the tissue structure (figure 4.13(a)). Now let's consider a more usual scan, i.e. voxels $1 \times 1 \times 3$ mm^3. The same slice location (figure 4.13(b)) will have a mixture of tissues within each voxel and it is obvious that fine structures cannot be resolved. This is known as the partial volume effect and introduces errors into the images. We cannot completely avoid partial volume effects as very small voxels take a long time to acquire (the scan in figure 4.13(a) took 8 min 23 s compared with 2 min 5 s for figure 4.13(b)), and have low signal-to-noise ratio. We have to reach a compromise between resolution, signal-to-noise ratio and scan time, as described in chapter 5 in more detail.

number of rows and columns (figure 4.12(b)), and then measure the MR signal from just one of the resulting voxels, that is the number held in the computer. The higher the MR signal, the higher number. The computer then uses this number to control the brightness of the corresponding pixel on the image display screen (previous section). Thus the larger the number, the brighter the screen. Working backwards, we can say that the brightness of the pixel on the (two-dimensional) screen represents the MR signal intensity from the three-dimensional volume of tissue in the patient, and we are just seeing the front face of the voxel.

The actual signal intensity depends on many factors, including the sequence timings and the intrinsic T_1, T_2 and PD of the tissues. If you scanned the same patient using the same parameters on a different scanner (even if it was made by the same manufacturer) you wouldn't necessarily get exactly the same pixel values in the images. Compare this with CT scans, where the pixel values are in Hounsfield units and we get pretty much the same values for each patient, even between scanners.

4.7 From 2D to 3D

As you now know, each image is a 2D representation of a 3D slice of the patient. You should always remember that your image has depth, due to the slice thickness. MR and CT images are known as cross-sectional imaging techniques to distinguish them from plain X-radiographs and DSA, which are both projection techniques where the final image has lost the 3D information about the patient. MR has the advantage over CT that slices can be produced in any orientation without moving the patient. So we can get the basic orthogonal slices, axial, coronal and sagittal, and both

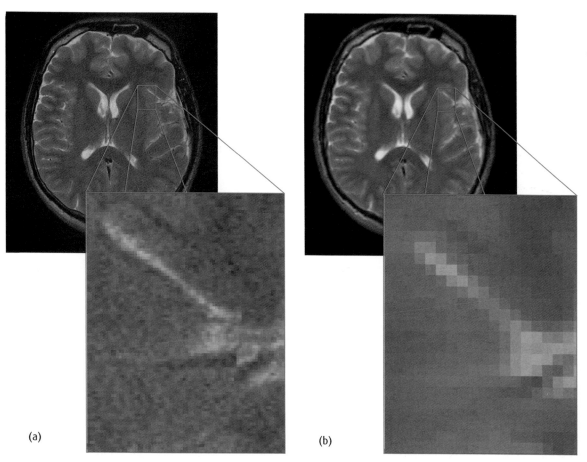

(a)

(b)

Figure 4.13 (a) High-resolution head scan with $0.25 \times 0.25 \times 3.00$ mm³ voxels. (b) The same slice position with $1 \times 1 \times 3$ mm³ voxels showing the partial volume effect.

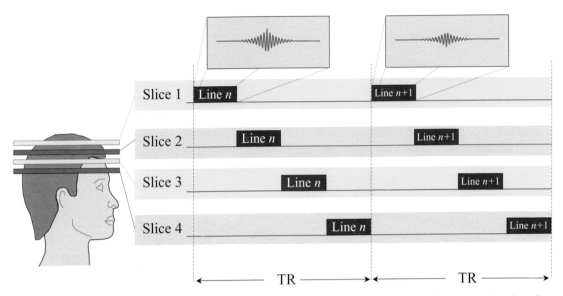

Figure 4.14 Multi-slice imaging. Once the spin echo has been collected, the scanner has plenty of time to excite other slices and collect their data, before starting to repeat the sequence with the first slice.

single and double oblique slices – tilted in just one direction or two respectively.

Since we have to repeat the imaging sequence many times to produce an image, and because we set the TR to get the appropriate image contrast (as described in chapter 3), scan times tend to be relatively long. If we were just producing one slice per scan, it would take all day to get enough information! Fortunately we can use most of the wasted time during the TR to image other slices.

Suppose we have a TR of 600 ms and a TE of 20 ms, to give T_1-weighted images. It takes about 30 ms to excite one slice, generate the spin echo and collect the data. That leaves $600 - 30 = 570$ ms before we have to re-excite that slice for the second time. While it's waiting, the scanner excites a second slice and collects the data from its echo, taking another 30 ms. This process can be repeated, exciting new slices and collecting data, until it's time to re-excite the first slice (figure 4.14). So during each TR, the scanner excites and collects echoes from many slices. The signals of different slices do not interfere with each other, thanks to the way slice selection works with gaps between slices to avoid cross-talk. A simple calculation ($600 \div 30$) shows us that we can get

20 slices within the TR. So for the same scan time as one slice, we can image up to 20 slice locations. This is known as *multi-slice* imaging.

Due to imperfections in the RF pulses we usually have to introduce a slice gap to separate the slices. This is measured as the distance between the slice edges, although sometimes it can be defined as the separation between slice centres (figure 4.15) – you just need to know which definition is used by your system. We generally try to keep the slice gap to a minimum, since tissues in the gap are not imaged at all. If the gap is too big, there is the possibility of completely missing a small pathological feature.

True 3D scanning, rather than 2D multi-slice imaging, requires a different kind of imaging technique. The scan times are increased, so the conventional spin-echo technique is much too slow: 3D images are acquired with gradient-echo sequences or fast spin echo. They have the advantage of very thin slices with no slice gaps (contiguous slices), and they can be reformatted on a workstation to produce images in any orientation. 3D scans are often used when high resolution is required, or when it is important not to miss anything in the slice gaps. We will discuss this technique in more detail in section 7.8.

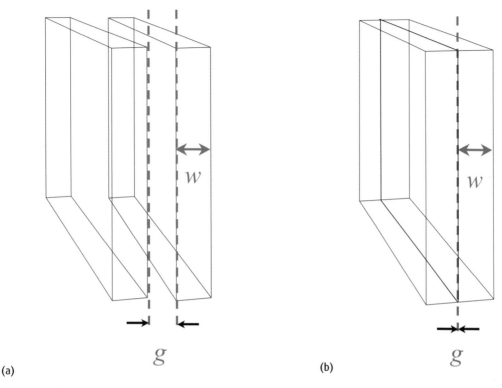

(a)

(b)

Figure 4.15 Definition of slice-to-slice separation: (a) distance factor 100% ($g = w$); (b) contiguous slices ($g = 0$).

Falling into the gaps

Different manufacturers have different ways of setting the gap between slices in a multi-slice sequence. General Electric systems let you set the edge-to-edge slice gap in millimetres.

Siemens scanners use a distance factor, which is the edge-to-edge gap as a fraction of the slice width. So if you have a slice width of 5 mm and you want a 1-mm gap, you set a distance factor of $1 \div 5 = 0.2$. A 3-mm slice with a gap of about 0.5 mm would be achieved with a distance factor of 0.15, and so on.

In Philips systems you also set the slice gap, the edge-to-edge distance between the slices. The system default is a gap of 10% of the slice thickness.

Having acquired a block of 3D data, we have more options for displaying the images. As mentioned already, the volume can be reformatted, i.e. re-sliced using any orientation and slice thickness (figure 4.16a). For complete freedom when reformatting, the 3D voxels should be isotropic or almost isotropic, with all three voxel sides the same length. If one dimension is much longer than the other two, you will see an unat-tractive blocky appearance on the reformatted slices (figure 4.16b), sometimes called a 'staircase artefact'. Curved reformats are also possible, popular for scoliotic spines or to produce a complete view of the optic nerve (figure 4.16c)

Another method is the maximum intensity projection or MIP, typically used for MR angiograms. The individual slices of an MRA show the blood vessels with

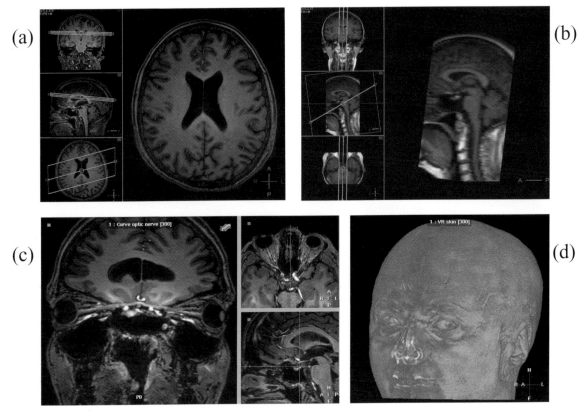

Figure 4.16. (a) Oblique slice reformatted from a 3D volume. (b) The "staircase" effect of having non-isotropic voxels. (c) Curved reformat of the optic nerve. (d) Shaded surface display. Note the crows-feet around the eyes!

much higher signal intensity than the static background tissues. As the name suggests, the display is a projection of the 3D data, much like a conventional X-ray angiogram, except that the MIP shows only the brightest voxel along the projection. More detail about MIP displays is given in chapter 13.

Less commonly, but growing in popularity, you can produce a display which looks very much like a 3D model of the anatomy. There are several different techniques, known as 'shaded surface display', 'volume rendering' or 'surface rendering'. There are subtle differences but in essence all these techniques produce a similar result (figure 4.16d) which can be spookily life-like!

See also:
• How frequency- and phase-encoding gradients work: chapter 7

• k-space and Fourier transforms: section 7.3
• 3D imaging: section 7.8
• Optimizing image resolution and signal-to-noise ratio: chapter 5

FURTHER READING

Elster AD and Burdette J (2001) *Questions and Answers in Magnetic Resonance Imaging*, 2nd edn. London: Mosby-Yearbook (ISBN: 0323011845), Chapter 4.

Hashemi RH and Bradley WG Jr (1997) *MRI The Basics*. Baltimore, MD: Lippincott, Williams & Wilkins (ISBN: 0683182404) Chapters 12 & 13.

Mitchell DG (1999) *MRI Principles*. London: WB Saunders Co. (ISBN: 0721667597), Chapters 7, 8 & 9.

What you set is what you get: basic image optimization

5.1 Introduction

We have seen that MRI is a digital, truly three-dimensional imaging modality of great flexibility with respect to image contrast and its spatial characteristics. However, one of the downsides of this flexibility is a greater complexity in terms of the choice of scanning parameters. This aside, does MR have any other weaknesses? Yes it does: in general scan times are not negligible and there is a certain tendency towards artefact (which we will investigate in the next chapter). However, most MR people would probably agree that the fundamental limitation in MRI is the signal-to-noise ratio (SNR). SNR is dependent upon the hardware, particularly the main field strength and radiofrequency (RF) coils, upon the relaxation properties of tissue and upon the choice of sequence parameters. SNR can be increased by injecting gadolinium or other paramagnetic contrast agents. But unlike X-ray imaging, there is no X-ray dose or milliampere-seconds (mAs) that can be increased to improve image quality. Good image quality depends upon making good scanning parameter choices. There are many parameters to tweak, buttons to press and dialogue boxes to click, and one way to learn about how each affects image quality would be to spend a lifetime tweaking! Alternatively you could read this chapter which will investigate the influence of various acquisition parameters and the practical trade-offs between SNR, contrast-to-noise, spatial resolution and scan time. You will see that:

- signal intensities and contrast are determined by the timing parameters TR and TE (also inversion time (TI) and flip angle (α) where appropriate);
- SNR is proportional to the voxel volume;
- signal scales with size parameters (field of view (FOV), slice width), and noise scales with averaging parameters (number of signal averages (NSA)), phase-encode matrix size (N_{PE}), frequency-encode matrix size (N_{FE})) with an 'inverse square root relationship' (some parameters affect both);
- judicious choice of receiver coil helps SNR;
- resolution is not usually the limiting factor;
- good contrast-to-noise ratio (CNR) is essential for diagnostic quality images;
- parameter juggling is often required to get a suitable scan time.

Knowledge of this chapter should enable you to predict the effect of changing the basic scan parameters: TR, TE, bandwidth, matrix, FOV, slice thickness and number of excitations (NSA or number of signal excitations (NEX)). Fundamental aspects of image quality will be discussed in chapter 11.

5.2 Looking on the bright side: what are we trying to optimize?

This section introduces the basic parameters: contrast, SNR, contrast-to-noise ratio (CNR) and resolution. These are illustrated in figure 5.1. Simple mathematical definitions are given in the box 'Here's the maths bit'.

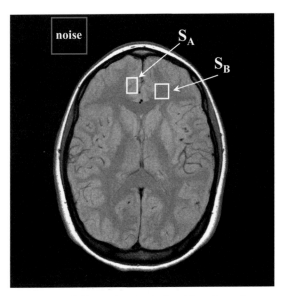

Figure 5.1 Definitions of contrast, signal-to-noise ratio (SNR) and contrast-to-noise ratio (CNR). See 'Here's the maths bit' box for mathematical definitions.

5.2.1 Contrast

Contrast was introduced in chapter 3 in terms of the image appearance, or relative brightness of different tissues and pathology. Image contrast arises (or doesn't) when tissues generate MR signals which have different intensities because of their physical properties, i.e. T_1 and T_2 relaxation times and proton density. You can refer to figure 5.2 or the box 'Try it for yourself 3: Predicting contrast behaviour' to estimate the relative MR signals for a given tissue (if you know its T_1 and T_2). Mathematical expressions are given in the box 'Signal Calculator'.

5.2.2 SNR and CNR

In using the term 'signal' in this chapter we mean the pixel or voxel brightness in the image. This is related to the NMR signal (i.e. what we measure from the coils). In any MR acquisition there is a finite amount of signal available dependent upon the MR characteristics of the tissue and the pulse sequence chosen. In chapter 4 we considered the image as being made up of a number of voxels, each with a particular volume. Since

Here's the maths bit

Mathematically we can define contrast as

$$C = \frac{S_A - S_B}{S_A + S_B}$$

where S_A and S_B are signal intensities for tissues A and B.

Signal-to-noise ratio (SNR) is defined as

$$SNR = \frac{signal}{noise}$$

Contrast-to-noise ratio (CNR) is defined for tissues A and B as

$$CNR_{AB} = \frac{S_A - S_B}{noise}$$

In the simplest terms spatial resolution of the voxels is related to the field of view (FOV) and matrix thus

$$\Delta x = \frac{FOV}{N_{FE}} \qquad \Delta y = \frac{FOV}{N_{PE}} \qquad \Delta z = \text{slice width}$$

the NMR signal that is returned from the patient during the scan has to be divided amongst the voxels that make up the image, the fundamental factor influencing the size of the signal is the number of protons within each voxel.

By 'noise' we don't mean the banging of the gradients (acoustic noise), but random differences in pixel values which give images a grainy, mottled look (like quantum mottle in a radiograph). Usually this noise originates mainly from the patient's tissues (see 'Who's making all that noise').

In a MR image the individual voxels that make up the image will contain a mixture of signal and noise. The ratio of signal intensity in the image to noise level is the *signal-to-noise ratio* (SNR). Images with a poor SNR will appear fuzzy. An important aspect of image optimization is to ensure that there is a high enough SNR for the images to be diagnostically useful. Low SNR may result in missing small details or the obscuring of subtle contrast changes. For this reason we often speak of a *contrast-to-noise ratio* (CNR). CNR is arguably the most

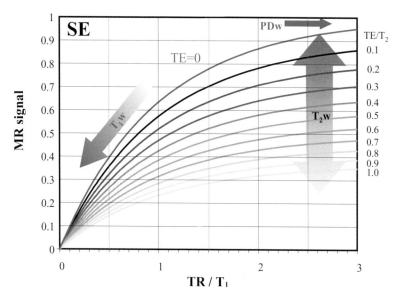

(a)

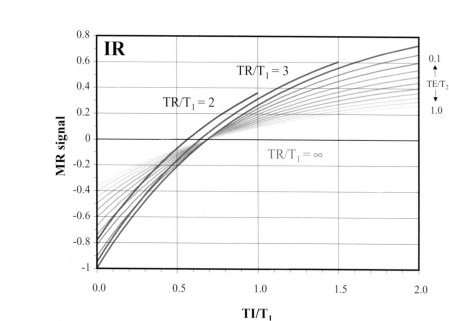

(b)

Figure 5.2 Normalized contrast behaviour. To use these graphs work out the ratio of tissue TR/T_1 and TE/T_2 or TI/T_1. Choose the nearest curve and read off the notional signal value. (a) Spin echo – blue line is for $TE = 0$. (b) Inversion recovery – blue line is for $TE = 0$, $TR = \infty$. The curves for $TR/T_1 = 2$ & 3 assume $TE = 0$ or that T_2 is very long. (c) Gradient echo (spoiled) all assuming $TE = 0$ or a long T_2^*.

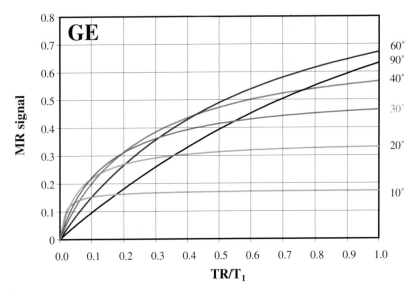

(c)

Figure 5.2 (*cont.*)

Try it for yourself 3: Predicting contrast appearance

Let's take two easily obtained substances: a saline bag and some cooking oil. The T_1 and T_2 of the saline are probably about 2000 ms and 1500 ms, and for the oil 200 ms and 180 ms. If we use a spin echo sequence with TR = 600 ms and TE = 20 ms, what will we see?

Looking at figure 5.2a, we have a ratio TR/T_1 of 0.3 and 2.5 for the saline and oil. For the oil the ratio of TE/T_2 is 0.1 so we should use the darkest of the grey curves. For saline TE/T_2 is 0.02. The blue curve is for TE/T_2 of zero, and as this is the closest value to the calculated ratio for saline, we should use the blue curve.

To calculate the oil signal you read off the value on the MR signal axis corresponding to TR/T_1 of 2.5, using the top grey curve. This gives about 0.83. For the saline, using the blue curve and the x-axis value of 0.4, we get 0.28.

So we predict that for this sequence oil will be brighter than water and that the contrast will be

$$C = \frac{0.83 - 0.28}{0.83 + 0.28} = 0.48$$

Now do the experiment on your scanner. Choose a single 5 mm slice which includes both substances and use a spin echo (not turbo or fast spin echo) with TR = 600 ms and TE = 20 ms. It doesn't matter what resolution you choose (256 × 256 will do fine). Check that the oil is indeed brighter and use regions of interest to measure the mean signal intensities in each container and calculate the contrast.

As a further test, using figure 5.2a, how should you change TR to make the saline and oil closer to the same signal? Looking at figure 5.2b, for inversion recovery, what value of TI should you use to get zero signal from the oil? How will this look in the image? Try it for yourself to check your predictions.

One point to note using these graphs and the maths is that although they let you predict the changes to image appearance when you vary the parameters (TR, TE, TI), they do not include any tissue differences in proton density. Nor do they give you absolute values, but they do serve as a guide to predicting the image contrast.

Who's making all that noise?

The noise comes from random fluctuations in electrical current. It therefore is called electronic noise, and exists in all electrical conductors. This obviously includes the MR coils with which we measure the signal, but it also includes the electrically conducting tissues of the patient. Human tissue contains many ions such as sodium, potassium and chloride which are electrically charged atomic particles carrying electrical currents within the body, e.g. in nerve conduction. These currents generate fluctuating magnetic fields which induce a noise voltage in the coil. The most effective way to reduce this noise is to use a small or dedicated anatomy coil. Where large fields of view are essential, array or phased array (synergy) coils are usually best (see section 9.4.6).

important aspect of image quality. Ways of measuring image quality are considered in chapter 11.

5.2.3 Resolution

The other important property of the images is spatial resolution. In MR we need to consider both the in-plane resolution, which may be different in each axis, and the through-plane resolution or slice width. Generally the latter is the largest dimension and is usually the more critical in visualizing a lesion.

5.3 Trading places: resolution, SNR and scan time

Just as compromises are common in real life, so too in MRI. Here we look at the trade-offs between the image quality parameters. For the mathematically minded, it's all in the box 'A complicated relationship: resolution and SNR'.

5.3.1 Resolution and SNR

Generally MRI resolution is pixel limited. That means that the smallest object or detail that you can visualize in the image has the dimensions of a single pixel. For a

Signal calculator

To calculate the relative signal strength in terms of relaxation effects, use the following equations for the sequence-dependent relaxation factor F. If you don't like the look of the maths, you can use figure 5.2 instead.

Spin echo

$$F_{SE} \propto \left[1 - \exp\left(\frac{-TR}{T_1} \right) \right] \cdot \exp\left(\frac{-TE}{T_2} \right)$$

provided $TE \ll TR$

Inversion recovery

$$F_{IR} \propto \left[1 - 2\exp\left(\frac{-TI}{T_1} \right) + \exp\left(\frac{-TR}{T_1} \right) \right] \cdot \exp\left(\frac{-TE}{T_2} \right)$$

also provided $TE \ll TR$, or if $TR > 5 \times T_1$ this simplifies to

$$F_{IR} \propto \left[1 - 2\exp\left(\frac{-TI}{T_1} \right) \right] \cdot \exp\left(\frac{-TE}{T_2} \right)$$

Gradient echo

$$F_{GE} \propto \frac{\sin \alpha \cdot (1 - \exp(-TR/T_1)) \cdot \exp(TE/T_2^*)}{1 - \cos \alpha \exp(-TR/T_1)}$$

for a 'spoiled' gradient echo (possibly called 'SPGR', 'FLASH' or 'T1-FFE' on your scanner). This will probably be the gradient-echo (GE) sequence you encounter most often. Other types of GE contrast are considered in section 12.4.

256 matrix and a 25 cm FOV this means that details of the order of 1 mm should be visible. In this MR is quite distinct from digital radiography, computed tomography (CT) and ultrasound, where other processes affect the ultimate resolution. In this section we consider the practical example illustrated in figure 5.3.

Three factors determine whether a particular detail or structure can be visualized in the image. Clearly there needs to be contrast between the structure and its surroundings. Second, if the resolution is insufficient,

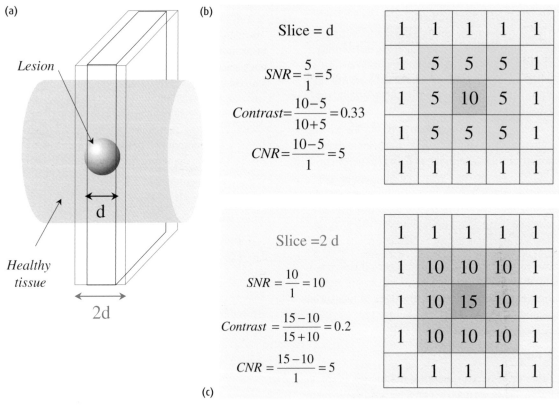

Figure 5.3 Contrast and CNR (a) example of changing slice thickness for a small lesion. The optimal contrast is obtained for a slice width less than or equal to the lesion d. (b) Simulated pixel values for a small lesion with slice thickness d and calculated SNR, contrast and CNR. The lesion has a signal value of 10, surrounding tissue 5 and background noise 1. (c) Pixel values and image quality calculated values when the slice thickness is 2d. SNR is better, but contrast is down. Ideally CNR is maintained.

Try it for yourself 4: FOV and matrix size

To see the effect of field of view (FOV) and matrix size, you need a phantom with some fine structure preferably with a range of sizes between 0.2 and 2 mm. These are commercially available, but you can make one of your own with a selection of plastic hair combs with different size 'teeth', including one designed to remove head lice (don't be embarrassed to buy this, you're going to use it for a scientific experiment!). Use a fairly deep plastic container and fill it with water, adding 1–2 ml of old gadolinium contrast to reduce T_1, and a few drops of detergent to break down the surface tension. Put the combs in the bottom making sure there are no air bubbles trapped between them.

Put the container in the head or knee coil, and perform a localizer scan. Use a T_1-weighted spin-echo sequence and keep the receiver gain constant in order to be able to measure changes in SNR related to the other parameters. Select a coronal slice at the bottom of the container, with a slice width of about 5 mm so that you can see the effect of various matrix sizes. Then start changing FOV and matrix size. Be sure to change only one parameter at a time, keeping all others constant.

information about the object will not be transferred into the image by the image-formation process. Third, if the SNR or CNR is too low, the details of the structure may be obscured by image noise.

In the example of figure 5.3 we see how the contrast and CNR are affected by the choice of slice thickness. If the slice is too thick, we get a good SNR but the contrast is reduced by a partial volume effect (mixing of the signals of the lesion and background). If the slice is too thin, the CNR may be too low to visualize the detail clearly.

The same argument is true for in-plane changes although the pixel dimensions are generally smaller. An important stage in image optimization therefore is to decide on the trade-off required between the voxel size required for an adequate SNR and the requirement for the voxel size to be small enough to permit the visualization of small anatomical or pathological details. Figure 5.4 shows similar images acquired with different resolution, but the same overall scan time.

5.3.2 Resolution and scan time

Spatial resolution in the frequency-encoding (FE) direction comes 'free' in terms of scan time (but not in terms of SNR) if the matrix is increased whilst keeping the FOV constant. To change the phase-encoding (PE) matrix, we have to acquire more lines of data, which takes time.

$$\text{Scan time} = \text{NSA} \times \text{TR} \times N_{PE}$$

In terms of the image slice, reducing the slice width will reduce the anatomical coverage unless slice gaps are increased. It is important to realize that changing the ratio of slice–slice increment to slice width in MRI is not like the 'pitch' in spiral CT. In MR the gaps are real gaps – and small lesions occurring exactly in a gap will be missed. The number of slices obtainable, in standard 2D mode, will be determined by the sequence timing parameters, particularly TR.

5.3.3 Predicting the effect on image quality

The relationships between SNR, CNR and spatial resolution are quite complicated, not the least in that many user-controllable scanner parameters affect them. How

A complicated relationship: resolution and SNR

The signal is proportional to the voxel volume and the appropriate sequence-specific relaxation factor (given in the 'Signal calculator' box).

$$signal \propto \Delta x \Delta y \cdot \Delta z \cdot F_{sequence}$$

where Δx and Δy are the in-plane pixel dimensions and Δz is the slice width. $F_{sequence}$ is the appropriate sequence dependent factor from Signal calculator. The noise is related to the bandwidth and "averaging parameters":

$$noise \propto \frac{\sqrt{BW}}{\sqrt{NSA \cdot N_{PE} \cdot N_{FE}}}$$

where BW is the bandwidth across the whole image. In terms of the 'bandwidth per pixel' (bw) we can write

$$noise \propto \frac{\sqrt{bw}}{\sqrt{NSA \cdot N_{PE}}}$$

Putting this together with the signal equation we get

$$SNR \propto \frac{\Delta x \cdot \Delta y \cdot \Delta z \cdot F_{sequence} \cdot \sqrt{NSA \cdot N_{PE} \cdot N_{FE}}}{\sqrt{BW}}$$

where BW is the total receiver bandwidth. In terms of the field of view, we can say

$$SNR \propto \frac{FOV_{FE} \cdot FOV_{PE} \cdot \Delta z \cdot F_{sequence}}{\sqrt{BW \cdot N_{FE} \cdot N_{PE}}} \sqrt{NSA}$$

For systems which utilise the "bandwidth per pixel" concept we get the following equation:

$$SNR \propto \frac{\Delta x \cdot \Delta y \cdot \Delta z \cdot F_{sequence} \cdot \sqrt{NSA \cdot N_{PE}}}{\sqrt{bw}}$$

A good rule-of-thumb is that if the scanning time is held constant, the achievable SNR is directly proportional to the voxel volume. So reducing the matrix from 256×256 to 128×128 and doubling NSA (to keep the same scan time) whilst maintaining the bandwidth per pixel will quadruple the SNR.

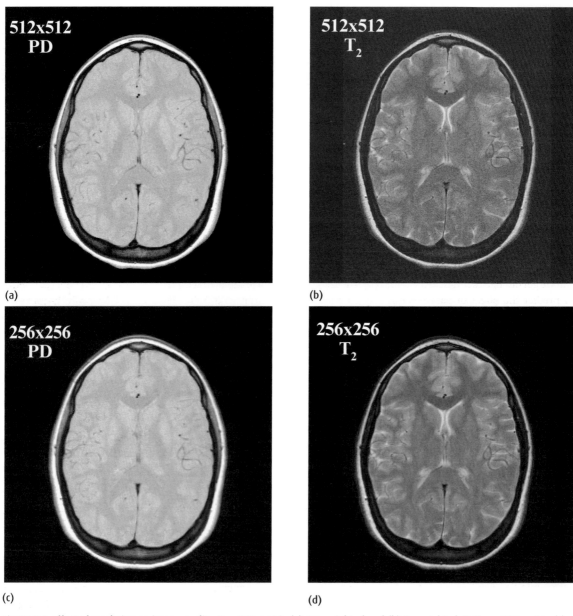

(a)

(b)

(c)

(d)

Figure 5.4 Effect of resolution on image quality. Top: 512 matrix (a) PD-weighted and (b) T_2-weighted. Bottom: 256 matrix (c) PD-weighted and (d) T_2-weighted. These all utilize the same overall scan time by changing NSA. The higher spatial resolution results in greater image noise (lower SNR).

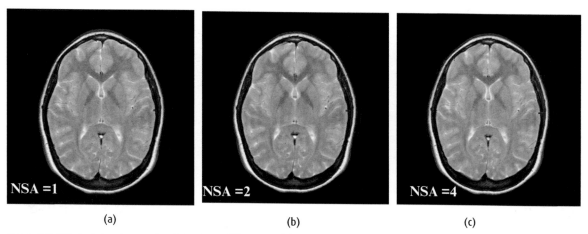

Figure 5.5 Effect of signal averaging (a) NSA = 1 (b) NSA = 2 (c) NSA = 4. Scan times increased proportionately. Image SNR improves with increasing NSA.

can we get our heads round what is going on sufficiently to predict the effect of parameter changes on image quality and, indirectly, diagnostic potential? It is clear that SNR and resolution are related. Throw in contrast and CNR and you have a recipe for potential confusion. One way is to understand the maths! Alternatively you could consider parameters as falling into two categories: *size parameters* determine how much signal is produced, *averaging parameters* reduce noise. Some parameters are a combination of both. Size parameters bear a linear relationship with SNR; averaging parameters have an inverse square root relationship.

FOV and slice width are size parameters only. They only affect the signal. Increasing them increases the signal and the SNR. Of course they affect resolution but

fortunately that is intuitive. So doubling the slice width doubles the SNR. Halving the FOV whilst keeping the same matrix will quarter SNR, as we have changed two dimensions, the FOV in the phase-encoding direction and in the frequency-encoding direction.

Signal averaging (NSA or NEX) is an averaging parameter. It does not affect resolution and reduces the noise. Going from NSA = 1 to NSA = 4 will double SNR. NSA obviously affects scan time. The effect of signal averaging is illustrated in figure 5.5.

N_{PE} and N_{FE} are combination parameters. They affect resolution and hence voxel volume, with a linear effect on signal. With standard two-dimensional Fourier transform (2D FT) MRI the acquisition of multiple 'lines' of data can be considered as a kind of averaging; therefore, they also affect the noise. So if we double N_{PE} we halve the number of protons in a voxel, producing half the signal, but we reduce the noise by $\sqrt{2}$ – so the net effect on SNR is a reduction of approximately 30%.

Changing N_{FE} affects the noise, but the effect depends upon what happens to the 'bandwidth' and field of view. It is a classic result of electronic theory that noise is proportional to the square root of total bandwidth ($\sqrt{BW}$). If the total bandwidth does not change, increasing N_{FE} has the same effect as increasing N_{PE}: doubling the FE matrix whilst maintaining FOV gives a two-fold reduction in signal (because the voxel size has halved), but a $\sqrt{2}$ reduction in noise, and hence a $\sqrt{2}$ reduction in SNR.

3D maths

The maths for 3D is the same as for 2D except that we have an extra 'averaging' term N_{PE2}.

$$SNR \propto \frac{\Delta x\, \Delta y\, \Delta z \cdot F_{sequence} \cdot \sqrt{NSA \cdot N_{PE1} \cdot N_{PE2}}}{\sqrt{bw}}$$

or on systems which use the total bandwidth instead of bandwidth per pixel:

$$SNR \propto \frac{\Delta x \Delta y \Delta z \cdot F_{sequence} \cdot \sqrt{NSA \cdot N_{FE} \cdot N_{PE1} \cdot N_{PE2}}}{\sqrt{BW}}$$

Which is more important, resolution or SNR/CNR?

Certain applications such as MR angiography work best with higher resolution, but in general you need a certain SNR whatever the resolution. How much? As a rule-of-thumb an SNR higher than 20:1 offers little image quality advantage to the observer and excess SNR would be best converted to either a larger matrix or reduced scan time. If SNR is adequate, high-resolution images will always look better but the diagnostic advantage of say 1024 matrix over 512 has not yet been established. Figure 5.4 shows the effect of different matrix sizes on image quality.

However, on systems which define bandwidth in Hertz per pixel, the noise is unaffected but the signal and therefore the SNR will be reduced by half.

5.3.4 2D versus 3D

We have seen from the simple example in section 5.3 that too thin a slice can ruin the CNR. What if we really want very thin slices, e.g. for multi-planar reformatting? The solution is to acquire a three-dimensional volume instead of interleaved multi-slicing. The way this works is described in section 7.8. The scan time is increased to

$$\text{Scan time} = \text{TR} \times \text{NSA} \times N_{\text{PE1}} \times N_{\text{PE2}}$$

where N_{PE2} is the number of 'slices' or partitions. Since these are acquired sequentially, TR must be reduced using one of the sequences described in chapter 12. The signal is reduced since the slice or 'partition' thickness is often very small. However, a reduction in the noise is achieved by using the extra dimension of phase encoding.

5.4 Ever the optimist: practical steps to optimization

Optimization is a complicated subject. In practice, however, certain physical constraints often apply. We offer the following guidance.

Try it for yourself 5: Predicting SNR

You can look at the maths in 'A complicated relationship: resolution and SNR' to predict the effect of changing parameters on image quality. Alternatively you can use figure 5.6, working from left to right. Each arrow indicates the effect of doubling or halving the parameter in each box. Read off the values on the left for the effect on SNR. Then multiply up for each parameter change.

Here is an example. Suppose you double the matrix size, keeping FOV and slice width unchanged. The first two boxes have no effect (FOV and slice are unchanged). Doubling N_{PE} halves the signal but lowers the noise – with an overall SNR reduction of 0.7.

Doubling N_{FE} will halve the signal and the SNR. However you need to consider what happens to the bandwidth. If the total bandwidth (BW) does not change, then the effect of doubling N_{FE} will be to halve the bandwidth per pixel (bw) and SNR will improve by $\sqrt{2}$. This will not affect systems which use a constant bandwidth per pixel.

As N_{PE} has increased, let's keep scan time the same by halving NSA, reducing SNR by a further $\sqrt{2}$ (0.7). Table 5.1 summarises what has happened.

Starting from the same original image, let's try halving the FOV and doubling the NSA but keep all other parameters unchanged. What do you get? You can now try it for yourself on the scanner using any phantom. Actually most scanners will do this calculation for you while you change the parameters, so you don't even have to do the scans – but do it anyway, it's good for your soul!

5.4.1 The golden rule: contrast first

Our golden rule for image optimization is first to set the required image contrast by choice of pulse sequence and basic timing parameters TR and TE (and α for gradient echo). In general for T_1 contrast using spin echo, a TR with a value intermediate to the tissue T_1 values of interest will produce the optimum contrast. The same is true for the choice of TE in terms of T_2 contrast. The situation for inversion recovery is more complex and is not considered here.

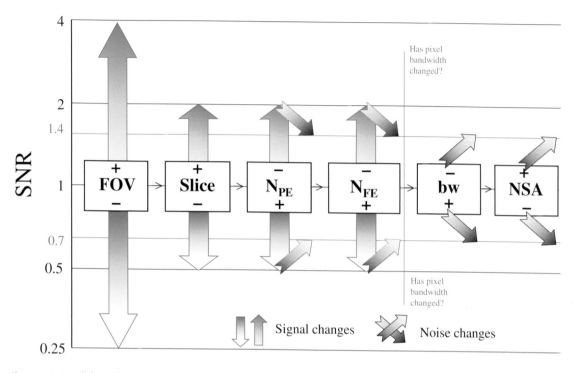

Figure 5.6 SNR "abacus" showing how parameter changes affect SNR, when each parameter value is either doubled of halved. To use the abacus, start at the left and work towards the right. For each parameter change follow the arrows to calculate the effect on SNR. To predict the overall effect on SNR multiply all the SNR changes together. Note that the arrow directions indicate the effect on SNR. An increase in either signal or noise is represented by the shading in the arrows, with a deeper colour indicating an increase in either signal or noise.

Table 5.1 Example of effect of parameter changes on SNR

Step	SNR (constant BW)	SNR (constant bw)
FOV unchanged	× 1	× 1
Slice unchanged	× 1	× 1
Double N_{PE}	× 0.7	× 0.7
Double N_{FE}	× 0.5	× 0.5
Check bandwidth per pixel. . . .	× 1.4 (bw halved)	× 1.0 (bw unchanged)
Halve NSA	× 0.7	× 0.7
TOTAL (multiplied)	**0.35**	**0.25**

5.4.2 Field of view and resolution

As a starting point choose a matrix of 256 for frequency encoding in the longer image direction, unless scanning sagittal or coronal whole spines or large FOV MRAs (in which case choose 512). Choose phase encoding in the other direction and use the smallest rectangular FOV factor to encompass the anatomy. Make the FOV fit the anatomy reasonably snugly, but make sure that it all fits within the phase-encode direction.

5.4.3 Adjusting the scan time

Even where scan time is not a major issue, shorter scans improve patient cooperation and reduce the opportunity for movement-related artefacts. They also improve your throughput. If the scan time is too long, a few tricks

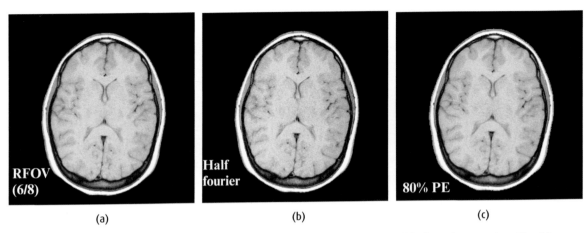

Figure 5.7 Images showing (a) rectangular field of view (RFOV): scan time 1 min 39 s, (b) half Fourier: scan time 55 s, (c) reduced matrix (80%), scan time 1 min 20 s. Full acquisition scan time would have been 2 min 8 s (spin echo, TR = 500 ms, TE = 15 ms). The half Fourier image is noisier, while the reduced matrix has less noise but reduced spatial resolution.

are available to help reduce scan time. One of the easiest ways is to reduce TR, but this will affect the contrast. The next easiest way is to reduce the number of phase-encode steps. Three ways of doing this are illustrated in figure 5.7: how they work will be considered in chapter 7.

Rectangular field of view

When the anatomical axes are dissimilar, e.g. in scanning the spine, it is possible to acquire with a smaller matrix in the physically shorter axis and to use this axis for phase encoding. This maintains resolution, keeping the pixels square, and reduces scan time but at a cost to SNR. Time savings of up to 50% are possible. It is known as 'reduced-phase FOV' or 'scan percent' depending on the scanner.

Half Fourier

In half Fourier (also known as 'halfscan' or 'half NEX') we acquire slightly more than half the phase-encode steps. This approximately halves the scan time and reduces SNR by 30% but does not affect resolution.

Reduced matrix

In reduced matrix the scanner acquires only the central phase-encoding steps and fills the outermost values of

k-space with zeroes. This reduces the scan time proportionately and reduces the resolution in the phase-encode direction. SNR is slightly improved.

Parallel Imaging

If you are using an array coil (see chapter 9) you may often be able to reduce the scan time without affecting the spatial resolution by using parallel imaging (see chapter 17). The use of parallel imaging reduces the image SNR and may result in image artefacts if applied too strongly. Reduction factors of up to 2 can usually be applied successfully without significant image quality degradation.

5.4.4 Check your slices

If you cannot get enough slices you may have to run the scan as two batches or acquisitions, i.e. the slices are split into two or more blocks and scans are run consecutively. To get a fixed z-axis coverage without increasing the number of slices, you could increase the slice thickness (at a cost of resolution loss and possible reduced contrast due to partial volumes), or increase the slice separation or gap (at a risk of missing a small lesion). If you are only one or two slices short, an increase in TR may help, but you will be changing the contrast which may have undesirable consequences. Bear in mind that any extra sequence options such as saturation bands (section 6.4.3, 7.4.4), fat suppression (section 6.5.3) and flow compensation (section 6.4.3) will all add to the time required to acquire each slice and should be used sparingly if scan time is a major constraint.

5.4.5 How to boost SNR

Above all make sure you choose the best coil. The simple rule-of-thumb is that ideally the receiver coil should encompass the whole of the anatomical region of interest and no more. Smaller coils 'see' less noise. Phased array coils allow the MR receiver to see more useful anatomy without seeing more noise.

The easiest way to improve SNR is to increase the number of signal averages (NSA). This also increases the scan time, so this may not be the most time-efficient way of improving the SNR. Five methods to improve SNR that do not affect scan time are listed below:

Increase the slice thickness
This improves the SNR in direct proportion to the slice thickness with no time penalty at all. One must consider the effect of reducing the resolution in the slice direction. Too thick a slice may result in reduced contrast in a lesion due to partial volume effects and there is a possibility that the lesion may be missed. If thin slices are essential, you should consider a 3D acquisition.

Increase the FOV
Increasing the FOV without changing the matrix size makes the in-plane pixels bigger, giving more signal without changing the noise. Spatial resolution is of course reduced and the desired part of the image will appear smaller, surrounded by more empty background. However, as you would normally match the FOV to the anatomy, this option may not be a terribly useful one.

Reduce the bandwidth
Reducing the bandwidth reduces the noise by a factor proportional to the square root of the reduction, e.g. halving the bandwidth reduces the noise by a factor of

---

Adjusting the bandwidth – a scanner guide
Some systems (e.g. General Electric) have the total MR receiver bandwidth in kilohertz (kHz) as a user-adjustable parameter. So to improve SNR you simply reduce the receiver bandwidth. For others (e.g. Siemens with Syngo software) the bandwidth per pixel is selectable.

For older Siemens scanners bandwidth is not adjustable. Instead each pulse sequence has a bandwidth per pixel in hertz (given as the last number in the sequence name following the letter 'b', e.g. se15_b130 has a pixel bandwidth of 130 Hz). So you must select the appropriate pulse sequence from the list.

For other scanners (e.g. Philips) the pixel bandwidth is presented as the 'fat–water pixel shift'. The meaning of this is explained in section 6.5. To improve SNR on these systems you must increase the fat–water pixel shift.

1.4. The way this is done in practice depends on your scanner. The side-effect of reducing the bandwidth is an increase in the chemical shift, which may create an unwelcome artefact (see section 6.5). Where chemical shift artefact is not a concern, the lowest bandwidth achievable is usually a good starting point. Your TE will determine the limit on how low you can set the bandwidth.

Select a preprocessing filter
Filtering of the MR signals prior to reconstruction improves SNR at a cost of reducing spatial resolution. Effectively we reduce the magnitude of the high spatial frequencies, where the noise is most apparent (because the signal here is low); in doing so, we attenuate genuine high spatial frequency information and thus reduce the resolution. Some manufacturers may apply filtering by default, in which case you are probably not told that it is happening, or as a user-selectable option. When should you filter? Basically, never, if you can avoid it. You would do better to reduce the number of phase-encode steps, which would improve SNR and save scan time. An exception to this is for certain so-called segmented sequences, e.g. fast or turbo

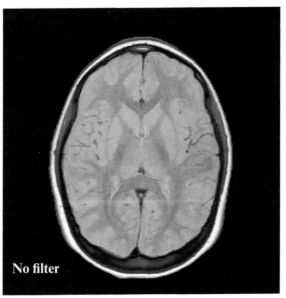

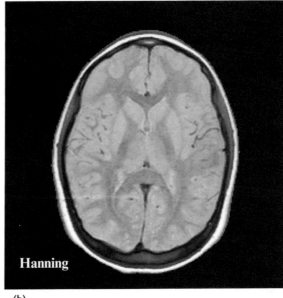

(a)   (b)

Figure 5.8 Effect of filtering: (a) no filtering; (b) strong (Hanning) filter. The filtered images are less noisy, but have slightly reduced spatial resolution.

spin echo where filtering reduces ringing artefacts (chapter 6). Filtered and unfiltered images are shown in figure 5.8.

5.4.6 Trying it out

To test your sequence you can apply the maths of this chapter or, alternatively, it's probably quicker just to do the scan! If you've done all the above and the images are still too noisy, then you need to work through the options in section 5.4.5. If scan time is no concern, simply increase the NSA. If water–fat shift is not an issue (e.g. your fat suppression is wonderful) reducing the bandwidth, if available, is a simple way of boosting SNR. As a last resort, you could always filter the images as a postprocessing step. The only other major consideration is the avoidance of artefacts . . .

See also:
- Image artefacts: chapter 6
- Spatial encoding using gradients: chapter 7
- Pulse sequences explained: chapter 12

FURTHER READING

Brown MA and Semelka RC (1999) *MRI Basic Principles and Applications*, 2nd edn. New York: Wiley-Liss (ISBN: 0471330620), Chapter 6.

Elster AD and Burdette J (2001) *Questions and Answers in Magnetic Resonance Imaging*, 2nd edn. London: Mosby-Yearbook (ISBN: 0323011845), Chapter 4.

Hashemi RH and Bradley WG Jr (1997) *MRI The Basics*. Baltimore, MD: Lippincott, Williams & Wilkins (ISBN: 0683182404), Chapter 17.

Rinck PA (2001) *Magnetic Resonance in Medicine*, 5th edn. Oxford: Blackwell Science (ISBN: 0632059869), Chapter 9.

Improving your image: how to avoid artefacts

6.1 Introduction

As we all know, real life is far from perfect and MRI is just as bad! MR scanners do not have absolutely uniform magnetic fields, the gradients don't produce exactly the pulse shapes programmed by the pulse sequence and patients don't keep still. These problems, and many others, produce artefacts in MR images. An artefact can be defined as any feature in an image which misrepresents the object in the field of view. This could be a bright signal lying outside the body, or lack of signal where there should be something. It might also be a distortion in the image, so that a straight line appears curved, or a certain area is artificially magnified or reduced. A large group of MR artefacts appear as 'ghost' images, where a faint copy of the anatomy appears in the image displaced in one direction or another. In general artefacts are most serious when they degrade the rest of the image.

In this chapter we will describe the most common artefacts encountered in MRI, along with ways to avoid or minimize them. The causes of artefacts can be broadly divided into three groups: motion, inhomogeneity and digital imaging artefacts:

- *Motion artefacts* tend to appear as ghosts along the phase-encode direction, and may be produced by physiological motion or involuntary movement by the patient. The most important physiological motion is probably flowing blood, which can affect images of all areas of the body, so it's important to understand this one.
- *Inhomogeneity artefacts* usually cause signal intensity changes and image distortions, and are due to hard-

ware imperfections and to the susceptibility effects within the human body; for example, air in the sinuses or blood breakdown products.
- *Digital imaging artefacts* have a variety of appearances, and include phase wrap-around artefacts and problems arising from the digital Fourier transform.

6.2 Keep still please: gross patient motion

Probably the commonest cause of artefacts on images is patient motion, causing a range of ghosting depending on the severity of the motion. Continuous movement during the scan causes a generalized blurring, often making the scan useless (figure 6.1), while a few twitches or only small movements cause a few subtle ghosts which may leave an acceptable image. Patients may move involuntarily if they are suffering from a movement disorder, or they may have difficulty understanding or remembering the instructions to keep still during the scan. In these cases it may be necessary to sedate the patient or even use a general anaesthetic in order to get a diagnostic scan.

More often patients become uncomfortable in the scanner and move to relieve pain or muscle cramps. Careful preparation for the scan should minimize the patient's discomfort. This should include a clear description of what they will hear and feel during the imaging, as well as using pads and immobilization straps to help them keep still. Visco-elastic foam cushions are particularly useful for making the patient comfortable and able to lie still for long periods. Immobilization often works particularly well with young babies who seem to like being well swaddled! It is also important to make sure patients can clearly hear breath holding and other instructions over the intercom even with ear protection.

If a scan is unacceptably degraded due to motion artefact, the only solution is to repeat the scan. Obviously it makes sense to check that the patient is as comfortable as possible and understands the need to

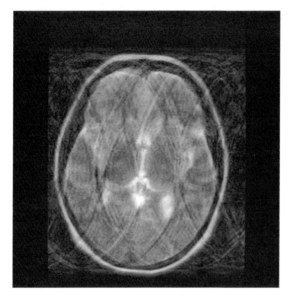

Figure 6.1 Gross motion artefacts due to patient moving continuously throughout the scan.

keep still before starting the repeat scan. If the scan is a particularly long one it is also worthwhile trying to reduce the scan time to improve the chances of an image without movement artefact, so long as the reduced SNR or resolution is still acceptable.

6.3 Physiological motion

Respiration, the beating heart and peristalsis can all cause motion artefacts on scans, appearing as multiple ghost images in the phase-encoding direction (figure 6.2). The number and severity of ghost images depends on the regularity of the motion, ranging from just a few high-intensity ghosts of the chest wall, to a generalized low-intensity blurring due to the nonperiodic motion of the bowels. For scans of the chest, heart and abdomen, these artefacts clearly must be minimized in order to produce diagnostic images, but there are also other situations where motion correction improves the scan. For example, a brachial plexus scan looks better with respiratory and cardiac gating, although the artefact may not interfere directly with the anatomy of interest.

Why are ghosts only produced in the phase-encode direction? The clue is in the timing of the scan process. Consecutive points in the frequency-encoding direction are measured close together, typically much less than 1 ms apart, whereas consecutive phase-encoding

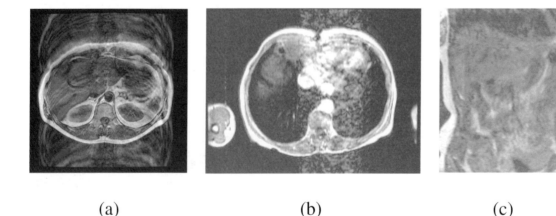

(a)   (b)   (c)

Figure 6.2 Motion artefacts due to (a) respiration, (b) cardiac motion, and (c) peristalsis.

steps are *TR* ms apart, often described as 'pseudo-time'. Motion such as respiration and blood flow occurs slowly compared with frequency encoding but much quicker than phase encoding. So between successive phase encodings, the anatomy moves and produces a ghost signal at a different PE position.

6.3.1 Respiratory motion

The best way of avoiding respiratory artefacts is to reduce the scan time to less than 25 s, so that the scan can be acquired during a single breath-hold. The acquisition can also be split up so that batches of scans are acquired in two or three breath-holds, using careful coaching of the patient's breathing technique before the examination so that the diaphragm is held in the same position for each batch. In general, breath-holding in expiration is more reproducible. However, patients can suspend breathing in inspiration for longer periods. Accordingly, if only one breath hold is necessary, inspiration may be preferable. But if multiple breath-holds are necessary, expiration is preferable.

If breath-holding is not suitable, a very simple way of reducing respiratory artefacts is to increase the number of signal acquisitions (NSA). The technique works because the static anatomy is always in the same place

in the field of view, while the ghosts due to moving anatomy are at random positions. Thus the averaging reinforces the signal intensity of the real image and reduces the signal-to-noise ratio (SNR) of the ghosts, although it must be said that it is not a very efficient way of avoiding artefacts. In order to work well at least four signal averages are required, and preferably six, which gives a long scan time.

There are three other techniques in common use; respiratory gating (or triggering), respiratory compensation (or phase re-ordering), and navigator echoes. The first two methods use a closed 'bellows' strapped around the patient's chest, which expands and contracts as the chest rises and falls. The changing volume creates a change in air pressure, which is detected and converted to an electrical signal that tracks respirations (figure 6.3). The success of both respiratory compensation and gating depends on the patient's breathing remaining regular throughout the scans. Although a few extra-deep breaths are not much of a problem, extremely irregular breathing may actually produce a worse image than an un-compensated one.

The respiratory gating technique uses the bellows waveform to start the imaging sequence at a regular place in each breathing cycle. As a result each signal is

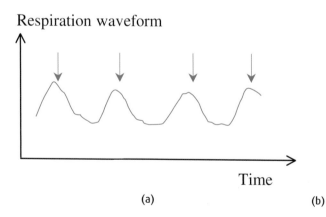

Respiration waveform

Time

(a)

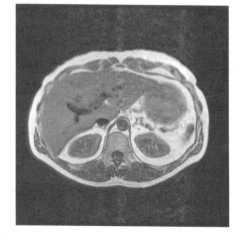

(b)

Figure 6.3 (a) The changing signal produced by respiratory bellows around a patient's chest. Respiratory gating triggers the scans so that all the acquisitions are synchronized to the same point in the cycle (small arrows). (b) Axial image of the abdomen acquired with respiratory-ordered phase encoding (ROPE).

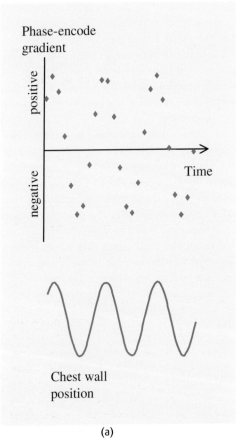

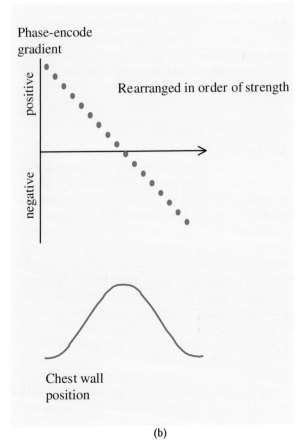

Figure 6.4 (a) Low-sort ROPE rearranges the phase encoding order to match the respiratory cycle. (b) When the data are arranged in order of phase encode gradient strength, neighbouring lines in k-space are close together on the respiratory waveform and it appears that the whole acquisition has taken place over one breathing cycle.

acquired when the chest wall is in the same position, so there are no ghost images. Instead of a regular TR, the sequence now uses the interval between two consecutive triggers, which at a normal breathing rate of about 10–15 breaths per minute gives an effective TR of at least 4000 ms. This means that respiratory gating is only useful for PD or T_2-weighted imaging, and scan times may be very long.

Respiratory compensation or phase re-ordering (also called **R**espiratory-**O**rdered **P**hase **E**ncoding, ROPE) also uses the waveform from the bellows to synchronize data acquisition with breathing. It makes use of the fact that all the signal and contrast information

is in the middle of k-space, which corresponds to the smallestphase-encoding gradients, while the large phase-encoding gradients fill the outer portions of k-space and therefore control the resolution of the image (see 'An easy introduction to k-space' in chapter 4). When the phase-encode gradient changes linearly from positive to negative through the imaging sequence, consecutive k-space lines are at very different places in the respiratory waveform. In ROPE the order of the gradients is matched to the respiratory cycle (figure 6.4(a)) so that neighbouring lines in k-space are acquired close together in the breathing cycle (figure 6.4(b)). ROPE is an efficient way of removing the breathing artefacts, although it does extend the scan time slightly since it may have to over-acquire data, and it has the advantage that it can be used for any type of image weighting.

Navigator echoes do not use the bellows, instead they use a rapid 1D imaging method to map the position of the diaphragm. A 15–30 mm thick column is defined in the superior-inferior direction across the right hemi-diaphragm (figure 6.5a), excited by an extra RF pulse and gradients in two directions. No phase encoding is used, the echo is simply frequency-encoded along the SI direction. The result is a single line of voxels, which you might think is pretty useless. However the strong contrast between the (dark) lung and the (brighter) liver

Breathe in, breathe out . . .

So in total there are five different ways of avoiding respiratory artefacts. How do you choose the right one for your application? We can start by saying that increasing the NSA is only useful if the resulting scan time is not too long. Respiratory triggering, where the TR is effectively the length of the breathing cycle, has such a long scan time that it is rarely used.

For cardiac imaging, the methods of choice are breath-hold for morphology and perfusion scans, and navigators for coronary arteries and high-resolution viability. Chapter 14 contains more details about cardiac imaging. Navigator gating is rather inefficient, since data cannot be acquired during large portions of the respiratory cycle, but it offers the best choice for breathless patients.

In abdomen imaging, a breath-hold is usually the best choice, but ROPE can also be used. However remember that long scan times may cause more blurring from peristalsis. ROPE has the big disadvantage that it cannot be used with fast spin-echo (FSE) sequences. FSE needs to control the phase-encode gradients with respect to the echo time required, whereas ROPE needs to control phase encoding relative to the respiratory cycle. These conflicting demands are currently not compatible, although in the future someone might work out a clever way of satisfying both requirements.

More about respiratory ghosts

The position and intensity of respiratory (or other motion) ghosts can be predicted by making some simple assumptions about the motion. Let us assume a sinusoidal translation with amplitude A and period T_m, described by

$$x(\tau) = x_0 + A \sin\left(\frac{t}{T_m}\right)$$

where T is the time from the start of the scan to the nth phase encoding step ($T = n \cdot TR$). It can be shown that the ith ghost has intensity $J_i(\gamma A \int G dt)$ where J_i is an ith order Bessel function, and the ghosts are located at separations of δy from the main static image, where

$$\delta y = \frac{TR}{T_m} \cdot FOV_{PE}$$

For example, if the breathing rate is 12 breaths per minute then T_m is 5000 ms; with a TR of 500 ms, and a field of view (FOV) of 32 cm, the ghosts will be 3.2 cm apart. Ghosts outside the FOV are wrapped back in due to phase aliasing, so they cannot be removed by simply increasing their separation.

Respiratory triggering makes the TR equal to T_m so that ghosts are separated by the size of the FOV; since they wrap back into the FOV the ghosts coincide with the original image. Respiratory-ordered phase encoding (ROPE) on the other hand increases the apparent T_m, or putting it another way it appears to reduce the breathing rate to one breath per scan time. To visualize this, consider a scan acquired with ROPE over several breathing cycles (figure 6.4(a)). When the k-space lines are rearranged in order of gradient strength they appear to occur over just one breath (figure 6.4(b)). This is called low-sort respiratory compensation. An alternative, called high-sort, can be combined with phase oversampling: in this case the phase encoding is re-ordered so that neighbouring lines in k-space are separated by half a wavelength on the respiratory waveform. Ghosts are produced at the edges of the larger phase FOV, which is then discarded. The choice of low-sort or high-sort is not under operator control, and is effectively invisible to the user.

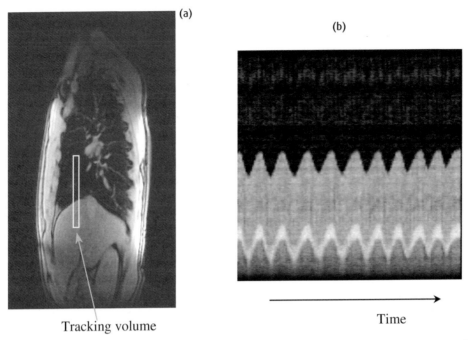

Tracking volume   Time

Figure 6.5 (a) Navigator echo imaging for respiratory motion correction excites a column of tissue over the diaphragm. (b) The navigator signal is frequency encoded in one direction, and the other direction becomes time. Courtesy of GE Medical Systems.

shows up clearly. When a series of linear navigators is acquired while the patient breathes normally, the changing position of the diaphragm can be visualised by displaying the 1D images side-by-side (figure 6.5b). The boundary can be automatically detected by the scanner software, and is used to 'gate' the acquisition so that the image data are only acquired when the diaphragm is within certain spatial limits, typically 2 – 4 mm. More details about navigator echoes can be found in chapter 14.

6.3.2 Cardiac motion

Removal of cardiac motion artefacts is achieved by gating the sequence to the cardiac cycle. Electrodes are attached to the patient's chest or back, in a similar way to normal ECG monitoring electrodes using sticky pads with conductive jelly. Note that MR compatible electrodes use carbon instead of metal to avoid causing artefact on the MR images. In addition, the MRI electrodes are larger with more conductive jelly to minimize

the possibility of burning the patient. The peak of the R wave is detected by the scanner and used to trigger the next imaging sequence (figure 6.6(a)). In this way each line of data is acquired at the same point in the cardiac cycle, and the ghosting is removed.

Scan time is determined by the heart rate. The faster the heart rate the faster the scan since one line of k-space data is collected for each heart beat. Advanced (sometimes called segmented) cardiac gating allows multiple lines of k-space data to be collected for each R-wave trigger. This can allow shortening the scan sufficiently to be acquired in a breath hold. Instead of a regular TR chosen by the operator, the TR is controlled by the R–R interval, which is typically 600–1000 ms, and images thus tend to be T_1-weighted (figure 6.6(b)). Longer TRs suitable for T_2 or PD weighted images are possible by gating to every 2nd, 3rd or even 4th R wave. Unfortunately this means that some slices will be acquired during systole of the inter-trigger heart beats, and these slices may be degraded by motion artefact.

ECG or peripheral gating?

Both methods are available on most modern scanners, although ECG gating may be a separate purchase option. What are the advantages and disadvantages of the two techniques?

ECG gating is a more accurate gating method, since the R wave is detected directly and the peak is usually sharp and easily recognizable by the scanner. This is particularly important for cardiac imaging since it allows as many multi-slice images as possible to be scanned within the R–R interval. Since all the other ECG peaks can be seen too, it is possible to acquire data selectively during diastole by setting a delay between the R wave and the sequence trigger (known as the trigger delay), to avoid systolic heart motion. In a multi-slice gated sequence, not only is each slice at a different location, it is also at a different point in the cardiac cycle. During systole the heart moves within the chest and so slices acquired during systole may be spatially mismatched with slices in the rest of the cycle.

In contrast peripheral gating only detects the arterial pulse and the peak is much broader than the ECG R wave (figure 6.6(c)). Thus peripheral gating is no good for cardiac imaging because it results in variability of the trigger position. In addition the trigger is delayed relative to systole due to the time it takes for the arterial blood to arrive in the finger, typically about 500 ms. Bear in mind that the arterial delay for the anatomy you are imaging may be different from that in the finger too, so there may be some residual ghosts. However, for the most common application, that of removing CSF pulsation artefact in neurological imaging, the delay times are actually quite similar, so peripheral gating is usually successful.

The advantages of peripheral gating are in the ease of preparing the patient and for safety. For ECG gating it is necessary for the patient to change into a hospital gown, and for electrodes to be carefully attached to the skin. A hairy chest may need to be shaved to allow adequate conduction. In comparison, placing the peripheral trigger detector on one of the fingers is very easy and more comfortable for the patient. Since it only uses a light detector (and the lead is made of optic fibre) the system does not pick up signals from the changing gradients, whereas the ECG wires and electrodes are very sensitive to the changing magnetic fields during imaging. MR scanners use electronic processing to reduce these spurious signals, which can otherwise produce false triggers for the sequence. From the patient safety point of view, high-impedance carbon-fibre ECG electrodes and leads should be used to avoid the possibility of skin burns. In addition the ECG lead wires must be carefully arranged to avoid loops which can absorb RF energy and also cause burns. With peripheral gating there is no possibility of an electrical skin burn since the electrical components of peripheral gating are far away from the patient.

ECG gating is obviously essential for imaging the heart and mediastinum, and is also useful for removing pulsatile flow artefacts in areas with large arteries. Specialist cardiac imaging including cine and perfusion imaging is covered in detail in chapter 14.

Cardiac gating can also be achieved by detecting the arterial pulse of blood in the patient's finger or toe. In these areas the blood vessels are very close to the skin, and an infrared light detector can pick up the increased volume of blood as the arterial pulse reaches the extremity. The signal only shows the arterial peak, not the other portions of the cardiac cycle, but this is sufficient to provide a trigger for the MR sequence. This technique is known as peripheral gating or photo-plethysmographic gating (rather a technical mouth-ful!). Peripheral gating is a useful way of removing pulsatility artefacts in the brain and spine and a good backup when ECG gating fails.

6.3.3 Peristaltic motion

Peristalsis causes a random continuous motion of the abdominal contents, and there is no physiological signal to trigger the MR acquisition. Acquiring multiple averages can reduce the ghost appearances, but a much more effective method, especially if it is necessary to image the small or large bowel, is to use an antiperistalsis drug such as hyoscine butylbromide (Buscopan®). This has the effect of freezing the peristaltic motion for a short time (usually around 15–20 min) which is just long enough to

(a)

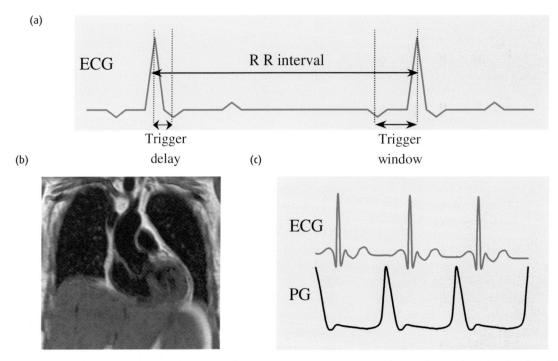

(b)

(c)

Figure 6.6 (a) The ECG waveform used to trigger the scan acquisitions to remove cardiac motion artefact, showing the effective TR (the R–R interval), the trigger delay and the trigger window. (b) Coronal view of the chest showing no artefact from cardiac movement. (c) Peripheral gating (PG) signal compared with ECG signal.

acquire the required images. Alternatively, images that have sub-second data acquisition times are fast enough to freeze peristaltic motion. Ultrafast pulse sequences such as HASTE (see section 12.3.7) or single-shot **F**ast **S**pin **E**cho (FSE) are able to freeze bowel motion and eliminate peristalsis motion artefacts (figure 6.7).

6.4 Motion artefacts from flow

Moving protons in blood vessels or the cerebrospinal fluid (CSF) cause a range of artefacts due to two effects. First there is an in-flow effect which increases signal within blood vessels on both spin-echo and gradient-echo images, as fresh protons flow into the imaging slice during the TR. Second there are velocity-induced phase effects, which decrease signal in blood vessels and create ghost images of arteries or veins in the phase-encode direction (figure 6.8(a)). Complete intra-

voxel dephasing occurs in areas of turbulent flow for example at a tight stenosis, leaving a dark appearance. Note that the direction of flow doesn't change the direction of the artefact; ghosts will appear along the phase-encoding direction even if the flow is through the slice or along the frequency-encoding direction. Degrading artefacts are a particular problem in gradient-echo imaging when the blood generally has a very high intensity due to the in-flow effect. In spin-echo sequences blood vessels usually have a 'dark-blood' appearance and phase-encode artefacts are less of a problem.

6.4.1 The in-flow effect on SE and GE sequences

The appearance of flowing blood depends not only on the type of sequence, but also on the TE or TR, the velocity of the blood, and the slice thickness. In this section a simple explanation will suffice, but for more details see chapter 13.

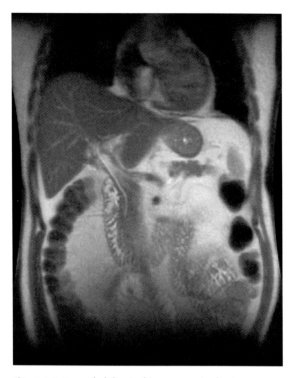

Figure 6.7 Coronal abdominal image acquired using singleshot FSE to 'freeze' the peristalsis motion.

Consider a blood vessel passing through an imaging slice (figure 6.8(b)), and assume that the blood flow is steady. In SE sequences, we use two RF pulses to create the echo. If the blood is moving fast enough, the bolus in the imaging slice will be replaced by another bolus during the gap between the two pulses. The first bolus receives a 90° pulse but not the 180°, while the second receives only the 180° pulse. Since both a 90° and a 180° pulse are required to create a spin echo, neither bolus will produce an echo. There will be a signal loss within the blood vessel, giving spin-echo images a characteristic dark-blood appearance. Remember that an artefact is any image appearance that does not accurately reflect the object, so these flow voids are considered to be artefacts even though they do not degrade the rest of the image.

During a GE sequence, the first RF pulse excites the bolus of blood within the slice, but that bolus immediately moves out of the slice. Unlike spin echo, the gradients which create the echo are not slice selective, so the excited blood still contributes a signal even though it is no longer in the image slice. For the next and every subsequent slice there is a fresh bolus of blood within the slice. Each bolus has not been excited before, so its

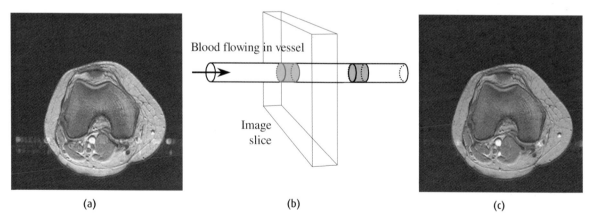

(a)   (b)   (c)

Figure 6.8 (a) Knee image showing artefact from flowing blood. (b) Blood vessel passing through an imaging slice. In a spin-echo sequence, the blood excited by the 90° pulse (coloured grey) moves on by the time the 180° pulse is applied (blue-coloured bolus), and neither bolus produces a signal. In gradient echo sequences, each bolus has fully relaxed magnetization M_0 when the excitation pulse is applied, and its signal is refocused by the gradients so that blood appears bright. (c) Axial knee image acquired with gradient moment nulling (flow compensation).

In the figure: Blood flowing in vessel / Image slice

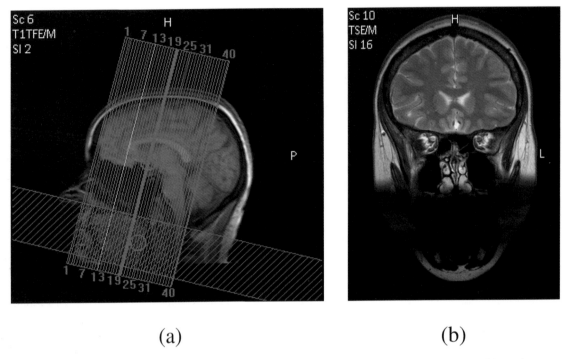

(a)   (b)

Figure 6.9 (a) Angled sat band within the FOV to eliminate artefacts from tongue movement and swallowing. (b) Resulting image.

magnetization is fully relaxed and the RF pulse creates a PD-weighted signal for the blood. Thus on GE images blood vessels have high intensity.

6.4.2 Velocity-induced phase effects

Apart from the in-flow or time-of-flight effects, phase-related artefacts arise because the blood protons are moving during the imaging gradients and so their resonant frequencies are changing continuously. Again, a simple explanation will suffice in this chapter and more detail will be found in chapter 13. The frequency differences induced by protons moving in a magnetic field gradient create a dephasing effect relative to the static protons in surrounding tissue. Since the phase angle of the signal is used for spatial encoding (in the phase-encoding direction), moving protons will not have the correct phase angle for their real position and they will produce ghosts at random positions along the phase-encoding axis.

The acquired phase angle depends on the velocity of the protons and the strength and duration of the gradient. If a single voxel contains protons moving at different velocities, for example in a region of turbulent flow, their signals will dephase rapidly and cause a signal dropout.

6.4.3 Avoiding flow artefacts

Perhaps the easiest way to avoid flow artefacts is to use spatial saturation bands just outside the field of view or in the slice direction. Saturation bands apply a 90° pulse to all the tissues within the band immediately before the RF excitation pulse for the imaging sequence. Blood flowing from the saturation band into the imaging slice will have no time to recover its z

magnetization, so it will give no signal. Spatial saturation bands take up pulse sequence time, thus reducing the number of slices possible for a given TR, and they also increase the SAR (specific absorption rate, see section 2.3.5) for the patient, which should be done with care in certain cases.

Saturation bands, also known as REST slabs or pre-sat bands, are simply slice selections, and can be used in many ways. They can be placed within the FOV, e.g. to saturate signal from the thoracic aorta for sagittal spines or reduce artefact from swallowing (figure 6.9), or at the edges of the FOV, e.g. to reduce phase wrap on coronal shoulders. Placed above and/or below the image FOV, sat bands can remove arterial and/or venous blood flow. In principle there is no limit to the number of sat bands you can use, but in practice most manufacturers restrict you to a maximum of 4 or 6.

It is also possible to correct for dephasing effects using a technique called *gradient moment nulling*, also known as *gradient moment rephasing* or *flow compensation*. Extra gradient pulses with carefully calculated strengths and durations are inserted into the pulse sequence, so that the net phase effect is zero for moving protons as well as for static ones. This reduces the velocity-induced phase angles so that a single image of the vessel will appear on the final image (figure 6.8(c)). In contrast to spatial saturation bands, gradient moment nulling doesn't increase the SAR, but the extra gradients will increase the minimum TE, which in turn has the disadvantage of reducing the number of slices possible.

6.5 Lose the fat!

Fat is often a source of problems in MR imaging. It tends to have high signal intensity at all contrasts, and that can mask pathologies. It also causes two types of artefact due to its structure, known as chemical shift artefacts.

In section 3.1 we subdivided tissues into fat-based and water-based tissues. In all MR images we are detecting signals from protons (the nuclei of hydrogen atoms), but fat and water have very different structures. Water has only two hydrogen atoms and an

oxygen atom, so it is a small molecule. Fat is made up of triglyceride chains, long backbones of 10–20 carbon atoms each with two hydrogen atoms on either side. Fat molecules are thus very large and each hydrogen atom is surrounded by many other atoms. The neighbouring electron clouds reduce the strength of the external magnetic field, so the hydrogen atoms in fat have a lower Larmor frequency than those in water, which do not have such a shielding effect. This difference is known as the chemical shift which is quoted in parts per million (ppm) and is independent of magnetic field strength. We can calculate the frequency difference by multiplying the chemical shift in ppm by the resonant frequency in megahertz of protons at a particular magnetic field strength. The chemical shift between fat and water is 3.5 ppm and at 1.5 T protons have a Larmor frequency of 63.855 MHz, so the frequency difference is approximately 220 Hz; at 1 T it is approximately 150 Hz and at 0.5 T roughly 74 Hz. If we look at the frequency spectrum from the human body we see two peaks, the larger one from water protons and the smaller one to the right from fats (figure 6.11(a)).

6.5.1 Chemical shift artefact

As we will see in chapter 7, we use frequency-encoding in one direction, i.e. we rely on the MR signal's frequency for spatial information. But fat naturally has a lower frequency than water, so the frequency encoding will be fooled into thinking that the fat is in a different position. Due to the frequency difference, the apparent position of fat signals is shifted by a number of pixels, but only in the frequency-encode direction. Depending on by how many pixels it is shifted, the artefact may appear as light and dark bands on opposite sides of a structure, or as an entire ghost image of the fat distribution in the anatomy (see figure 6.11(b)). This is called the chemical shift artefact or chemical shift misregistration artefact. The severity of the pixel shift depends mainly on the receive bandwidth used: the lower the bandwidth the worse the problem. So to avoid an artefact you should ideally use a higher bandwidth. However, increasing the bandwidth also reduces the signal-to-noise ratio in the image, so it is not always desirable.

Gradient moment nulling

To understand how gradient moment nulling works, let us imagine just two protons, one stationary within the field of view and the other moving at constant velocity in the direction of the slice select gradient, which is switched on during an excitation pulse (figure 6.10(a)). We can ignore the part of the gradient before the RF pulse, as the protons are not yet excited. Immediately after the excitation pulse the two protons will be in phase. While the gradient is switched on the stationary proton changes its frequency to match the field strength at position x, and precesses at that frequency until the gradient is switched off. It therefore acquires a phase angle relative to protons at the isocentre (figure 6.10(b)).

We need to remove this phase angle before applying the phase-encode gradient, so that the final phase angle will depend only on the proton's position in the phase-encode direction. This can be achieved by adding a negative lobe, equal in strength and duration to the slice select gradient, to 'rephase' the static protons. Thus at the end of the rephase gradient all static protons will be back in phase.

The moving proton starts off at the same frequency as the stationary proton in position x, but as it moves in the direction of the gradient it experiences a changing magnetic field (let's assume it is increasing). Its resonant frequency will also increase to match the field at each position, and as the frequency changes the moving proton will acquire a phase difference relative to the static proton (figure 6.10(b)). The rephase gradient doesn't correct this effect because (in simple terms) the moving proton starts from a different position during this gradient.

It turns out that to correct the velocity-induced phase shift we have to make the rephase lobe twice as strong as the initial slice select lobe, and add a third positive lobe after it (figure 6.10(c)). Notice that the phase of static protons is zero halfway through the second, negative lobe, but that the moving protons are not properly refocused until the end of the final lobe. The gradient lobes have areas (strength × duration) in the proportion 1:2:1. The gradient area is more properly called the first-order gradient moment, hence the term 'gradient moment nulling' or 'gradient moment refocusing'. This scheme for flow compensation works well provided the protons are flowing at constant velocity.

Constant velocity is known as first-order motion ($v = dx/dt$), and is a reasonably good model of blood flow in peripheral arteries and veins. However, in the larger arteries the blood is also accelerating and decelerating due to the heart beat, and has both second-order (acceleration, d^2x/dt^2) and third-order motion, known as 'jerk' (d^3x/dt^3). Similar analysis of the second-order gradient moments (for accelerating protons) shows that four lobes are required with moments in the proportions 1:-3:3:-1, while for third-order motion six lobes with moments in the ratio 1:-2:1:-1:2:-1 are necessary. Thus it is possible to fully compensate for pulsatile blood flow using gradient moment nulling, but at the expense of a delayed echo time in order to fit in all the gradient pulses. For this reason, most scanners only have first-order motion compensation, but some have options for higher-order gradient moment nulling.

6.5.2 Phase cancellation artefact

The chemical shift artefact occurs with both spin-echo and gradient-echo sequences. There is a second type of artefact, also caused by the chemical shift between fat and water, which only occurs with gradient-echo imaging. Some texts call this 'chemical shift of the second kind', 'black line' artefact, 'India ink' or the 'phase cancellation artefact', which is the term we will use. The phase cancellation artefact appears as a black outline (figure 6.12(b)), especially noticeable in the abdomen where water-based tissues are surrounded by peritoneal fat. It occurs in any voxel containing both fat and water, and depends on the fat–water chemical shift and the TE used.

Why does it occur? Immediately after the excitation pulse of the sequence fat and water signals are in phase with each other, but due to the small difference in their Larmor frequencies they begin to dephase. If the echo is acquired when fat and water are exactly

(a)

(c)

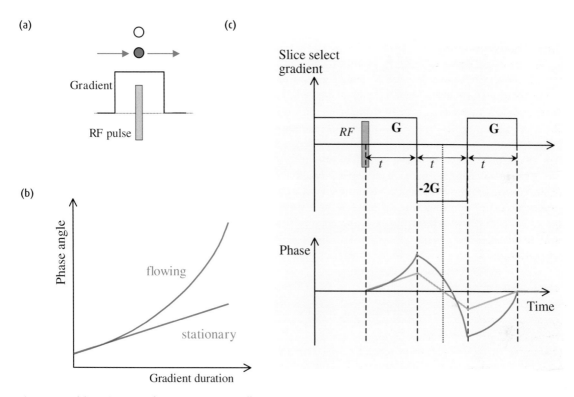

Figure 6.10 (a) Stationary and moving spins, initially at the same position when a gradient is switched on. (b) The moving spins continuously change frequency as they move along the gradient, and acquire a phase angle relative to the static spins. (c) Gradient moment nulling for a single gradient lobe. *G*, amplitude of the gradient; *t*, its duration.

out of phase (at 180° to each other), voxels with a mixture of tissues will have a reduced signal since the fat signal subtracts from the water. This gives the characteristic dark outline at fat/water interfaces, due to all the mixed voxels around the edge. If the TE is increased so that fat and water are back in phase with each other, the signals will add together instead of subtracting, and no black line occurs (figure 6.12(a)).

So there are specific TEs in gradient-echo imaging which give the phase cancellation artefact, and others which don't. Some manufacturers list 'in-phase' and 'out-of-phase' as options for the TE, which makes life easy! Some radiologists find the black outline distracting, others don't mind it. Whether you want to avoid the artefact or not, it's simply a case of choosing the right TE. The phase cancellation artefact is not a

problem in spin-echo imaging because the fat–water phase shift between the 90° and 180° pulses is inverted by the 180° pulse, so that at the echo time they are back in phase.

Deliberately creating images with the phase cancellation artefact has been called **O**ut-**O**f-**P**hase **S**canning OOPS) and this can be useful as a way of reducing signals from fat. However, the signal is not completely removed, just reduced. Better fat suppression can be achieved either by frequency-selective saturation of only the fat protons, or using STIR (short TI inversion recovery). A good example is for time-of-flight MR angiography of the Circle of Willis, where choosing an out-of-phase TE noticeably reduces the periorbital and subcutaneous fat signal, improving the quality of the maximum intensity projections (see figure 6.12(c) and (d)).

How many pixels is it shifted?

You need to know how much the fat image is shifted with respect to the water in order to know if the chemical shift artefact is a problem. The severity of the chemical shift effect depends on two things: the field strength of the magnet and the receive bandwidth used for imaging. Some manufacturers quote the receive bandwidth in terms of the number of pixels by which fat will be shifted; this is the easiest way for operators to avoid the artefact! Others use 'hertz per pixel' for the receive bandwidth; again this makes life easy as you just have to divide the chemical shift for your magnet strength by the bandwidth. For example at 1.5 T the chemical shift is 220 Hz, so if you choose a bandwidth of 100 Hz/pixel the fat signals will be shifted by about two pixels relative to water, whereas a bandwidth of 500 Hz/pixel will give a negligible shift of $220 \div 500 \approx 0.5$ pixels.

Lastly, some manufacturers quote the receive bandwidth directly in kilohertz. Working out the chemical shift is a little more long-winded, so you might like to work it out for a range of bandwidths and either memorize them or have them in a handy notebook when you are at the console. Start by checking carefully in the manufacturer's manuals whether the bandwidth is exactly as quoted or is it $\pm$ the value. For example, is 10 kHz actually 10 kHz or ± 10 kHz? In the latter case you need to double it in your calculation, as we will do in the following example.

First work out the bandwidth in hertz per pixel; multiply by 1000 to get it into hertz, then divide by the frequency matrix. At the moment 256 is the commonest frequency matrix (although 512 is becoming much more popular), so in this example we will use 256.

$$\frac{10 \times 2 \times 1000}{256} = 78.2 \text{ Hz/pixel}$$

Now divide the chemical shift for your scanner's field strength by this number. We will use the example of 1.5 T, so

$$\frac{220}{78.2} = 2.8 \text{ pixels}$$

So at this field strength a ± 10 kHz bandwidth with a 256 frequency matrix gives a moderate chemical shift artefact. If the matrix is increased to 512, the shift will be more than five pixels and will be more of a problem. However, a ± 10 kHz bandwidth at 0.5 T gives the following shift:

$$\frac{74}{78} = 0.95 \text{ pixels}$$

which is insignificant.

6.5.3 MRI liposuction: removing fat signals

There are two ways of suppressing fat signals more or less completely. The first we have already met: the STIR sequence which uses the inversion recovery pulse sequence with the TI set at the null point of fat as described in section 3.9. This technique depends on the T_1 of fat, which is considerably shorter than that of most other tissues. The TI varies slightly with field strength, from 110 ms at 0.5 T to 150 ms at 1.5 T. The initial ('inversion') 180° pulse inverts all the equilibrium magnetization, which then begins to recover towards the equilibrium value, M_0, with T_1 recovery. When the 90° pulse is applied at the null point of fat, fatbased tissues produce zero signal as they have nothing to tip into the xy plane. At an appropriate TE a refocusing 180° pulse is applied to generate a spin echo and create an image with no signal from fat. Since we use 'magnitude' reconstruction in MRI, all the other tissues give bright signals, with fluids (with the longest T_1s) having the highest signal.

The alternative technique is frequency-selective fat saturation, often known simply as 'fat sat' or 'chemical sat'. This takes advantage of the chemical shift

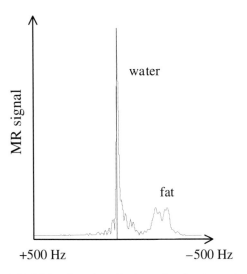

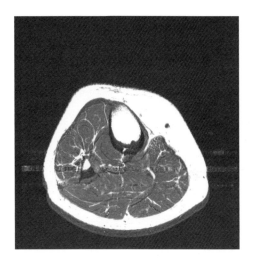

Figure 6.11 (a) Spectrum from the lower leg showing water and fat peaks with a separation of 3.5 ppm. (b) Chemical shift artefact in the lower leg.

between fat and water to excite only the fat protons. A narrow range of RF frequencies centred on the fat Larmor frequency is used (see figure 6.13(a)) to give a 90° pulse to protons in fat, leaving the water protons

In-phase and out-of-phase TEs

If your scanner doesn't show 'in-phase' and 'out-of-phase' as TE options, you need to work out some appropriate values. As with the chemical shift artefact, you might find it useful to keep this information in a handy notebook. We start with the chemical shift in hertz between fat and water, for example at 1.5 T the shift is 220 Hz. Fat and water are in phase immediately after the excitation pulse, but we can't acquire the signal immediately. The next time they are in phase will be 1/220 s later, i.e. 4.55 ms. So a TE of 4.55 or 9 ms will have fat and water in phase, avoiding the black line artefact. Halfway between these two echo times fat will be exactly 180° out of phase with water, so a TE of 6.9 ms (or 2.3 ms if the gradients allow it) will give the phase cancellation artefact. To get a T_2^*-weighted gradient echo with in-phase TE, you need to go to 22.7 or 27.3 ms, while an out-of-phase T_2^*-weighted TE would be halfway between these values at about 25 ms.

Dixon method for fat/water separation

Dixon suggested in 1984 that in-phase and out-of-phase gradient-echo images could be combined to create images of just fat or water, known as fat/water separation. The idea is that in the first (in-phase) image, the signal (S_{ip}) is the sum of fat (S_f) and water (S_w) signals:

$$S_{ip} = S_w + S_f$$

while in the second out-of-phase image (S_{oop}) it is the difference:

$$S_{oop} = S_w - S_f$$

By adding the two images, only the water signals remain, while the subtraction of the out-of-phase image from the in-phase image produces a fat-only image:

$$S_{ip} + S_{oop} = (S_w + S_f) + (S_w - S_f) = 2S_w$$

$$S_{ip} - S_{oop} = (S_w + S_f) - (S_w - S_f) = -2S_f$$

In practice it is necessary to correct for T_2^* differences since the two images have different echo times. A refinement, called the three-point Dixon method, uses a third image with an in-phase TE to correct for main field (B_0) inhomogeneities.

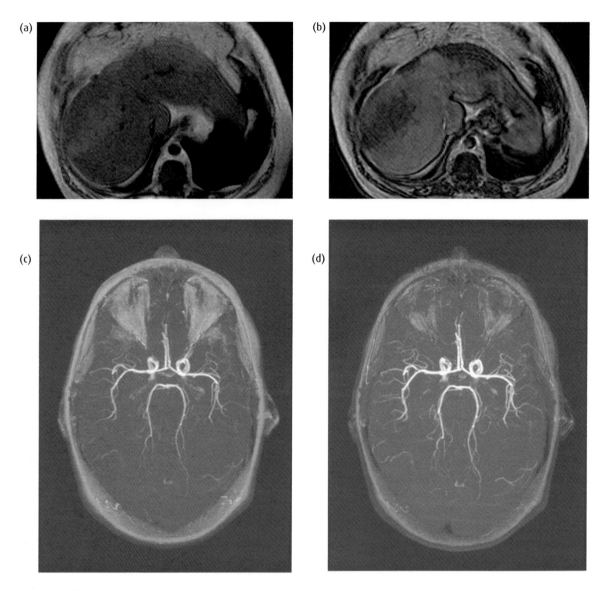

Figure 6.12 Phase cancellation artefact. (a) At a TE of 4.2 ms the fat and water signals are in phase and no phase cancellation artefact is seen. (b) At a TE of 2.1 ms, a black line appears at boundaries between fat and water, because the fat and water signals within the voxel are out of phase with each other. (c) Cranial time-of-flight (TOF) MR angiography with TE for fat and water in phase, and (d) out of phase. Notice how much the periorbital fat intensity is reduced.

unexcited. This is known as a CHESS (**CHE**mical **S**elective) pulse. The imaging sequence is started immediately after the CHESS pulse, so that fat has no time to recover its z magnetization and the image is produced with a suppressed fat signal. Typically crusher gradients are applied immediately after the CHESS pulse to dephase the transverse fat magnetization, which otherwise tends to produce an echo due to its rapid relaxation. There has to be some compromise over the fat sat pulse; it needs a bandwidth wide enough to saturate all the fat protons, but shouldn't excite any water protons. At lower field strengths (e.g. 0.5 T) the chemical shift is only 74 Hz which makes it rather difficult to achieve good fat suppression without losing signal from the water peak (figure 6.13(b)). At field strengths of 1 T and higher, the chemical shift is bigger and that improves the separation between the fat and water peaks.

A slight modification of fat sat combines frequency-selective excitation with STIR. This is known as SPIR (**SP**ectral **I**nversion **R**ecovery) by Philips or SPECIAL (**SPEC**tral **I**nversion **A**t **L**ipid) by General Electric. A frequency-selective pulse is applied to the fat protons, fol-

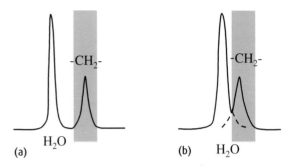

Figure 6.13 (a) Frequency-selective saturation uses a narrow-bandwidth RF pulse to excite only fat protons. (b) At low field strengths the peaks overlap, making it impossible to saturate all the fat without affecting the water protons.

Which is better, STIR or fat sat?

If your scanner has a field strength higher than 1 T, fat sat or SPIR is almost always better than STIR. At these fields it is possible to apply a good suppression pulse to just the fat, leaving the water protons unexcited, thanks to the higher chemical shift. Frequency-selective fat saturation pulses can be inserted before almost any pulse sequence, so the image contrast can be controlled independently of the fat suppression. In comparison, STIR can only produce fat-suppressed T_2-weighted-like images. The exceptions for high-field scanners are when a large field of view (FOV) is required. A large FOV includes a bigger range of magnetic field inhomogeneities, either in the main magnet or in the RF field. Under these circumstances it is not possible to get a frequency-selective pulse to adequately saturate all the fat protons, and STIR tends to be preferred because it is independent of these inhomogeneities.

Conversely at low fields, especially 0.5 T and lower, fat sat doesn't work well because the fat and water peaks are so close together (often overlapping in fact). In addition the magnetic field inhomogeneities tend to be worse on lower-field magnets, so even moderately sized FOVs show patchy fat suppression. STIR is often the only choice for fat-suppressed imaging at these field strengths.

Try it for yourself 6: chemical shift effects

The chemical shift artefacts and methods to avoid them are easily shown using a cooking oil and water phantom. Fill a deep plastic container one-third full with water, adding a drop of gadolinium to reduce the T_1, then carefully pour on some cooking oil until the container is two-thirds full. The oil will float in a separate layer on top of the water, but you have to handle it carefully to avoid making a salad dressing at the interface! Put the container into the head coil or knee coil, do a localizer scan and start changing parameters one at a time. For instance, use several different receive bandwidths (fat/water shifts on Philips systems) to see the chemical shift artefact, or try gradient-echo scans with echo times for fat and water in and out of phase.

A couple of things to look out for:
• Use a T_1-weighted spin-echo sequence to see the chemical shift effect, and make sure the frequency-encode direction is across the fat–water boundary not parallel to it.
• To compare STIR and fat sat, use the fat sat with a T_2-weighted spin-echo scan to get similar contrasts in the final images. Try both techniques at large and small FOVs (you might want to devise a larger phantom for the big FOVs).

Calculating the partial volume effect

In general partial volume artefacts occur in the slice-select direction when the voxel size is rather large compared with the in-plane resolution. Whenever a voxel contains two or more tissues, the final signal intensity in that voxel is simply a proportional sum of the individual tissues. For example a 50/50 mixture of fat (high intensity) and bone (zero intensity) will give a mid-range grey level. We can calculate this for any mixture of n tissues as

$$S = f_1 \cdot S_1 + f_2 \cdot S_2 + \cdots + f_n \cdot S_n$$

where f_n is the fraction of the voxel filled with tissue giving signal intensity S_n and $\Sigma f_n = 1$. Bear in mind that air may be one of the 'tissues', for example in the sinuses and the lungs. In figure 6.14, you can see two adjacent thin slices, compared with a single image of double the slice thickness. If the two thin slices are averaged together using the signal intensity equation (figure 6.14(d)), the result looks almost identical to the acquired thick slice. Unfortunately we can't do the opposite to the thick slice, because we don't know the fractions for the various tissues. So the only cure for partial volume artefact is to re-scan the area with a higher resolution.

lowed by crusher gradients to dephase any signal produced in the transverse plane by inaccuracies in the 180° pulse. At an appropriate TI (depending on field strength) the rest of the imaging sequence is started, producing an image with better fat suppression than the simple CHESS pulse.

To avoid incomplete fat suppression due to RF inhomogeneities, a particular problem at 3.0 T, adiabatic pulses may be used. These RF pulses are quite different from normal excitation pulses and understanding them is rather tricky (when you are ready, turn to chapter 12). For normal use, you just need to know that they create more uniform fat suppression especially over large fields of view, but with the slight disadvantage of higher SAR.

An alternative to CHESS for fat saturation is a family of composite RF pulses known as binomial pulses. Good fat suppression can be achieved even at low field strengths because the binomial pulses rely on dephasing effects rather than RF bandwidth. Full details are given in chapter 12. This type of fat suppression is called 'Proset' on Philips scanners. In principle binomial pulses can be used to saturate either fat or water, but not all systems allow this.

6.6 Partial volume artefact and cross-talk

Partial volume artefacts occur wherever a voxel contains a mixture of tissue types. Considering that the typical voxel is 1 mm × 1 mm × 5 mm, it is easy to see that in a structure as complex as the human body, most voxels in any given slice will have a mixture of tissues. We can consider this as a digital imaging artefact, since we are representing a lot of information in a relatively small number of voxels (yes, 256 × 256 = 65 536 does sound like a lot, but it's not enough!). Chapter 5 deals with the question of optimum resolution; in this section we are only concerned with the artefacts, i.e. what happens when the mixture of signals causes misleading pixel intensities in the image.

Fortunately it is not too difficult to avoid the problem, by selecting a slice thin enough for the area being scanned. For example, we use 3 mm slices for the internal auditory meatus (IAMs), because we know that the nerve is only about 4 mm in diameter and lesions may be only 2 or 3 mm in diameter. Conversely 7 or 10 mm slices are appropriate for the liver, because it is a much larger organ and clinically significant pathology is likely to be at least 5 to 10 millimetres across.

A related problem with multi-slice imaging is cross-talk between adjacent slices, also known as cross-excitation or (erroneously) cross-relaxation. Cross-talk appears as a reduced intensity on all but the first slice of a multi-slice set, which is often only detectable when comparing the end slices with their neighbours. It happens because the slices are not straight-edged, like a sliced loaf of bread, but have a curved profile (see figure 6.15(a)) due to imperfections in the selective excitation pulse. The slice width is defined by the full-width at half-maximum (FWHM), so if the slice gap is too small the edges of the slice may overlap with its neighbours (figure 6.15(b)). Tissue in the overlapping section

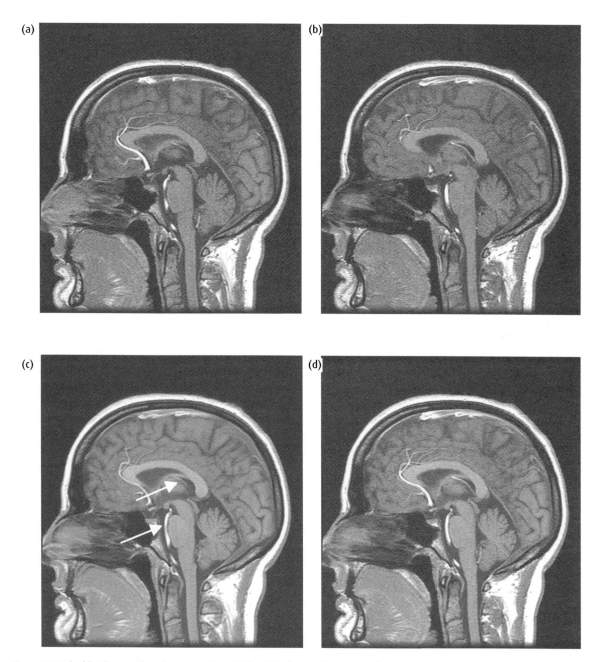

Figure 6.14 (a, b) Adjacent thin slices near the middle of the brain. (c) A single slice covering the same volume as the two thin slices, showing intensity changes (arrows). (d) A mathematical average of the two thin slices shows the same changes as the thick slice.

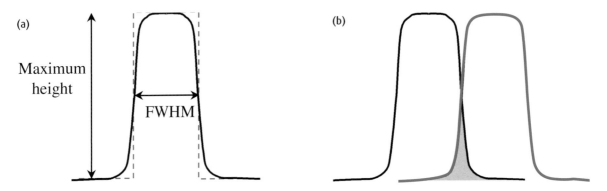

Figure 6.15 (a) The slice excitation profile, ideally rectangular (dotted line), is in reality a curved shape (solid line) whose full-width half-maximum (FWHM) defines the slice width. (b) When the slice gap is too small the edges of neighbouring slices overlap.

is excited by both slices, and experiences a very short effective TR instead of the TR set by the user. It doesn't have time to relax between the pulses, so its signal intensity is reduced. A similar effect occurs with multi-angle oblique acquisitions, e.g. in the lumbar spine, where you may see horizontal black bands across neighbouring slices.

The cure for cross-talk is to avoid small gaps, especially in IR sequences since the slice profiles are worse for 180° pulses. However, you should bear in mind that large gaps reduce resolution, as tissues in the gap are not imaged at all. If very thin gaps or contiguous slices are required, it may be better to do an interleaved or 3D acquisition.

6.7 Phase sampling artefacts

6.7.1 Phase wrap-around artefact

The phase wrap-around artefact arises whenever the anatomy continues outside the field of view (FOV). It causes images of the tissues just outside the FOV to be produced at the opposite edge of the scan in the phase-encode direction (see figure 6.17(a)). The wrapped-in image can overlay the real anatomy being scanned and interfere with the diagnosis. Although it is most common in the phase-encode direction, it also occurs in the slice direction in 3D imaging (when the slice-select axis is also phase encoded) and causes the end slices of the volume to wrap into each other.

Why isn't the slice profile straight-edged?

The reason for nonrectangular slice profiles is the nature of selective excitation. The frequency spectrum of the RF pulse, with the strength of the slice-select gradient, defines not only the slice width but also its profile. To get a perfectly rectangular excitation profile, where all protons within the slice receive exactly a 90° pulse and all protons outside the slice are unexcited, the amplitude of the excitation pulse must be a sinc $(\sin(x)/x)$ function (figure 6.16(a) and Appendix). However, a sinc function is infinitely long in the time domain, and we obviously have to truncate the pulse. In the simplest case, truncating the sinc corresponds to multiplying by a top-hat (see figure 7.5 and Appendix) in the time domain, and the excitation profile becomes a rect function convolved with a sinc, with significant ripple at the edges of the slice (figure 6.16(b)). A better approach is to apodize the sinc, i.e. multiply it by a smoothly varying function such as a Hanning filter or a Gaussian. The excitation profile then has much less ripple (figure 6.16(c)), although its FWHM is slightly greater than the original width.

One way of reducing phase wrap-around is to saturate the signals just outside the FOV using spatial saturation bands. These are simply broad slices excited with a 90° pulse immediately before the main imaging

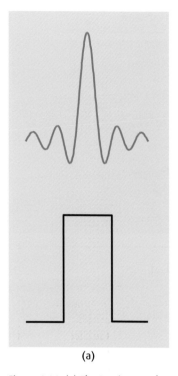 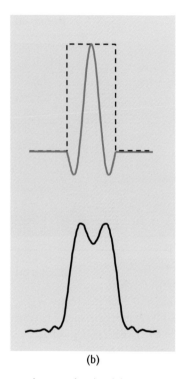 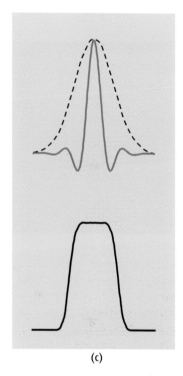

(a)   (b)   (c)

Figure 6.16 (a) The Fourier transform of a rectangle or top-hat (rect) function is a sinc $(\sin(x)/x)$. (b) Simply truncating the sinc produces large ripples on the slice profile. (c) An apodized sinc RF pulse produces a cleaner excitation profile, although the FWHM is slightly wider.

sequence. Thanks to the versatility of the MR gradients, they can be any thickness and oriented in any direction. However, it's not very successful because sat bands don't fully suppress the signal.

A more reliable method is to use phase oversampling, also called the 'no phase wrap' or 'foldover suppression' option. This technique increases the FOV in the phase-encode direction and also increases the number of phase-encode steps so that the pixel size remains the same. The simplest implementation of phase oversampling is to simply double the size of the phase-encode matrix (N_{PE}) and also double the acquired FOV, but many scanners allow phase oversampling to be specified as a percentage of the FOV, which optimizes the technique. The anatomy just outside the desired FOV is now properly phase encoded, and the unwanted edges can simply be cut off by the computer leaving a clean image (figure 6.17(b)).

Increasing the phase-encode matrix also extends the scan time and slightly increases the signal-to-noise ratio.

6.7.2 Gibbs' artefact

The Gibbs' artefact, also known as truncation or ringing artefact, is another consequence of undersampling in the phase-encode direction (and it can sometimes be seen in the frequency-encode direction too). It occurs at high-contrast boundaries, where the intensity changes from bright to dark, and appears as a series of alternating light and dark lines superimposed on the image. The intensity of the lines fades away from the boundary, and they follow the contours of the interface. A common example is on T_1-weighted images of the cervical spine (figure 6.18(a)), where it can mimic the appearance of syringomyelia.

Required PE field of view

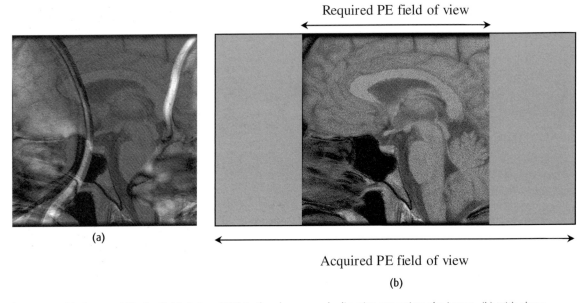

(a)

Acquired PE field of view

(b)

Figure 6.17 (a) Tissue outside the field of view (FOV) in the phase-encode direction wraps into the image. (b) With phase oversampling the reconstructed image is larger than the required FOV, and the computer just throws away the unwanted regions.

Gibbs' artefact is caused by having the acquisition matrix too small, i.e. the pixel size is too large to represent accurately the high-contrast boundary. It is most often a problem with the phase-encode matrix, which is generally smaller than the frequency-encode matrix to reduce scan time. As a rule-of-thumb the phase-encode matrix should never be less than half the frequency-encode matrix. If the artefact reduces the diagnostic quality of the image the scan should be repeated with a larger phase-encode matrix (figure 6.18(b)).

6.7.3 Ringing artefact in CE-MRA

Ringing artefact, also known as 'Maki artefact', is similar to Gibbs' artefact but occurs on MRA studies when gadolinium is arriving in the arteries just as the centre of k-space is being acquired. Rapidly changing gadolinium concentration causes the phase-encode steps to have different contrast weighting that can overly emphasize high spatial-frequency information. This causes ringing of vessel edges on the images. Ringing is especially prominent when the

> **Try it for yourself 7: Phase wrap and Gibbs' artefacts**
>
> You can show the phase-wrap artefact with almost any phantom, although to see the Gibbs' artefact you need something with a sharp high-contrast boundary. Set up the phantom in the head coil or knee coil and scan a localizer. To show phase-wrap, set up a really small FOV in the middle of the phantom, or deliberately move it off-centre in the phase-encode direction. Gibbs' artefact is best seen with a very low matrix of 128–192 on a medium-sized FOV. When you increase the matrix size you probably won't be able to see it visually, but you can measure the pixel intensities across the boundary to see if it is still there: it shows up as 'ringing' on either side of the boundary.

bolus is late while acquiring with elliptic-centric-ordered k-space. In this instance there is minimal gadolinium when the middle of k-space is acquired and high gadolinium concentration when the edges are acquired.

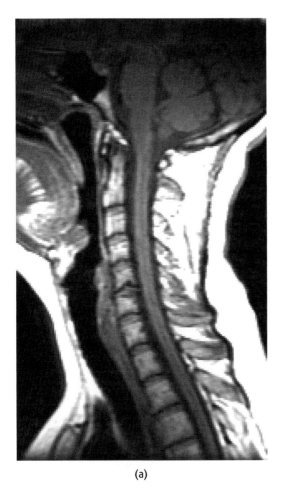
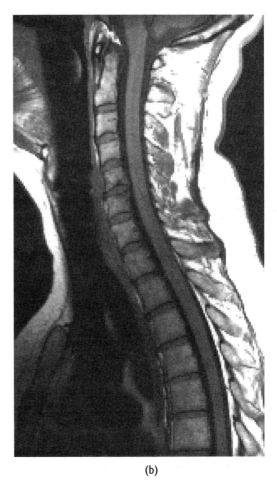

(a)   (b)

Figure 6.18 (a) A low phase-encode matrix can cause Gibbs' artefact, alternating light and dark bands near a high-contrast interface. (b) Increasing the phase-encode matrix avoids the artefact.

6.8 Susceptibility and metal artefacts

Susceptibility and metal artefacts are closely related, having essentially the same appearance on images except that susceptibility artefacts are more subtle than metal ones. Typically a metal artefact consists of an area of zero signal, often with a very high intensity rim on one or two edges (figure 6.19(a)) and with neighbouring regions showing significant geometric distortion. Susceptibility artefacts may just have reduced rather than zero intensity, and may not show any geometric distortion (figure 6.19(b)).

As described in chapter 3, different tissues become magnetized to a different extent when placed in the scanner's magnetic field due to their susceptibility differences. These microscopic field changes increase the dephasing of protons around boundaries between these tissues, reducing the signal intensity of voxels in the area. Most metals have much higher susceptibilities than the body tissues creating large magnetic field inhomogeneities around the object. Since metals are good conductors, they also absorb energy from the RF excitation pulses very easily, and can pose a safety hazard if they heat up.

Susceptibility

Magnetic susceptibility is defined as the extent to which any material becomes temporarily magnetized when it is placed in a large magnetic field (see 'Magnetic properties of tissues' in chapter 3). Among the body tissues, bone has the lowest susceptibility, similar to air, most tissues have mid-range susceptibility, while iron-containing molecules such as haemoglobin and blood breakdown products have the highest. At the boundaries between these tissues, the slightly different magnetic fields within the tissues create micro-gradients which speed up the dephasing between protons on either side of the boundary. The phase change caused by susceptibility is given by

$$\Delta\phi = \gamma \cdot G_i . \Delta r \cdot TE$$

where G_i is the internal magnetic field gradient, Δr is the voxel size. This equation shows that susceptibility artefacts are worst with large voxels and at long TEs, and can be minimized by reducing TE or increasing the resolution. Often there is not just one simple boundary but many tiny boundaries on a microscopic level, for example in trabecular bone or the mastoid processes. Thus the T_2^* is reduced over a large area, giving the characteristic low signal of susceptibility artefacts.

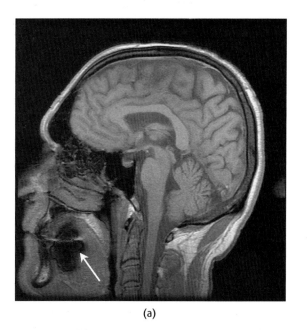

(a)

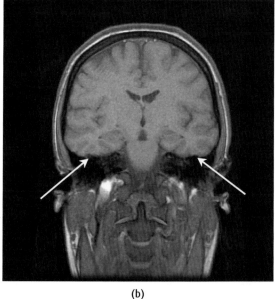

(b)

Figure 6.19 (a) Metal artefact from dental work on a spin-echo image. (b) Susceptibility artefact in the temporal lobes on a gradient-echo image.

Because they are caused by inhomogeneities, metal and susceptibility artefacts are generally worse on gradient-echo images (figure 6.19(b)) than spin-echo images, and they can be particularly marked on echo planar images. Spin-echo images may not show susceptibility artefacts at all. Susceptibility and metal artefacts can be minimized by using a very short echo time (provided T_1-weighted or PD-weighted contrast is required), but they cannot be completely avoided. If the images are severely degraded by metal artefacts, only spin-echo sequences should be used to acquire the data.

RF inhomogeneity effects

Larger metallic implants also cause distortion of the radiofrequency field generated by the transmit coil. The implants tend to preferentially absorb RF energy, and thus neighbouring tissues don't receive a proper flip angle. The signals will be reduced and the artefacts are very similar to those produced by the susceptibility inhomogeneities. In practice you cannot separate the effects of RF and static field inhomogeneities just by looking at the images. Both gradient-echo and spin-echo sequences are affected by the RF inhomogeneity problem, and there is no way to avoid it.

Another common artefact caused by RF inhomogeneity is known as 'Moiré' fringes or 'zebra stripes'. These effects are usually seen at the edges of large FOVs, especially where the patient's elbow or sides are very close to the transmitting body coil. Be aware that true-FISP-type sequences can also cause alternating stripes, because these scans are very sensitive to static field inhomogeneities, but these tend to be thicker stripes and are not necessarily at the edges of the FOV.

Metal artefacts also raise the question of safety for the patient, since the preferential absorption of RF can cause a local temperature rise. We don't provide a list of MR-compatible implants in this book, and there are other texts and web sites that can be consulted. Rather we hope to give you an understanding of the potential interactions between implants and the various fields used in imaging, which will help you to work out for yourself whether or not a particular implant is safe to scan. Chapters 2 and 10 include other aspects of safety advice.

6.9 Equipment artefacts

6.9.1 Zipper artefact

The so-called zipper artefact, due to RF breakthrough, is probably the most common equipment artefact. It appears as a line of alternating light and dark pixels, sometimes two or three pixels wide, extending across the image in the phase-encode direction (see figure 6.20(a)). Occasionally there will be multiple ghost zippers, regularly spaced across the image, but usually there is just one, most often in the centre of the FOV.

The cause of the zipper is external RF radiation finding its way into the magnet room and being picked up by the imaging coils. This may be due to a break in the RF screened room – the metal shield built into the walls, floor and ceiling of the scan room. In this case the artefact will be present on all images and the manufacturer's engineers should be called to investigate the problem.

A more common cause is anaesthetic monitoring equipment, especially if it relies on metallic leads or mains leads going through the waveguides into the scan room. The leads pick up RF waves from the environment and carry them through the Faraday cage, then transmit them into the room where they are picked up by the RF imaging coils. Even if there are no leads going through the waveguides, some pulse oximeters use radiofrequency noise-reduction processing, which may also be picked up by the imaging coils if the equipment has defective RF shielding. These problems can be particularly difficult to track down. Although it is more expensive, all monitoring equipment used should be the specially MRI-compatible type – it saves a lot of heartache over zipper artefacts!

More RF interference

Generally the zipper artefact is the result of external RF, which is not coherent with the phase-encode gradient and it thus appears across the whole image. In rare circumstances the RF may be coming from faults within the MR system, in which case it may be coherent. If this is the case, the artefact will be a very intense spot at the centre of the image. Another rare possibility is RF being carried on the mains electricity, which creates a 50 Hz modulation and a regularly spaced series of fairly faint zipper artefacts. Providing the anaesthetic and monitoring equipment has been eliminated as a possible cause, any of these problems needs investigation by the system engineers.

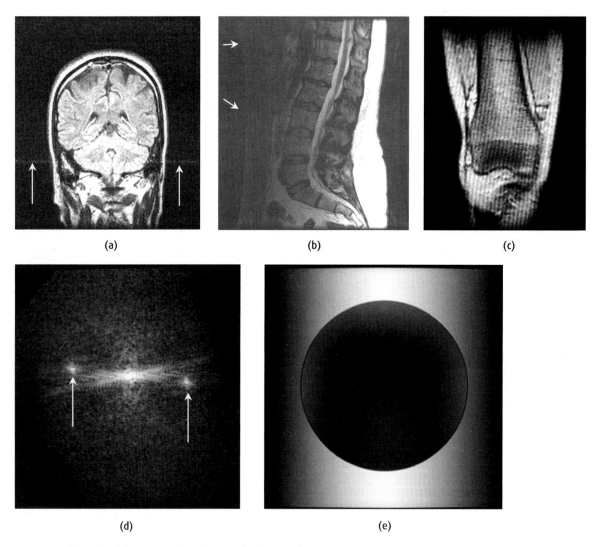

(a) (b) (c)

(d) (e)

Figure 6.20 (a) RF breakthrough artefact. (b) Curved edges on a large FOV after compensation for gradient inhomogeneities. (c) Corduroy or herring bone artefact is caused by (d) a noise spike in k-space. (e) Halo effect caused by overflow on the analogue-to-digital converters.

6.9.2 Gradient nonlinearities

The gradients only produce linear magnetic field gradients over a limited distance, and very large FOVs may include regions of gradient nonlinearity; for example, whole spine images. The effect of nonlinearities is to distort the image, tending to compress the image information at the edges of the FOV. Many systems apply a correction to the images to stretch out the pixels, and on rectangular FOV a curved edge can be seen (figure 6.20(b)). This is quite normal and also unavoidable; if necessary the area should be re-imaged using a smaller FOV.

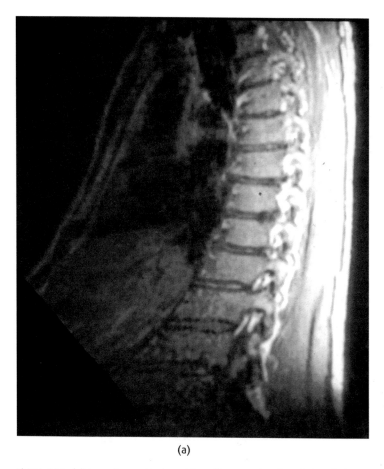

(a)

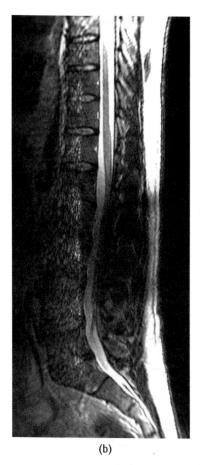

(b)

Figure 6.21 (a) Loss of a gradient or shim coil causes skewing of the whole image. (b) Shading caused by an RF coil fault.

6.9.3 Herring-bone artefact

The 'herring-bone' or 'corduroy' artefact is a regular series of high- and low-intensity stripes extending right across the image (figure 6.20(c)). The intensity variation, the angle and the spacing of the stripes are all variable, and it often appears on just one or two images in a multi-slice set. It is caused by spike noise in the raw data (figure 6.20(d)), whose Fourier transform (a series of spikes) is then convolved with all the image information. In theory the bad data points can be removed and the image reconstructed again, and this is indeed an option on some clinical scanners, but for many the only solution is to re-scan the image. A single image with a corduroy artefact is probably just bad luck, but problems

with several different scans is a symptom of breakdown of either the RF coils or the decoupling system. Multiple bad data points in a single image give more severe artefacts which can be easily confused with motion artefacts. This is a clear sign of trouble with the RF system.

6.9.4 Halo artefact

A halo effect can be produced if the receiver gains are incorrectly set (figure 6.20(e)). When this happens the signal is too large for the range of the digitizer and information in the centre of k-space is lost, known as data clipping. It is a rare artefact with modern automatic prescan systems, and is more likely to occur when receiver gains are manually set.

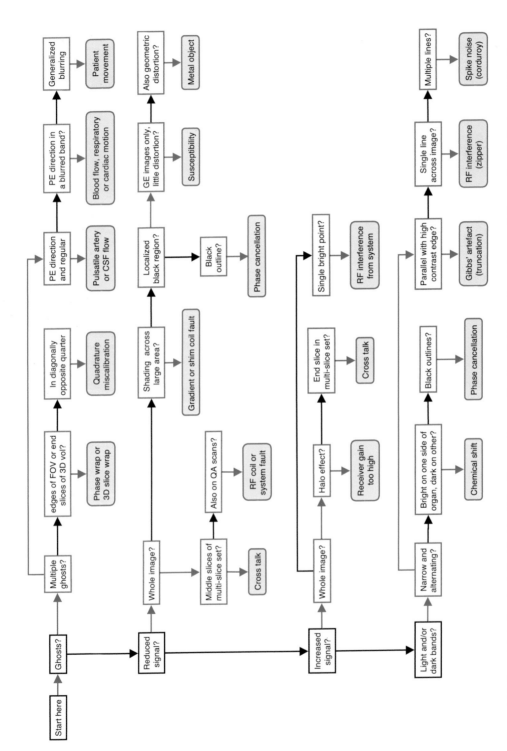

Figure 6.22 The artefacts flowchart. Start by identifying the symptoms on the degraded image, then ask yourself the questions in the boxes. Follow the blue arrows if the answer is "yes" and the black ones if it's "no". You should arrive at one of the blue boxes which will tell you the most likely cause of your artefact.

Artefacts due to equipment failure

In general equipment failures are becoming less and less common, although some systems may have persistent problems due to the vagaries of the manufacturing process. A skewing of the whole image can be caused by a malfunctioning gradient coil or amplifier, or more rarely by a failure of one of the shim coils (figure 6.21(a)). If it is one of the gradients, images in the three orthogonal directions can be used to identify the faulty direction. Discrete image ghosts in various quadrants are theoretically possible due to quadrature imbalance but are highly unlikely with digital RF systems. Reduced intensity or shading across the image can be caused by faults in the RF transmit or receiver coils (figure 6.21(b)), which could be mechanical breakage or electrical problems.

6.10 What's causing this artefact?

We hope this flow chart (figure 6.22) will help you to decide the most likely cause of your artefact, but we can't guarantee it! Bear in mind that serious system artefacts are rare and most problems are due to the patients, either by motion or metallic implants.

See also:

- Flow appearances and MR angiography: chapter 13
- Cardiac MRI: chapter 14
- Safety of metal implants: chapters 2 and 10
- Optimizing SNR and resolution: chapter 5
- Phase encoding: section 7.5.2

FURTHER READING

Haacke EM, Brown RW, Thompson MR and Venkatesan R (1999) *Magnetic Resonance Imaging: Physical Principles and Sequence Design.* London: Wiley-Liss (ISBN: 0471351288), Chapters 13, 17 & 23.

Mitchell DG (1999) *MRI Principles.* London: WB Saunders Co. (ISBN: 0721667597), Chapter 19.

Woodward P (ed.) (2000) *MRI for Technologists*, 2nd edn. New York: McGraw-Hill Professional Publishing (ISBN: 0071353186), Chapter 14.

MR Technology Information Portal, artefacts section: http://www.mr-tip.com/serv1.php?type=art [accessed 5th January 2005]

MR Tutor web site: http://www.mritutor.org/mritutor/artifact.htm [accessed 5th January 2005]

Spaced out: spatial encoding

7.1 Introduction

By now you are probably a regular user of the MR scanner and are familiar with the appearance of images, in terms of brightness or contrast (as seen in chapter 3) and with the digital nature of the image, as pixels or voxels (chapters 4 and 5). In this chapter we will examine how the scanner produces these voxels from MR signals.

An understanding of the image-formation process is particularly helpful for obtaining the optimum diagnostic information from an examination, modifying or creating new protocols, recognizing common image artefacts and taking measures to overcome or avoid them. It will also help as a basis for understanding the diverse data-acquisition strategies examined in chapter 12. It should be stressed here that understanding image formation in MRI is neither simple nor obvious and most people struggle to conceptualize it. There are a number of ways of understanding this and what matters is that you find a way that makes sense to you. Persistent students also find that eventually the penny always drops, a light bulb inside their brain suddenly switches on and usually, like the current in a superconducting magnet, it stays on forever.

In this chapter you will see that:

- magnetic field gradients form the basis of MR signal localization;
- 2D slices are produced by the combination of an excitation RF pulse and simultaneous slice-select gradient;
- the in-plane MR signal is encoded in terms of the spatial frequencies of the object using phase-encoding and frequency-encoding gradients;

- we collect or sample every spatial frequency that can exist within the image before we Fourier transform these data (known as 'k-space') to produce the image directly;
- inadequate or erroneous k-space sampling leads to certain image artefacts.

7.2 Anatomy of a pulse sequence

You will have noticed by now that some scans, particularly spin echo, may take a long time to acquire, that the progress of the scan involves a loud banging sound from the MR system and that sometimes (if not many slices are required) there is more silence than banging. Each sound is produced by *gradient* pulses applied to interrogate every possible spatial frequency that may contribute to the image. In MR the static magnetic field B_0 ('B-nought') is constantly present. The gradients are not. They are applied in a controlled fashion to form an MR *pulse sequence*. MR pulse sequences do a number of things; however, in this chapter we will only consider a basic gradient-echo pulse sequence from the point of view of how it manages to localize the MR signal. An MR *pulse sequence diagram* is a simple means of showing how the RF and gradients are applied. The vertical axis represents amplitude and the horizontal axis is time. Figure 7.1 shows a basic gradient-echo MR imaging sequence. For the present we will only say what each bit *does*.

First (top line) an RF pulse is applied simultaneously with a slice-selective gradient G_{SS} (line 2). The RF pulse stimulates the MR interactions in tissue which

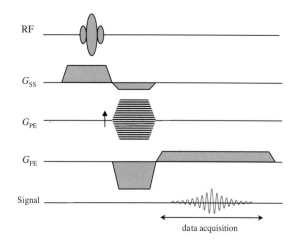

RF

G_{SS}

G_{PE}

G_{FE}

Signal

← data acquisition →

Figure 7.1 Basic gradient-echo MR imaging sequence. Amplitude is shown vertically, time horizontally. G_{SS} is the slice-selective gradient, G_{PE} the phase-encoding gradient and G_{FE} the frequency-encoding gradient.

lead to the MR signal. By combining the RF excitation with a gradient the MR interactions are restricted to a two-dimensional plane, slab or slice. Any physical gradient G_x, G_y or G_z or combinations of these can be used for this purpose, allowing us to produce transverse, sagittal or coronal, oblique or double oblique slices.

Next, in line 3, *phase encoding* is applied in a direction orthogonal to the slice selection. This encodes the MR signal in the phase-encode direction. In line 4, the *frequency-encode* or readout gradient is applied in the third direction and finally line 5 shows the time when the MR signal is measured or *acquired*. Note that this is during the frequency-encode gradient but after the phase encoding. The whole sequence pattern has to be repeated for every 'line' of data, corresponding to a different value of phase-encode gradient until the data or *k-space* matrix is filled. A time period, TR, occurs between the application of one RF excitation and the next.

The total scan time is

Scan time $= \text{NSA} \times N_{PE} \times \text{TR}$

where NSA is the number of signal averages and N_{PE} the size of the phase-encoding matrix.

Once all the data are acquired a two-dimensional Fourier transform is applied. This converts the data, already encoded as spatial frequencies, into an image. Reconstruction in MRI is generally simpler than in X-ray CT; most of the hard work has been done during the acquisition by the gradients.

Although this is the simplest possible MR imaging sequence, once you have grasped the purpose of each element, it is relatively easy to make the jump to more complicated sequences as they all have the same basic elements. We will describe three of the steps towards localization, slice selection, phase encoding and frequency encoding, in some detail. First, however, it is important to make sure you understand some underpinning principles.

7.3 From Larmor to Fourier via gradients

The basic groundwork for this chapter is a knowledge of the Larmor equation to describe the behaviour of excited nuclei ('spins'), an understanding of the effect of magnetic field gradients and familiarity with the concept of spatial frequencies. Mathematical skills that would be useful include an understanding of sine waves and an awareness of Fourier transforms (see Appendix). If you already know about sine waves you can skip to section 7.3.1.

A purely sinusoidal signal or waveform has three basic properties: amplitude, frequency and phase. Amplitude describes how large the signal is, measured in volts or arbitrary 'signal units'. Frequency, measured in hertz (Hz), describes how rapidly in time the instantaneous magnitude of the wave is changing: 1 Hz equals one cycle or rotation per second. Phase describes the instantaneous position within the cyclic variation in terms of an angle. It is measured in degrees or radians, and can vary from 0° to 360° (0–2π radians), thereafter repeating itself. It is sometimes helpful to think of a phase as the angle displayed on a 'clockface'.

7.3.1 Larmor equation

Sir Joseph Larmor was an Irish physicist who died 4 years before the discovery of NMR but who nevertheless predicted the relationship between the *precession* frequency of spins and the magnetic field strength (he also has a crater named after him on the Moon). In a simple picture we can think of the spins as rotating at the *Larmor* or *resonance frequency* which is also the frequency of the MR signal given approximately by the equation

Frequency $\approx 42 \times$ magnetic field

where frequency is in megahertz (MHz) and magnetic field is in tesla (T). The good news is that this is the *only* equation you need to know to understand spatial localization, although you do need to develop a thorough understanding of its consequences. The number 42 is called the gyro-magnetic ratio (which has the symbol γ, pronounced 'gamma') and is a property of the nucleus in question. Its value more exactly is 42.56 MHz T^{-1} for hydrogen (water or fat protons). Other nuclei (e.g. phosphorus) have a different value of gamma, as described in chapter 15.

So, if the magnetic field strength of the MR magnet is 1.5 T, the MR signal obtained has a frequency of

$1.5\,T \times 42\,MHz\,T^{-1} = 63\,MHz$.

Similarly at 0.5 T the Larmor frequency becomes 21 MHz. An RF pulse applied at 63 MHz in a 1.5-T MR

Where's the bar?

Conventionally, the Larmor equation is written as

$\omega_0 = \gamma B_0$

where ω_0 is the angular frequency of the protons ($\omega = 2\pi f$). Using this scheme gives γ a value of 2.67×10^8 radians s^{-1} T^{-1}. We find this number unmemorable and angular frequencies are not as intuitively understandable as regular (scalar) frequencies. When the use of scalar frequency is helpful or important for understanding, we will use the symbol $\bar{\gamma}$ ('gamma bar'), which is equal to $\gamma/2\pi$ (i.e. 42 MHz T^{-1}). The use of gamma and gamma bar only affects the material in the advanced boxes.

---

system will result in MR signals of a periodic (sinusoidal) nature also at 63 MHz. These can be detected by a coil and receiver tuned, in the same manner as a transistor radio, to this frequency. The proportionality of field and frequency underlies all of the image-formation process.

This signal alone is insufficient to produce an image of a patient lying within the magnet bore because we would have no way of assigning parts of the signal to where in the patient they originated. To achieve this localization we now need to introduce the concept of magnetic field gradients, or in short 'gradients'.

7.3.2 Gradients

In MRI the term 'gradient' refers to an additional spatially linear variation in the static field strength in the z direction, i.e. along B_0. For example an 'x gradient' (G_x) will add to or subtract from the magnitude of the static field at different points along the x axis or x direction. Figure 7.2 shows representations of the main field (a) and the field plus an x gradient (b) with the total field represented by the spacing of the 'field lines'. Gradient field strength is measured in millitesla per metre (mT m^{-1}).

In figure 7.2(a) all the protons (spins) experience the same field and have the same frequency. When a gradient is added (b) the magnetic field produced by the gradient adds to the main field B_0. At the centre ($x = 0$) the total field experienced by the nuclei is simply B_0, so these spins resonate at the Larmor frequency. As we move along the x direction, however, the total either increases or decreases linearly and thus these protons resonate faster or slower depending upon their position. Faster or slower precession is detected as higher or lower frequencies in the MR signal, and so frequency measurements may be used to distinguish between MR signals at different positions in space. Gradients can be applied in any direction or orientation. Three sets of gradient coils, G_x, G_y and G_z, are included in the MR system. They are normally applied only for a short time as pulses. It is these three sets of gradients that give MR its three dimensional capability.

The effect of gradients

Mathematically the three orthogonal spatial gradients of B_z are defined as

$$G_x = \frac{\partial B_z}{\partial x} \qquad G_y = \frac{\partial B_z}{\partial y} \qquad G_z = \frac{\partial B_z}{\partial z}$$

When a gradient (e.g. G_x) is applied the total field in the z direction experienced by nuclei will be dependent upon the position in space, e.g.

$$B(x) = B_0 + x \cdot G_x$$

When a gradient is applied the Larmor frequency will depend upon the total z component of the magnetic field and thus becomes spatially dependent, e.g. for the x gradient.

$$f(x) = \gamma (B_0 + x \cdot G_x)$$

where we are using $\gamma \approx 42 \, \text{MHz} \, \text{T}^{-1}$.

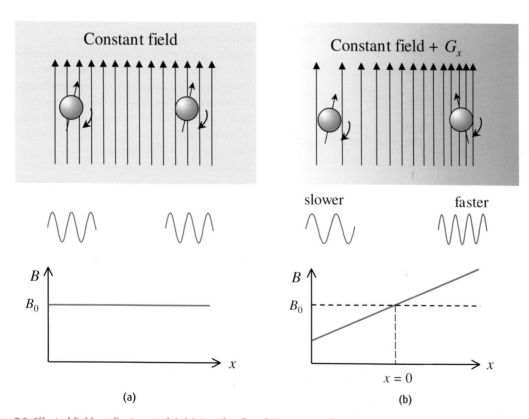

Figure 7.2 Effect of field gradient on nuclei. (a) B_0 only, all nuclei precess at the same frequency. (b) B_0 plus gradient G_x – precession frequency now depends upon position.

7.3.3 Dephasing and rephasing

If we have a uniform distribution of water producing an MR signal and we apply a gradient G for a given time, what will happen to the MR signal? There will be variations in frequency of the MR signal, either faster or slower, depending upon position as in figure 7.2. The spins which are precessing faster, because of the action of a gradient, appear to move apart or dephase (see figure 7.3), and those which are precessing slower dephase in the opposite direction. The combined effect is often thought of as a 'fanning out' due to dephasing. The speed at which this happens depends upon the gradient amplitude or strength. The total angle of dephasing depends upon the product of the gradient strength and its duration, also known as the gradient moment.

If we now apply another gradient with a reversed sign or polarity (i.e. negative amplitude) as shown in figure 7.4, the signals which sped up before now will start to precess slower and the ones which had travelled with a

---

Gradient dephasing

In the rotating frame (see 'My head's in a spin!') we can view the action of the gradient as a dephasing of components of transverse magnetization in the xy plane. The phase change at any time and place is

$$\phi(x,t) = \exp(i\gamma \cdot x G_x \cdot t)$$

and it evolves for as long as the gradient is applied. Once the gradient is switched off, the accumulated phase changes remain encoded until the transverse magnetization decays to zero or further gradients are applied. A gradient echo results from the application of gradient of equal moment but with the opposite polarity. The echo time TE occurs for

$$\int_0^{TE} G^-(t)\,dt = -\int_0^{TE} G^+(t)\,dt$$

where the plus and minus signs refer to the positive and negative lobes of the gradient waveform. Signal loss due to main B_0 field inhomogeneity is not restored. The MR signal decays exponentially with time constant T_2^*.

My head's in a spin!

What's the rotating frame? It's a set of x-y-z axes that rotates around the z axis at the Larmor frequency. In this frame of reference, a proton at exactly the Larmor frequency is static, which makes all the maths a bit more straightforward. We're not going to say any more than that for now, because it's easy to get confused. Once you have come to the end of this chapter and read the next ('Getting in tune: resonance and relaxation'), you will realize that all along in this chapter we have been subversively operating in the 'rotating frame of reference'. You don't need to worry about this at all; in MR we tend to naturally adopt this frame of reference, after all we live on one! The rotating frame is fully explained in the box 'The rotating frame of reference' in chapter 8.

---

slower rotation will now speed up. The spins will start to rephase until, when the gradient moments are equal, the components of the MR signal will all be pointing in the same, original direction. At this point in time we get a measurable MR signal, known as a gradient echo. Each gradient pulse is known as a lobe and is described as dephasing if it occurs first, or as rephasing if it corrects for an earlier dephasing.

7.3.4 Fourier transforms

Joseph Fourier was a French mathematician who enjoyed a colourful life spanning science, politics and high society during the time of the Emperor Napoleon Bonaparte. His lasting achievement was the invention of the Fourier transform, a concept which met with much resistance from the scientific establishment of his time, but one which entirely underpins the theory of MR imaging. Fourier's great idea was that any signal or waveform in time could be split up into a series of 'Fourier components' each at a different frequency. For example, the sound of a musical instrument could be described either by the actual pressure waveforms it produced in the time domain, or by the appropriate magnitude of its constituent frequencies or its spectrum in the frequency domain. An acoustic signal, such as

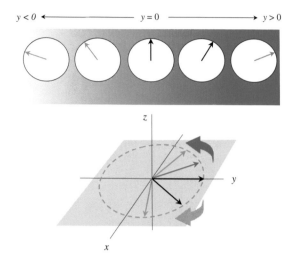

Figure 7.3 Effect of gradient on MR signal (transverse magnetization). Signal originating from different positions along the y-gradient axis will have a position dependent phase change. These are shown as clock-face diagrams in the upper part of the figure. It is usual in the MRI literature to "collapse" or superimpose these all on the same xyz axes as in the lower portion.

that produced by a musical instrument, is an example of a one dimensional waveform and when Fourier transformed gives a one-dimensional spectrum. In MR we use two or three-dimensional Fourier transforms. Variables which relate to each other in their respective domains are called Fourier transform pairs. Examples are shown in figure 7.5. One of the key features of the Fourier transform is that 'less is more': if a shape is small in one domain, its transform will be large in the other.

7.4 Something to get excited about: the image slice

Slice selection or selective excitation is the process whereby MR signals are restricted to a two-dimensional plane or slab within the patient. The position, width and orientation of the slice can all be controlled by the operator.

7.4.1 Selective excitation

In selective excitation we apply a specially designed RF excitation pulse at the same time as a gradient (the

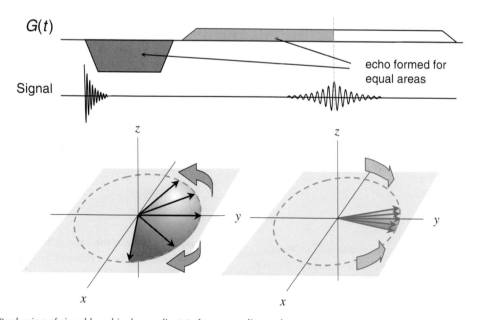

Figure 7.4 Rephasing of signal by a bipolar gradient to form a gradient echo.

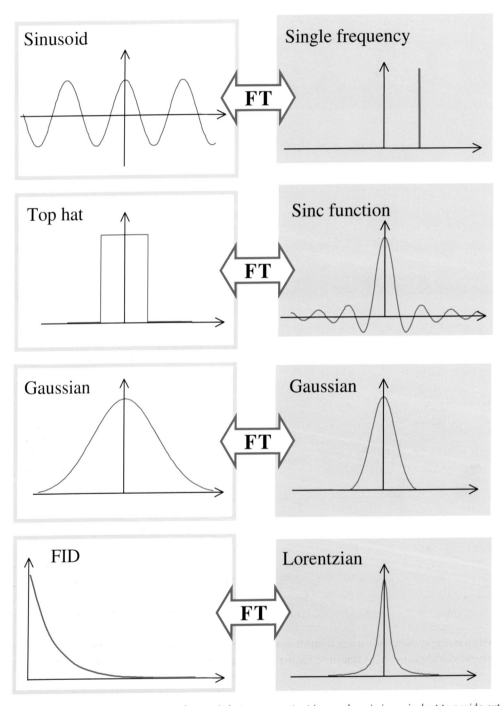

Figure 7.5 Spectra and waveforms (Fourier transform pairs). A narrow extent in one domain is equivalent to a wide extent in the other. FID stands for free induction decay.

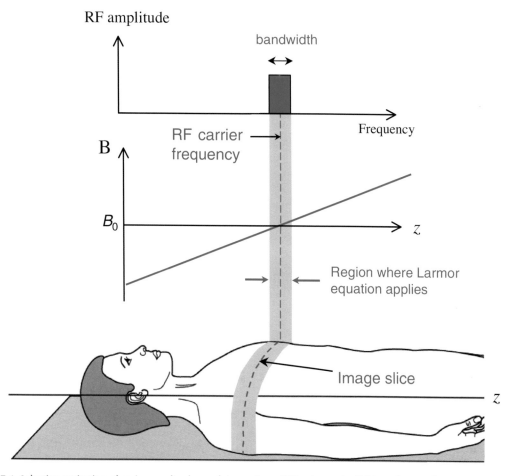

Figure 7.6 Selective excitation of an image slice by applying a shaped RF pulse and a field gradient at the same time.

slice-selective gradient) as shown in the top two lines of the pulse sequence diagram in figure 7.1. The designer RF pulse contains a narrow range of frequencies of RF, centred about the Larmor frequency. In technical terms we say it has a 'narrow bandwidth'. (Note that this is different from the receive bandwidth: the transmit bandwidth is not operator-controlled.) In contrast, an RF pulse which is simply switched on and then off again has a wide bandwidth because it is a sinc function in the frequency domain (see figure 7.5).

The principle of slice selection is illustrated in figure 7.6. The presence of the gradient causes the resonant frequency (required for producing MR signals) to vary with position in the gradient direction. At the isocentre where the effect of the gradient is zero, the normal Larmor frequency will apply. Further away along the selection axis, either a higher or lower RF frequency will be needed. If the required frequency is present within the RF pulse's transmit bandwidth then resonance will happen, i.e. protons will be excited. Thus excitation will only take place at or close to the isocentre. At more extreme points along the gradient axis the frequency required for resonance will not be present within the RF pulse bandwidth; in this case resonance does not happen and no MR signal is produced. If the slice-select gradient is applied along the z axis, the resultant slab of excited nuclei or slice will form a transverse plane. Further along the z axis the additional gradient will have added sufficient field to not fulfil the resonance condition and thus no signal will be produced from these regions.

In the advanced box 'Slice selection maths' (which is for those who wish to know more about the maths), we show that the shape of the physical slice is related to the shape of the spectrum of the RF pulse. We could use figure 7.5 to give an indication of the distribution of flip angle in the slice-select direction (the slice profile) for various RF waveforms. Commonly a version of a 'sinc' or 'sin$x$/x' pulse (an apodized or truncated sinc) is used for the RF, which gives an approximately rectangular slice profile.

7.4.2 What's your orientation? Manipulating the slice

All features of the slice can be manipulated by adjusting the gradient or RF waveform properties, i.e. electronically, rather than having to move the patient as required in X-ray CT. These include position, orientation and thickness. The box 'Slice selection maths' contains a more mathematical description of these features.

First, the position of the slice can be varied simply by changing the basic (or carrier) frequency of the RF pulse but using the same gradient strength. The region which now fulfils the MR resonant condition will have moved. Second, the thickness of the slice can be controlled by

---

Slice selection maths

For a selective pulse the magnetic field gradient introduces a position-dependent spread Δf in the Larmor frequency about the carrier frequency f_0 such that

$$\Delta f(z) = \gamma z G_z$$

using the z gradient for excitation (to produce a transverse slice). Let us apply an amplitude-modulated RF 90° pulse with a form

$$B_1(t) = A(t)\cos(2\pi f_0 t)$$

where A is the pulse envelope or shape and f_0 is the 'carrier' frequency. Applying a result which will be derived in section 8.3 the resultant flip angle will be (approximately)

$$\alpha(z) = \gamma \int A(t) \cdot \exp(i\gamma z G_z \cdot t)\mathrm{d}t$$

$$= \gamma \int A(t) \cdot \exp(i2\pi \cdot \Delta f t)\mathrm{d}t$$

The integral is the Fourier transform of $A(t)$, i.e. $\alpha(z) = \gamma A(f)$. So the shape of the RF pulse's spectrum determines the shape of the slice with regard to the selection direction (in this case z).

The position of the slice is given by

$$z = \frac{f_1 - f_0}{\gamma G_z}$$

where f_1 is the shifted carrier frequency. Thus for a slice shift of 100 mm, using a 5 mT m^{-1} gradient an RF carrier frequency shift of about 20 kHz is required. The slice width or thickness is given by

$$\text{slice width} = \frac{\text{RF bandwidth}}{\gamma G_z}$$

So for a 5-mm thickness with a 5 mT m^{-1} gradient the RF bandwidth needs to be approximately 1 kHz. This implies an RF pulse duration of the order of 1 ms.

An oblique view

Oblique slices may be obtained by driving two orthogonal gradients in proportion to the sine and cosine of the angle required, e.g. to obtain a transverse slice rotated through an angle ϕ from the x axis requires the simultaneous application of

$$G_x = G_{SS} \cos \phi \qquad G_y = G_{SS} \sin \phi$$

whilst the generation of a double oblique angulation of ϕ from x and θ from z requires the application of

$$G_x = G \sin \theta \cos \phi, \quad G_y = G \sin \theta \sin \phi, \quad G_z = G \cos \theta$$

changing either the shape of the designer RF pulse (changing its bandwidth) or the strength of the gradient. A stronger gradient will result in a thinner slice (figure 7.7(a)). Alternatively we can use a narrower RF pulse bandwidth. According to Fourier theory, this means using a longer duration RF pulse. Notice the 'less is more' principle again: you can have a thinner slice but it will take longer to excite (figure 7.7(b)).

Third, the orientation of the slice can be varied by using a physically different gradient axis. The selected slice is always orthogonal (perpendicular) to the gradient applied. So far we have assumed the application of G_{SS} in the z axis, along the patient, giving a transaxial or transverse slice. If we use G_x as a slice-select gradient we get a sagittal slice. For a coronal slice we use G_y (as was shown in figure 4.8). Oblique and double oblique slices can be created using combinations of G_x, G_y and G_z.

7.4.3 Multiple slices

It doesn't take very long to excite a slice and collect its echo, typically much less than the TR needed to control the image contrast. We can use the 'dead time' within the TR period to acquire multiple interleaved slices (see section 4.6). By applying a slice-select gradient and changing the central frequency of the RF pulse we can move the position of the slice (figure 7.8). This is the standard means of image acquisition. A multi-slice interleaving scheme is shown in figure 7.9. It is possible to acquire the slices in any order. Normally an 'interleaved' slice order is used, e.g. for an eight-slice sequence acquiring the following positions in this order: 1, 3, 5, 7, 2, 4, 6, 8 (see section 4.6).

7.4.4 Rephasing

In figure 7.1 you will have noticed a negative portion of the slice-select gradient. This is necessary to rephase the MR signal in order to get the maximum possible amount. Whilst the selective excitation process is occurring, the signal being generated is also being dephased by the gradient. We normally consider the action of the RF pulse to occur at its centre in time. In this case, a rephasing gradient moment of half the slice-selection gradient is required to leave all the spins in phase throughout the slice.

7.5 In-plane localization

In MRI we use the gradients to measure the two- (or three-) dimensional spectrum of the object being imaged. This spectrum is what we call k-space and consists of an array or matrix of individual spatial frequencies.

7.5.1 Spatial frequencies demystified

The concept of spatial frequencies is not just a theoretical abstraction dreamt up to torment students of MRI. In real life the brain makes use of spatial frequencies to

Spatial saturation slabs

The concept of spatial saturation was introduced in section 6.4.3 to help to remove signals from flowing blood. More generally 'sat bands' can be used to selectively remove any area of signal which would otherwise cause artefacts. A saturation band or slab is created in exactly the same manner as the image slice, except that it is followed by very large dephasing gradients ('spoilers') to ensure it contributes no signal. The spatial saturation pulses will be applied for each TR period, prior to slice selection.

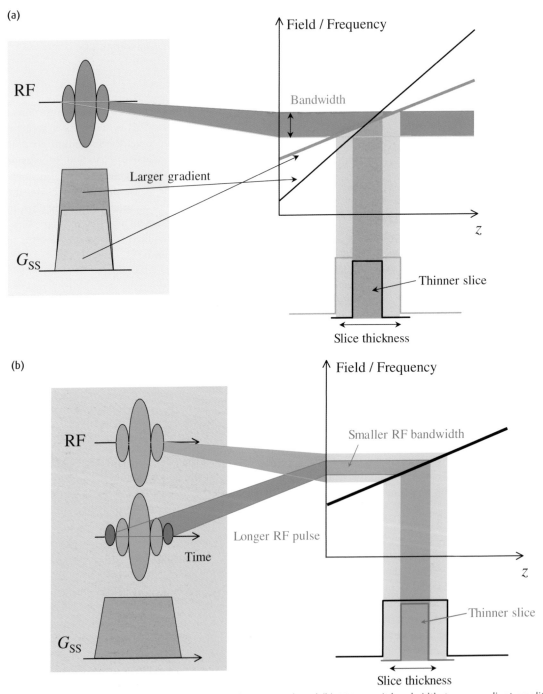

Figure 7.7 Dependence of slice thickness on (a) gradient strength and (b) RF transmit bandwidth. Larger gradient amplitude and longer RF pulses both result in thinner slices.

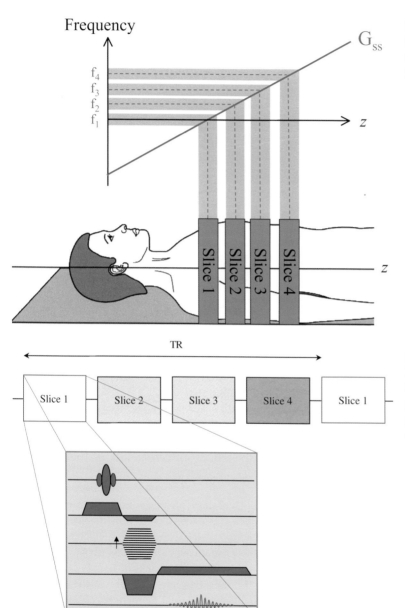

Frequency

G_{ss}

f_4
f_3
f_2
f_1

z

Slice 1
Slice 2
Slice 3
Slice 4

z

Figure 7.8 By changing the RF centre frequency multiple slices may be acquired at different locations quite independently of each other.

TR

Slice 1 Slice 2 Slice 3 Slice 4 Slice 1

Figure 7.9 Multi-slice sequence. Different slices can be selected and lines of data acquired within each TR period. The expanded section is repeated for each slice position using a different RF carrier frequency.

construct the visual images that you see. Spatial frequencies may be hard to conceptualize but they are very natural and we'd all be in the dark without them!

One of the easiest ways of understanding spatial frequencies is to think of a line pair test object, such as those used for testing X-ray imaging systems. These consist of alternate light and dark bands or *line-pairs* of differing spacings. Suppose we have five line-pairs per centimetre. This means that five dark-light patterns are contained within a centimetre. The pattern of image brightness produced by this line-pair pattern is like a spatial frequency. In MR a spatial frequency is a

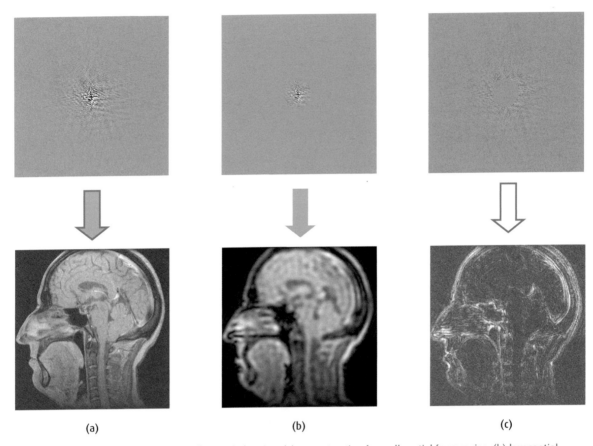

Figure 7.10 Images and their 2D spectra (k-space) showing: (a) reconstruction from all spatial frequencies, (b) low spatial frequencies, i.e. the centre of k-space only and (c) high spatial frequencies, i.e. the edges of k-space only.

periodic variation in signal spatial distribution or image brightness, measured not as line-pairs per centimetre but as 'cycles per centimetre' (which are very similar).

Applying the theory of Fourier, any image (not just MRI) may be decomposed into a spectrum of periodic (sinusoidal) brightness variations or spatial frequencies. In a digital image with a matrix of 256×256 pixels there are 256×256 possible spatial frequencies, allowing for positive and negative values. If we know the spatial frequencies we can calculate an image of the object that formed them. The purpose of MR localization by gradients is to manipulate the MR signal so that it gives all the spatial frequencies necessary to form an image. Each point of data or k-space is a spatial frequency component.

Figure 7.10 shows an image and its constituent spatial frequencies (k-space). If we remove the high spatial frequencies we are left with an image which has the right brightness but no detail. Removing the low spatial frequencies leaves the image with details of edges and sharp features but low intensity elsewhere. So big objects have low spatial frequencies. Small objects or sharp edges have high spatial frequencies.

7.5.2 Totally fazed: phase encoding

Most people find phase encoding the hardest part of MR image formation to understand, but gaining a conceptual grasp of it will pay dividends in terms of your overall understanding. Consider the following in

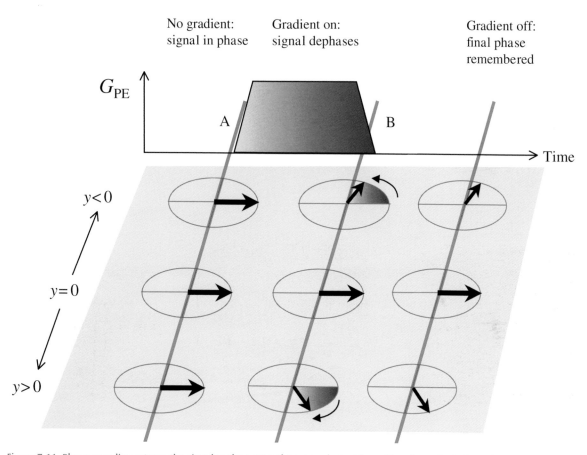

No gradient:
signal in phase

Gradient on:
signal dephases

Gradient off:
final phase
remembered

G_{PE}

A

B

Time

$y<0$

$y=0$

$y>0$

Figure 7.11 Phase encoding returns the signal to the Larmor frequency but with position-dependent phase changes.

conjunction with figure 7.11, which shows the effect of the phase-encoding gradient on the transverse magnetization at three different locations and times.

Suppose we already have an MR signal with all the spins in phase. If we apply the phase-encode gradient (G_{PE}) at time A in the y direction, then the precession of the nuclei will speed up or slow down according to their position along the y axis. As we saw in section 7.3.3 this causes the spins to dephase or fan out to a progressively greater degree for as long as the gradient is applied. When we switch off the gradient at time B, all the nuclei will revert to their original frequency or speed, but will keep their different phase angles. They are said to be phase encoded. The relative phase differences between

signals in different locations remain until either another gradient is applied or the MR signal decays due to T_2 relaxation.

Figure 7.12 shows the phase encoding generated by three different gradient amplitudes on a column of protons in the phase-encode axis. We see that without any applied gradient, the spins are all in phase and a large signal is obtained, but that the dephasing or twisting of the spins increases with gradient strength until the dephasing is large enough for all the spins to cancel each other out and no signal is obtained.

How is this measuring spatial frequencies? Referring to figure 7.13, suppose we have a uniform distribution of protons and we apply a sufficient phase-encode

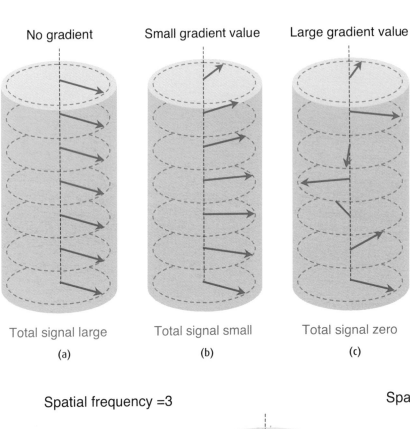

No gradient   Small gradient value   Large gradient value

Total signal large   Total signal small   Total signal zero

(a)   (b)   (c)

Figure 7.12 Effect of three different strengths of phase encoding on a uniform distribution of signal-producing material. The MR signal detected is given by the sum of all the vectors. (a) No gradient, (b) small gradient, (c) large gradient.

Spatial frequency =3   Spatial frequency = 0

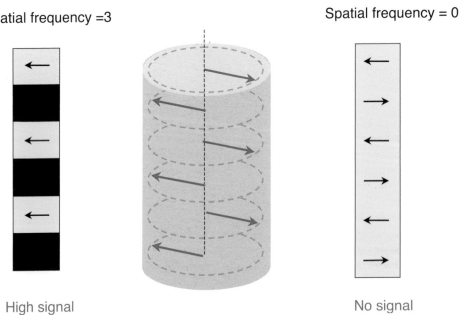

High signal   No signal

Figure 7.13 Picking out a single spatial frequency for a given phase-encode gradient amplitude. Black represents an area which produces no signal (i.e. with zero proton density).

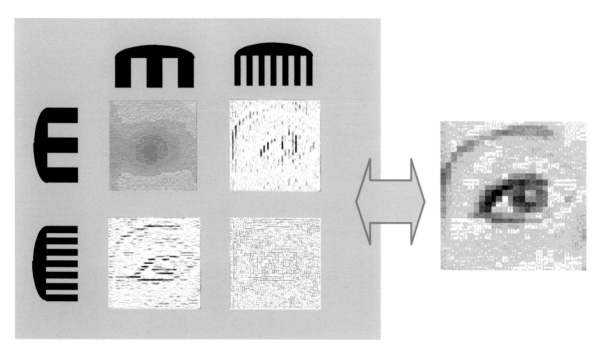

Figure 7.14 The "MR eye": picking out spatial frequencies in two dimensions by applying spatial frequency "combs" or filters. The thumbnails show the parts of the overall image selected by each comb. Like understanding MRI, the eye is not always obvious at first.

gradient to cause the phase of the spins to vary by $3 \times 360°$ (6π radians). When we add up the MR signal from this column we get zero as the spins are evenly distributed throughout each direction. We can say that this object contains no information at the spatial frequency of three cycles per unit length.

Consider now a line-pair object with alternating sections containing protons or nothing with a spatial frequency of three cycles per unit length. Obviously only the sections containing protons can contribute to the signal. In this instance due to their distribution in space they are in phase and thus add up to give a net positive signal. That is to say, this particular value of phase-encode gradient is sensitive to objects containing the spatial frequency three cycles per unit length, but not to others.

In general, however, an object (i.e. the patient) will have a range of spatial frequencies. Each value of phase encoding can be considered as a template or a comb (technically, a filter) that only responds to one spatial distribution of MR signal or spatial frequency. To build up a whole picture, the entire range of possible spatial frequencies has to be interrogated in this way as illustrated in figure 7.14. When no gradients are applied, we get a signal from the whole object, and this is referred to as the zero spatial frequency or zero k.

So the MR sequence consists of multiple repetitions of the excitation process followed by a different phase-encode gradient until all possible spatial frequencies are interrogated. Once all these signals are collected the application of a Fourier transform converts the spatial frequency distribution into a spatial distribution of the excited nuclei, i.e. an image of the patient. In pulse sequence diagrams the phase-encode steps are represented by a series of parallel lines as shown in figure 7.1.

7.5.3 Frequency encoding

There is no reason why this phase-encode process should not be re-applied to obtain the full image in the

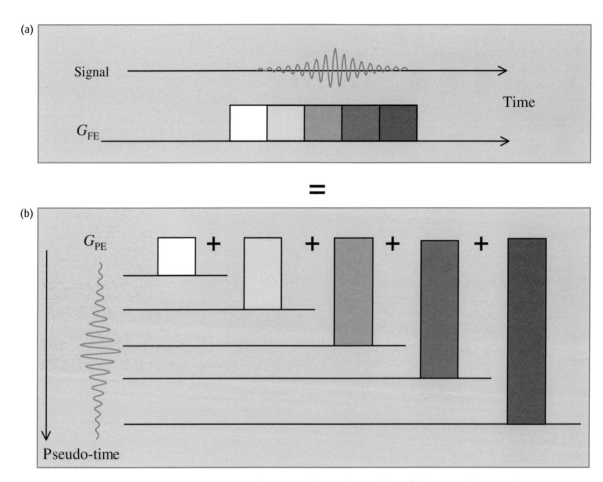

Figure 7.15 Equivalence of frequency encode acquired continuously in real time (a), and phase encode acquired step-wise in "pseudo-time" (b).

other directions. The only practical difficulty is that for every value of G_{PE} (or spatial frequency in the PE direction, k_{PE}) we have to collect ALL the values of k_{FE} (apply all the G_{FE} gradient steps). This would take a long time, but it is possible, and three-dimensional imaging or three-dimensional Fourier transform (3D FT) does something similar. Fortunately there is a quicker, more convenient and conceptually simpler method of encoding the second in-plane direction: *frequency encoding*.

In frequency encoding we can acquire all the spatial frequency information needed from one MR signal following one RF excitation. In phase encoding we

required one MR excitation (RF pulse) for every line of data (i.e. every value of k_{PE}). For a 256-pixel image we thus required 256 MR excitations, and this will take 256 $\times$ TR ms. Figure 7.15 shows a gradient being applied for a certain time, giving a certain gradient moment and phase change, after which, the signal strength is measured. The next data point is measured after a different gradient step (and gradient moment and phase change). We then have data points corresponding to the strength of the MR signal after a whole range of gradient moments.

Suppose however that we apply a gradient continuously and measure or sample the MR signal at different

Frequency encoding: an alternative story

Another way of understanding this process is to consider the effect of this gradient on the frequency of the MR signal. This is the more conventional treatment covered in other texts and is illustrated in figure 7.17.

Because the frequency-encode gradient is present at the same time as the MR signal is being measured, the signal's frequency will now depend upon the position of the material from which it originated within the gradient field. It will not be a single sinusoid wave but a mixture of many frequency components. We then have a signal which is frequency encoded. It is easy to determine the frequency components; we simply perform another Fourier transform. Applied in one dimension this produces a spectrum which represents a one-dimensional projection of the object.

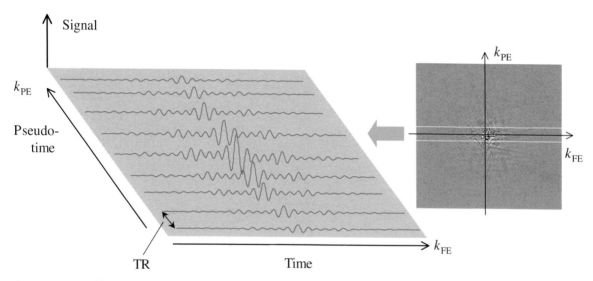

Figure 7.16 Central lines of k-space (magnified) showing the equivalence of phase and frequency axes. Signal strength is shown in the vertical direction in the magnified portion and as a greyscale in the thumbnail. Each PE line is separated by time TR.

time points during the application of that gradient. At each point, the MR signal is affected by a different amount of gradient moment and has a different amount of phase change. Each data point therefore reflects a different amount of 'phase encoding' and thus corresponds to a different spatial frequency. We can therefore collect all the spatial frequencies for that direction from the evolving MR signal in real time following a single RF excitation. This is analogous to the phase-encode acquisition which works in 'pseudotime', with a sampling separated by TR, as shown in figure 7.16. The resulting raw data matrix is sometimes referred to as k-space.

So if we can do frequency encoding all at once, why waste all that time with multiple excitations and phase

encoding? The answer is that frequency is a scalar parameter, i.e. it is described by a single number. If we applied frequency-encoding gradients in two directions at the same time we would have no way of knowing whether a particular frequency in the signal originated from one or the other (or both) of the applied gradients. By combining phase encoding and frequency encoding in two orthogonal directions we can collect all the spatial frequencies unambiguously that we need to make the image.

7.5.4 Spatial encoding: a musical analogy

You can think of MRI in-plane localization in terms of playing a multi-stringed musical instrument such as a

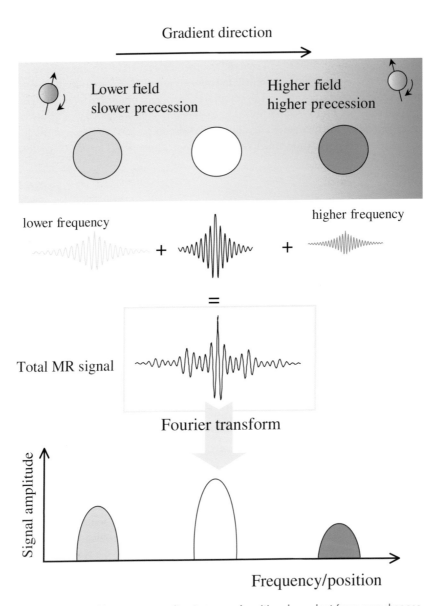

Figure 7.17 Alternative description of frequency encoding in terms of position-dependent frequency changes.

guitar. Suppose you wish to play every possible note (or frequency) distinctly, you first have to pluck a string. This is like the RF excitation. The sound it makes is like the MR signal. It is then relatively easy to play every note available on that string by running a finger up the fretboard. As one does this the length of the string is in effect shortened (this is like a gradient) and the pitch of the note (or frequency) changes. All the while the sound can be heard. This is like frequency encoding.

However, there are other strings. To hear them we have to pluck one of them (perform another RF excitation)

Imaginary

Real

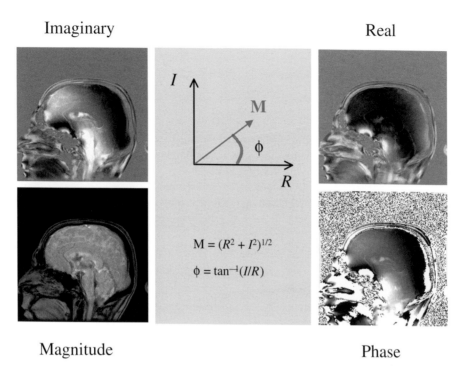

Magnitude

Phase

Figure 7.18 Reconstruction of a magnitude (M) image from real and imaginary parts following Fourier transformation. A phase (ϕ) image can also be calculated.

and repeat the pitch changing action. The action of changing to a different string is analogous to the operation of phase encoding in MRI.

7.5.5 2D FT reconstruction

To reconstruct the image we do a 2D FT on the raw data matrix or k-space. Usually the image is then displayed as a 'magnitude' image. The result of the 2D FT is actually a complex image with 'real' and 'imaginary' parts as shown in figure 7.18, or with amplitude and phase (see the Appendix for a reminder about complex numbers). We usually combine these as a complex magnitude (this gets round some problems with the B_0 field) and the images only contain positive values. Sometimes a phase image can be optionally produced too.

Certain types of scan may require 'real' reconstruction, which allows the image to have positive and negative values. In this case the image background is mid-grey. True inversion recovery is an example of this (see section 12.3.5).

7.5.6 Resolution and field of view

For a 2D FT MR acquisition the resolution is normally pixel limited provided the signal-to-noise ratio (SNR) is adequate. So if the pixel size is 1 mm, then you should be able to see details of this size clearly. To increase the resolution for a fixed field of view (decrease the pixel size) you can do one of three things: increase the gradient strengths, increase the matrix or increase the sampling time (for the FE direction only). In practice you cannot get arbitrarily small pixels as sooner or later you will run out of gradient power and SNR.

To decrease the field of view (zoom in) whilst maintaining the matrix size you can either increase the gradients or increase the sampling time (in the FE direction only).

Encoding for 2D FT imaging

Following the excitation of a localized slice, frequency- and phase-encoding gradients are applied to manipulate the MR signal to encode spatial frequencies. The effect of a gradient G_{FE} applied along the x direction following the initial excitation on a discrete signal element ∂s is

$$\partial s(t) = \rho(x) \cdot \exp\left(\frac{-t}{T_2^*}\right) \cdot \exp(i\gamma x G_{FE} t) \cdot dx$$

where $\rho(x)$ is the proton density along x, and i is the square-root of -1, denoting complex notation (see Appendix). This gradient is applied continuously during the signal acquisition (sampling). A dephasing gradient is usually applied prior to sampling in order to generate a symmetrical echo.

The phase encoding is applied (along the y direction for our example) through a gradient G_{PE} with a duration of τ prior to the signal measurement (sampling). The signal from a small element following the application of both gradients is

$$\partial s(t) = \rho(x,y) \cdot \exp\left(\frac{-t}{T_2^*}\right) \cdot \exp(i\gamma x G_{FE} t) \cdot \exp(i\gamma y G_{PE} \tau) \cdot dx dy$$

In words this is,

signal = spin density $\times$ T_2^* decay $\times$ phase change due to G_{FE} $\times$ phase change due to G_{PE}

The total MR signal is the integral of this with respect to x and y. In a complete MR acquisition the signal is sampled M times at intervals Δt, and the pulse sequence repeated N times, each time incrementing the PE gradient amplitude such that

$$G_{PE}(n) = \Delta G \cdot n \qquad \text{for } n = -\frac{N}{2} \text{ to } \frac{N}{2} - 1$$

Now *define* quantities k_{FE} and k_{PE} such that

$$k_{FE} = \gamma \cdot G_{FE} \cdot \Delta t \cdot m$$

$$k_{PE} = \gamma \cdot \Delta G \cdot n \cdot \tau$$

(See box 'Where's the bar', section 7.3.1 for a reminder of γ.) The total signal S acquired in two dimensions time t and 'pseudo-time' $n \cdot \tau$ is found by integrating over x and y

$$S(m,n) = \iint \rho(x,y) \cdot \exp\left(\frac{-t}{T_2^*}\right) \cdot \exp(i2\pi x k_{FE}) \cdot \exp(i2\pi y k_{PE}) \cdot dx dy$$

which (except for the T_2^* term) is the form of an inverse Fourier transform of the spin density $\rho(x, y)$, i.e..

$$S(m,n) = \rho(k_{FE}, k_{PE})$$

Thus the 2D FT of the encoded signal results in a representation of the spin density distribution in two dimensions. An alternative way of viewing this is that the spatial frequency components are given by the discrete signal elements $S(m,n)$, the raw k-space data. Position (x, y) and spatial frequency (k_{FE}, k_{PE}) constitute a Fourier transform pair.

To summarize, by applying the gradients, we have encoded the MR signal in terms of the spatial frequencies of the original object as shown in figure 7.10.

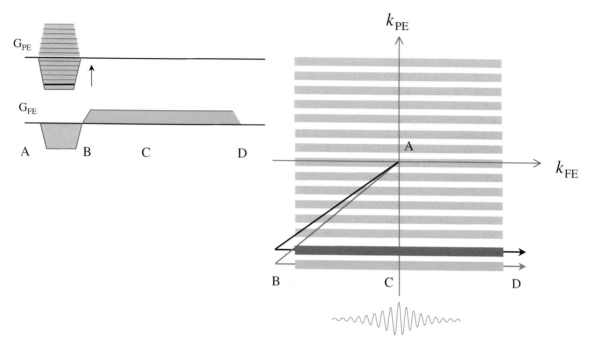

Figure 7.19 k-space path for a pair of frequency- and phase-encode gradients, showing echo formation. Following the RF pulse, and before the gradients are applied, the signal is at the centre of k-space. This means that it represents the total image brightness irrespective of spatial localization.

Resolution and field-of-view maths

The maximum resolution is given by the pixel size

$$\Delta x = \frac{1}{\gamma G_{FE} M \Delta t} \qquad \Delta y = \frac{1}{\gamma \Delta G N \tau}$$

The size of the image or the field of view (FOV) is given by the inverse of the minimum spatial frequency step

$$FOV_{FE} = \frac{1}{\gamma G_{FE} \Delta t} \qquad FOV_{PE} = \frac{1}{\gamma \Delta G_0 \tau}$$

Notice that the Fourier transform principle of 'less is more' applies: it is the maximum size of the gradient which controls the pixel size, while the time between samples or phase-encode step size controls the FOV.

7.6 Consequences of Fourier imaging

The consequences of Fourier imaging relate to the properties of k-space, the determination of resolution and field of view and the generation of typical artefacts.

7.6.1 Adventures in k-space

In simplest terms k-space is the raw data matrix which stores the already-encoded MR signals (figure 7.16). We can think of the application of the gradients as defining a path or a trajectory through k-space, as shown in figure 7.19. At time A, the application of the frequency- and phase-encoding gradients, the signal is at the centre of k-space (corresponding to a summation of the total MR signal from the object). The dephase portion of G_{FE} gradient combined with the maximal negative G_{PE} step moves it to the bottom left corner at time B. The

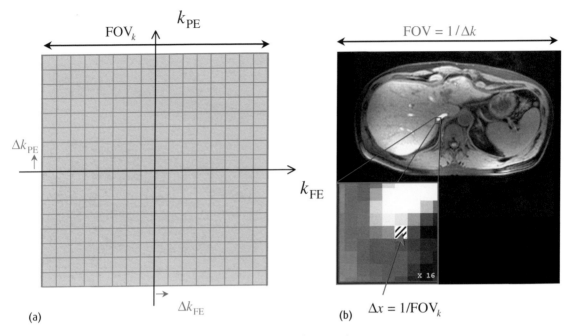

Figure 7.20 Relationship between (a) k-space and (b) image resolution and FOV.

readout part of G_{FE} moves it along a line of k_{FE} from left to right. The peak of the gradient echo occurs on crossing the k_{PE} axis (time C). Provided the MR signal has totally decayed before the next excitation we will start at the centre again. This time G_{PE} moves us to the second bottom line of k-space. By the end of the scan we will have acquired N_{PE} gradient echoes, each corresponding to a different k_{PE} position. This gives us a full sample of the spatial frequencies in the image.

The pixel size is defined by the total length of the kspace axes. The FOV is determined by the separation of the k_{PE} lines and of the samples along each k_{FE} line as shown in figure 7.20. We have already seen that central portion of k-space determines the overall brightness or contrast of the image whilst the outer regions determine the fine detail (figure 7.10).

7.6.2 T_2^* blurring

We have seen how the gradient-encoded MR signal represents the matrix of spatial frequencies. However, a glance at the maths shows that this equivalence is not exact – there is a term which depends upon T_2^*. This affects some spatial frequencies more than others and can lead to loss of resolution and blurring of the image. This is explored in section 11.4.2.

7.6.3 Artefacts

Fourier imaging is susceptible to specific artefacts, e.g. phase wrap and Gibbs' ringing (see section 6.7). Aliasing occurs because the anatomy being scanned exceeds the FOV in the PE direction causing image wrap round. In Fourier terms this means that the sampling interval Δk is insufficient. Phase encoding will occur as in section 7.5.2 and figure 7.12, but as the gradient field is physically larger than the selected FOV, the twisting of the columns of vectors outside the FOV will be too tight. This will exceed the Nyquist criterion and is therefore interpreted erroneously. Phase-encode oversampling reduces the problem. Aliasing is not commonly a problem in the frequency-encode direction as the signal from outside the FOV is encoded as a real frequency which can be removed by electronic filtering.

k-space exploration

For a 2D object represented by the function $f(x, y)$, the spatial frequencies k_x, k_y are given by

$$F(k_x, k_y) = \iint f(x,y) \cdot \exp(i2\pi(xk_x + yk_y)) \cdot dxdy$$

and the object expressed in terms of the spatial frequencies is

$$f(x,y) = \iint F(k_x, k_y) \cdot \exp(-i2\pi(xk_x + yk_y)) \cdot dk_x dk_y$$

The functions f and F are a Fourier transform pair. The quantities x and k_x bear a reciprocal arrangement, i.e. small spatial objects (little x) have big k values and vice versa. Less is more again! Thus the highest spatial frequency represents the smallest object detectable (i.e. the pixel size)

$$\Delta x = \frac{1}{N\Delta k} = \frac{1}{FOV_k}$$

and the largest object (i.e. the field of view)

$$FOV_x = \frac{1}{\Delta k_x}$$

For example, in the phase-encode axis if the maximum gradient strength is 8.6 mT m^{-1} applied for 0.7 ms with 256 steps

$$\Delta k = \frac{8.6}{128} \times 0.7 \times 42.56 = 2 \text{ m}^{-1}$$

(remember we step through G_{PE} from $-N/2$ to $N/2-1$) so the FOV is 0.5 m or 500 mm. Hint: if you use units of mT m^{-1}, ms and use γ in MHz T^{-1}, you get k in m^{-1}.)
 Similarly,

$$FOV_k = 2 \times 8.6 \times 0.7 \times 42.56 = 512 \text{ m}^{-1}$$

The pixel size in mm is therefore

$$\Delta y = \frac{1000}{512} = 1.95 \text{ mm}$$

For a read out gradient of amplitude 5.87 mT m^{-1} and a total data sampling time of 2.048 ms

$$FOV_k = 42.56 \times 5.87 \times 2.048 = 512 \text{ m}^{-1}$$

giving the same pixel size $\Delta x = 1.95$ mm. If 256 samples are taken (a sampling time of 8 μs) Δk will be 2 m^{-1} and the frequency-encode FOV will be 500 mm again.
 The MRI image-formation process can be thought of as a sampling of k-space. If sampling conventions (i.e. the Nyquist criterion) are not fulfilled with regard to the spatial frequencies in the object, then artefacts will occur as shown in section 7.6.3.
 In a generalized form for an arbitrarily shaped gradient we can write

$$k = \gamma \int_0^t G(t)dt$$

which defines any k-space trajectory.

Haunted by Fourier

It can be argued that the fundamental weakness of Fourier transform encoding and reconstruction is its suscepti-bility to modulation artefacts which produce 'ghost' replications of the image displaced relative to the true image and often aliased in the phase-encode direction. Any interaction which results in a modulation of either the fre-quency (FM) or amplitude (AM) of the MR signal will result in ghosting artefacts.

Consider a one-dimensional example of a signal $s_0(t)$ giving an image $i_0(\omega)$ by its FT

$$i_0(\omega) = \mathfrak{F}\mathfrak{I}\{s_0(t)\}$$

Suppose we have a temporal modulation of this signal such that

$$s = s_0(1 - m \cdot \cos\omega_m t)$$

where m is the modulation amplitude and ω_m is the modulation frequency (i.e. this is amplitude modulation or AM). We can then apply the Fourier modulation theory to predict the image in terms of modulation frequency ω

$$i(\omega) = i_0(\omega) + \frac{m}{2}i_0(\omega - \omega_m) + \frac{m}{2}i_0(\omega + \omega_m)$$

The encoding produces an equivalence between frequency (or 'pseudo-frequency') and position giving a resultant image

$$i(y) = i_0(y) + \frac{m}{2}i_0(y - \Delta y) + \frac{m}{2}i_0(y + \Delta y)$$

This is a combination of the true image plus two shifted ghost images with intensity m. Converting the modulation frequency in terms appropriate to k-space (PE) we get a distance shift Δy given by

$$\Delta y = \frac{1}{p\Delta k}$$

$$\Delta y = \frac{FOV_{PE}}{p}$$

where p is the periodicity of the modulation in numbers of PE lines. In real time this becomes

$$\Delta y = \frac{FOV_{PE} \cdot TR}{T_m}$$

where T_m is the real time period of the modulation, the same result we saw in section 6.3.1. The effect of signal aver-aging is to change the periodicity of the modulation relative to the phase-encode time scale. If $TR = T_m/n$ there will be n ghosts, separated by FOV/n.

Gibbs' artefact is a ringing of signal on sharp edges in the image. In k-space terms it is a truncation effect; that is, there are not enough k-values to repre-sent the detail. In basic Fourier theory the transform of a sharp (high frequency) detail will involve spectral components at all frequencies, theoretically extend-ing infinitely over k-space. Obviously an infinite k-space is impossible. The ringing occurs because of the abrupt ending, or truncation, of k-space. Filtering the data by multiplying it by a smooth func-tion prior to Fourier transformation helps to reduce ringing at the cost of spatial resolution. The best remedy is more k-space samples, i.e. to increase the PE matrix.

Ghosting is slightly different in that it arises from a modulation, i.e. a variation in amplitude or time, of the MR signal over the lines of k-space (k_{PE}) possibly arising from physiological motion or equipment imperfections. The shift of the ghost images is inversely proportional to the period of the unwanted modulation. The fastest perceptible modulation is from one line to the next (period = $\Delta k/2$). This gives a ghost separation of half the FOV. Slower modulations, covering several TR intervals, will result in less shifted ghosts. The size (or depth) of the modulation determines the amplitude of the ghost images.

7.7 Speeding it up

There are three things we can do to speed up the data acquisition which involve tricks in k-space: they are half Fourier, reduced matrix and rectangular field of view (RFOV). We also encountered these in chapter 5. Some are illustrated in figure 7.21, along with a fourth option, partial echo. Partial echo is like half Fourier but applied to frequency encoding (see box 'Real or imaginary').

7.7.1 Half Fourier

The most radical trick we can do is called 'half Fourier', 'halfscan' or 'half NEX', in which we only acquire slightly more than half the data, i.e. we omit half the phase-encoding gradient steps (either the positive or negative ones). In terms of k-space we acquire just the lower (or upper) half (figure 7.21(a)) and then estimate the other half of the data using a mathematical trick called complex conjugate synthesis. This is a property of Fourier transform of 'real' functions. This produces a time saving of approximately 50%, does not significantly affect spatial resolution but loses about 30% in signal-to-noise ratio (SNR).

7.7.2 Reduced matrix

Secondly we can apply a reduced matrix, or reduced acquisition, i.e. just not bother to acquire the largest phase-encoded lines of data (k-space) (figure 7.21(c)). Instead we replace the omitted k-space data with zeros

Real or imaginary

A property of 'real' functions is that their Fourier transforms possess complex conjugate symmetry. In a perfect magnetic field we would expect the encoded MR signal to be real, i.e.

$$S(k_{FE}, k_{PE}) = S^*(-k_{FE}, -k_{PE})$$

where S^* denotes the complex conjugate of S (see Appendix). We can say that signals in k-space have 180° rotational symmetry about the origin (zero), so that values in the top-right hand corner of k-space should be equal to those in the bottom left-hand corner.

This means that we can synthesize one-half of k-space from the other, simply by making a copy of the acquired data and swinging it through 180° to fill the other half. In half Fourier we use this property to reduce the number of phase-encode steps. However, since the magnetic field is never perfect we actually have to collect slightly more than half the data in order to apply phase corrections to the synthesized part. Another application of complex conjugate symmetry is in partial or fractional echo techniques where up to about 40% of the k_{FE} data are not acquired directly, but synthesized (figure 7.21(b)). Once again field imperfections prevent a reduction of exactly 50% in the data. Fractional echo is used in rapid imaging to reduce TE and TR.

(zero-filling). The time saving will be proportional to the number of PE lines missed out. The downside of this technique is a loss of spatial resolution in the phase-encode axis. Small improvements in SNR are made.

A 'k-space shutter' is similar except that it chops off the corners of k-space and thus affects resolution in both frequency and phase-encode directions. This offers no time-saving in 2D scanning, but it can help in 3D acquisitions and in single-shot acquisitions such as echo planar imaging.

7.7.3 Rectangular field of view

Finally, sometimes we can acquire a rectangular field of view. In the explanations above we have assumed a

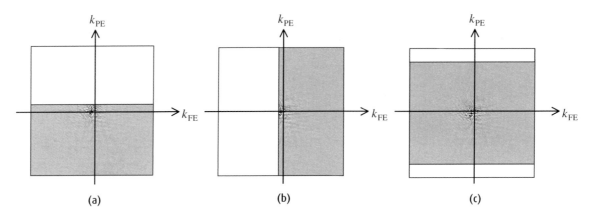

Figure 7.21 Fourier transform speed tricks: (a) half Fourier, (b) partial echo, which can be used to reduce TE and TR but does not reduce the number of PE lines, and (c) reduced matrix.

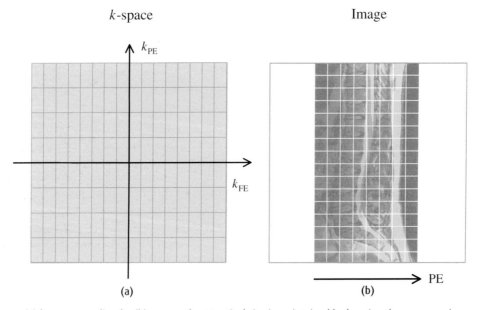

Figure 7.22 (a) k-space sampling for (b) rectangular FOV. Pixel size is maintained by keeping the same maximum and minimum k. The PE field of view is changed by altering the spacing between k_{PE} lines.

square field of view (FOV) with an equal matrix size in both directions, e.g. 256×256. Often the anatomical region to be scanned is not of similar dimensions in either axis of the image plane, so we can reduce both the phase-encode FOV and the PE matrix. Typical examples are for sagittal or coronal scanning of the knee or spine, where an unequal number of phase-encode to frequency-encode points gives a more efficient coverage of space. To save time (and avoid phase wrap) we always choose the phase-encode axis to be the smaller of the two physical dimensions, i.e. for a sagittal spine we would choose posterior-anterior for phase encoding,

It looks good, but is it real?

'Zero-filling' is a very common feature of MRI. Since computers like to work in powers of 2, any non-square matrix (where $N_{PE} \neq N_{FE}$) must be filled up with zeroes before it can be Fourier-transformed. The zeroes are added at the edge of k-space, which corresponds to the high spatial frequencies. This means a smaller pixel size, which is equivalent to interpolating the pixels in the image. However the zeroes do not contain any signal information about the high spatial frequencies, so it is not real data.

It is also possible for the user to decide to add extra zeroes to improve the apparent resolution of the final image. Remembering that the edge of k-space contains information about high spatial resolution, adding zeroes all around the edge of the acquired k-space can artificially reduce the pixel size. On GE scanners these are the 'zip512' and 'zip1024' options, on Siemens it is the 'interpolate' box, and on Philips you set the reconstruction matrix separately from the scan matrix.

The extra zeroes contain no signal, but also no noise, so they have no effect on the SNR of the image. The acquired pixel resolution is unchanged but the displayed pixels are smaller. As with reducing the phase-encode matrix, the rule of thumb is that you shouldn't zero-fill by more than a factor of two.

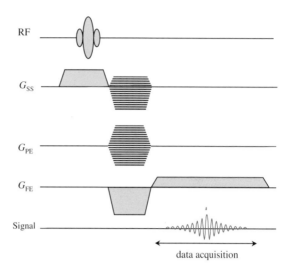

Figure 7.23 Simple 3D FT pulse sequence.

while for a transverse head we would commonly chose left-right for the phase-encode direction.

In k-space the effect of a rectangular field of view is to 'space out' the lines in the PE axis (figure 7.22). Only the field of view is affected as the value of k_{max} remains the same. A time saving of up to 50% is achievable with no resolution loss and only a slight loss of SNR.

7.8 3D FT

A fully three-dimensional technique may sometimes prove advantageous over two-dimensional multiple slice acquisition. The principle is simply to apply a second phase-encode axis, ensuring that for every gradient step in the new axis we apply the whole set of other axes steps: i.e. for a $L \times M \times N$ 3D matrix, we acquire $L \times M$ MR signals. The scan time for basic 3D acquisitions is then

$$\text{Scan time} = \text{NSA} \times \text{number of "slices"} \times N_{PE} \times \text{TR}$$

where, as before, NSA is number of signal averages and N_{PE} the size of the phase-encode matrix.

In practice multiple slabs are often acquired, with excitation being restricted to a slab or group of slabs by selective excitation and within-slab resolution being produced by stepped rephase gradients (figure 7.23). In multi-slab or multi-chunk 3D FT we combine

2D versus 3D: which is best?

The advantages of 3D acquisitions are that you obtain thinner and more slices with better profiles, and better SNR for an equivalent slice thickness. The disadvantages are longer acquisition time and possible ringing artefacts from slice to slice and aliasing. 3D FT is usually only applied for gradient-echo sequences. As a rule-of-thumb, if the desired slice thickness is 3 mm or more, use 2D multi-slice. For thinner slices use 3D FT.

interleaved slab or thick-slice selection with additional slice phase encoding to obtain multiple 3D volumes in a single scan. This is a popular technique for producing high axial resolution images of the spine through the vertebrae.

See also:

- Image artefacts: chapter 6
- Optimizing SNR and resolution: chapter 5
- Acronyms anonymous: a guide to the pulse sequence jungle: chapter 12

FURTHER READING

Bracewell RN (1986) *The Fourier Transform and its Applications*. London: McGraw Hill (ISBN: 0070664544).

Edelstein WA, Hutchison JMS, Johnson G and Redpath T (1980) Spin warp NMR imaging and applications to human whole-body imaging. *Phys Med Biol* **25**: 751–6.

Elster AD and Burdette J (2001) *Questions and Answers in Magnetic Resonance Imaging*, 2nd edn. London: Mosby-Yearbook (ISBN: 0323011845), Chapter 4.

Haacke EM, Brown RW, Thompson MR and Venkatesan R (1999) *Magnetic Resonance Imaging: Physical Principles and Sequence Design*. London: Wiley-Liss (ISBN: 0471351288), Chapters 9, 10 & 11.

Kumar A, Welti D and Ernst RR (1975) NMR Fourier zeugmatography. *J Magn Reson* **18**:69–83.

Mansfield P and Maudsley AA (1977) Medical imaging by NMR. *Br J Radiol* **50**:188–94.

Smith H-J and Ranallo FN (1989) *A Non-mathematical Approach to Basic MRI*. London: Medical Physics Publishing Corp. (ISBN: 0944838022), Chapter 19.

Twieg DB (1983) The k-trajectory formulation of the NMR imaging process with applications in analysis and synthesis of imaging methods. *Med Phys* **10**: 610–23.

Getting in tune: resonance and relaxation

8.1 Introduction

MRI involves three kinds of magnetic field: the main field of the scanner, the gradients which are used for spatial localization, and the oscillating magnetic field of the RF pulses. There must be something in the body which has magnetic properties in order to interact with all these fields. So far we have deliberately avoided a detailed discussion of these properties, since we believe it's easier (and more useful practically) to understand the images first. However, the time has come to explore the protons which are essential for MRI, and on the way we will tackle some difficult concepts from quantum mechanics. We will discuss the relaxation mechanisms T_1 and T_2 in more detail, including a molecular model of tissues that is used to explain effects such as magnetization transfer. We will find that:

- hydrogen nuclei have a magnetic moment which interacts with the main field of the scanner;
- quantum mechanics controls the behaviour of the individual protons, but classical mechanics is used to describe the changes in a large collection of nuclei;
- excitation and relaxation of a collection of protons is described by the Bloch equations;
- spin-spin and spin-lattice relaxation mechanisms are due to dipole interactions and relaxation times depend on molecular motions within the tissues;
- relaxation times can be measured using special pulse sequences (but these are not commonly used in the clinical setting);
- we can use contrast agents to modify the relaxation times of tissues, usually to create a brighter signal from pathological tissues.

8.2 Spinning nuclei

At school, we all learned that atoms consist of electrons orbiting a central nucleus composed of neutrons and protons, and electrons, protons and neutrons are known as fundamental particles. As you probably know by now, MRI is derived from NMR, nuclear magnetic resonance, so we're only interested in the nucleus. In particular we want to look at the nucleus of the hydrogen atom, because it's abundant in the human body in water and other molecules. The nucleus of the hydrogen atom is a single positively charged proton. Something you probably didn't learn at school is that all fundamental particles spin on their own axes, and the hydrogen nucleus is thus a continuously rotating positive charge. Basic electromagnetism tells us that a moving charge (i.e. a current) has an associated magnetic field, and so the proton generates its own tiny field known as its magnetic moment.

8.2.1 Classical mechanics explanation of NMR

If the proton is placed in a strong external magnetic field, it experiences a turning force, known as a torque. This is similar to a compass needle which experiences a force in the Earth's magnetic field and turns so that it is aligned with the direction of the field. The proton tries to align itself with the external field, but it is constrained by the laws of quantum mechanics. Quantum mechanics (QM) is a branch of physics which explains the rather odd behaviour of very small particles such as protons and electrons, which sometimes act like particles and sometimes like waves. Classical mechanics (CM) on the

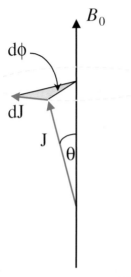

Figure 8.1 Geometric representation of the precession of the magnetic moment μ around the main field B_0.

other hand works for normal-sized ('macroscopic') bodies, and for large numbers of small particles where their quantum mechanical behaviour is averaged out. Although we have to do a bit of QM to understand why the protons don't simply align with the field, we will find that CM is quite capable of explaining almost everything else (sigh of relief!).

Since it can't align exactly with the external field, the proton continues to experience a torque which makes it precess around the direction of the field. This precession is analogous to the wobbling of a spinning top (gyroscope) tilted slightly off axis so that it experiences a torque due to gravity. If you've never seen this, it's worth while buying a gyroscope from any toy store and trying to make it precess. All serious MR specialists have a gyroscope!

The precessional frequency of the protons is found to be proportional to the external magnetic field, given by the Larmor equation

$$\omega_0 = \gamma B_0$$

where γ is a constant called the gyromagnetic ratio, equal to 2.7×10^8 rad s^{-1} T^{-1}. We use γ to denote angular frequencies which are vectors, but we are more used to scalar frequencies denoted f; in these terms the gyromagnetic ratio is 42.57 MHz T^{-1}. (All the

Derivation of the Larmor frequency: classical mechanics

We use vector notation in the boxes in this chapter because direction is important. Vectors are written in bold upright font, while their corresponding magnitudes are in italics, with subscripts to show component magnitudes where appropriate.

The magnetic moment μ is directly proportional to the angular momentum J

$$\mu = \gamma J$$

where γ is the gyromagnetic ratio. When this moment is in an external field B it experiences a torque and precesses about the field, its angular momentum changing according to the equation

$$\left|\frac{d J}{dt}\right| = |\mu \times B| = |\gamma J \times B| = \gamma J B \sin\theta$$

where θ is the angle between the magnetic moment and the main field. From basic geometry (figure 8.1) we can see that dJ is given by

$$dJ = J \sin\theta\, d\phi$$

Combining these two results we can show that the precessional frequency is given by

$$\omega = \frac{d\phi}{dt} = -\frac{d\phi}{dJ} \cdot \frac{dJ}{dt} = \frac{1}{J \sin\theta} \cdot -\gamma J B \sin\theta$$

$$\omega_0 = \gamma B_0$$

The minus sign, which we quietly dropped just before the last line, is there to make sure that ω_0 defines a clockwise rotation about the z axis. So the magnetic moment precesses clockwise about B_0 at an angular frequency of ω_0 or a scalar frequency of f_0 if you prefer to use $\gamma = 42.57$ MHz T^{-1}.

equations in this chapter use angular frequencies, but you could simply replace ω with f and use $\gamma = 42.57$ MHz T^{-1} to get the frequencies in MHz. See also 'Where's the bar?' in chapter 7.) So the protons in a magnetic field all precess at the same Larmor frequency, not any old frequency. This is known as a resonance condition.

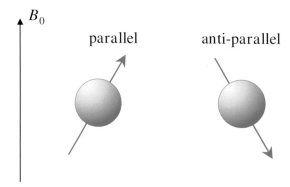

Figure 8.2 Two possible orientations for the proton in an external magnetic field.

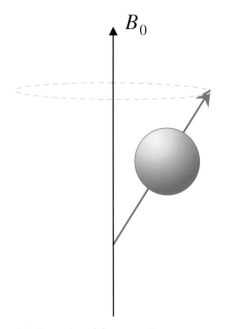

Figure 8.3 Precession of the magnetic moment.

8.2.2 Quantum mechanics explanation

So here's the QM bit. The proton's spin is said to be quantized in the presence of an external field, and the torque it experiences makes it precess in one of only two orientations, known in QM as states. One state is almost aligned with the main field, and is known as spin-up or parallel. The other state is aligned almost opposite to the external field, known as spin-down or

anti-parallel (see figure 8.2). Since the magnetic moment is at an angle to the external field, the tip of its vector traces out a circle around the direction of the field (figure 8.3) whichever orientation it is in.

How does the proton choose which orientation to precess in? It just depends on how much energy it has, since the anti-parallel direction requires slightly more energy than the parallel direction. Both states are stable, so protons are quite happy to stay in either position. However, protons can swap between the two states simply by gaining or losing a certain amount of energy in the form of a photon (a packet of electromagnetic radiation). It turns out that the energy difference

Derivation of the Larmor frequency: quantum mechanics

The magnetic moment of the proton is related to the quantized angular momentum

$$\boldsymbol{\mu} = \gamma \mathbf{J} = \gamma \hbar I$$

where I is the spin angular momentum quantum number, equal to ½ for protons, $\hbar$ is Planck's constant divided by 2π and γ is the gyromagnetic ratio. In an external magnetic field there are $2I + 1$ possible values for the angular momentum, ranging from I, $I - 1$, …0, …, $-(I - 1)$, $-I$. Thus for the proton there are only two possible states, with values of $\pm$½. The energy of each state (ε) is given by

$$\varepsilon = \boldsymbol{\mu} \cdot \mathbf{B} = \gamma \hbar I \cdot B$$

and thus we can calculate the energy difference as

$$\Delta \varepsilon = \left(\frac{1}{2} - -\frac{1}{2} \right) \gamma \hbar B = \gamma \hbar B$$

De Broglie's wave equation tells us that the frequency associated with this energy is

$$\Delta \varepsilon = \hbar \omega$$

and so we can find the precessional frequency (using the subscript 0 to indicate the Larmor frequency and applied external field)

$$\hbar \omega_0 = \gamma \hbar B_0$$

$$\omega_0 = \gamma B_0$$

between the two states is directly proportional to the strength of the external magnetic field, and from QM we can calculate exactly what the energy difference is, and thus the frequency of electromagnetic radiation required. We will find that the frequency is the Larmor frequency, just as we found from classical mechanics,

$$\omega_0 = \gamma B_0$$

So we can have a link between the classical and quantum mechanical pictures, showing that the precessional frequency of the proton in a magnetic field is the same as the frequency of radiation required to cause transitions between the two states.

In the human body there are many millions of protons; after all we are about 75% water. So although an individual proton obeys QM, we should expect to measure their average behaviour with CM. There is a statistical distribution of protons between the two states and we find that the lower-energy state is slightly favoured, so that there are more protons spinning parallel than anti-parallel. The ratio depends on both the main magnetic field strength and (inversely) on temperature. At body

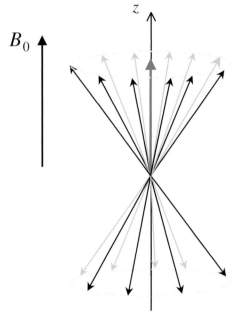

Figure 8.4 Average of many protons produces the net magnetization M$_0$.

Population of energy states

Whether a proton is in the parallel or anti-parallel direction depends on its internal energy. For a large collection of protons, the number in each state is given by the Boltzmann distribution:

$$\frac{N_{up}}{N_{down}} = \exp\left(\frac{\Delta\varepsilon}{k_B T}\right)$$

where k_B is the Boltzmann constant, 1.38×10^{-23} JK^{-1}. Since $\gamma\hbar B_0 \ll k_B T$ at body temperature and clinical field strengths, we can write this as

$$\frac{N_{up}}{N_{down}} = 1 + \frac{\gamma\hbar B_0}{k_B T}$$

$$\Rightarrow N_{excess} = N_{up} - N_{down} = \frac{N_{total}}{2} \cdot \frac{\gamma\hbar B_0}{k_B T}$$

This difference creates the net magnetization M$_0$. If we replace N$_{total}$ with proton density ρ we will get M$_0$ per unit volume. We also know that the magnetic moment of the proton has a magnitude of $\frac{1}{2}\gamma\hbar$ thus can calculate

$$M_0 = \frac{\rho\gamma^2\hbar^2 B_0}{4 k_B T}$$

Now we can calculate that water contains 6.67×10^{22} protons ml^{-1}, so we can show that at body temperature and 1.5 T we get M$_0 \approx 0.02$ μT ml^{-1}. Assuming that the human head has a volume of approximately 1500 ml and is about 80% water, M$_0 \approx 20$ μT which is small, but measurable!

temperature (37°C) and in a 1.5-T scanner, this works out at about 1.000004, which means that for every million protons in the spin-down direction there are a million-and-four protons in the spin-up direction.

In equilibrium the protons are all out of phase with each other, so the tips of the magnetic moment vectors are evenly spread out around the circles (see figure 8.4). Since there are so many protons, we can make each vector represent the average magnetic moment of a large group of protons all precessing at exactly the same frequency, rather than an individual proton's magnetic moment. This is sometimes called an 'isochromat' of protons, but we will use the term 'spin'. This may seem like an unnecessary complication but it means that we can drop QM and just use CM from now on! The vector sum of all these spins is called the net magnetization M_0, which is aligned exactly with the main field B_0 (conventionally shown as the z direction). M_0 is a measurable magnetization which can be calculated to be of the order of microtesla (μ T).

8.3 Measuring the magnetic moment

As we've just seen, the magnetization in the body is very small (e.g. 1 μ T) compared to the main magnetic field (e.g. 1.5 T). It is virtually impossible to measure it while it is at equilibrium, lying parallel with B_0, and much easier to tip it through 90° into the x-y plane (known as the transverse plane). Using a detector which only measures magnetic fields in the transverse plane, M_0 is now a significant signal which can be recorded.

The rotating frame of reference

In order to explain the effects of RF pulses and relaxation mechanisms, it is helpful to use a rotating frame of reference. However, many people automatically think about the protons in a rotating frame, and may actually find it confusing to have it explained. Physicists should read this section, but others may like to skip it for now. Refer to the Appendix if you're unsure about vector notation and the cross product.

We choose a frame rotating at the Larmor frequency about the z axis, which is defined by the direction of B_0 (figure 8.5). In the rotating frame, spins at exactly the Larmor frequency are stationary, while those at higher or lower frequencies gain or lose phase respectively. We can describe the motion of the magnetization **M** in the new rotating frame as

$$\left(\frac{d\mathbf{M}}{dt}\right)_{rot} = \left(\frac{d\mathbf{M}}{dt}\right)_{fixed} - \boldsymbol{\omega} \times \mathbf{M}$$

where $\boldsymbol{\omega}$ is the frequency of the rotating frame. We already know that a magnetic moment precesses in an external field **B** (see 'Derivation of the Larmor frequency: classical mechanics'), with its motion described by

$$\left(\frac{d\mathbf{M}}{dt}\right)_{fixed} = \gamma \mathbf{M} \times \mathbf{B}$$

Thus we can write

$$\left(\frac{d\mathbf{M}}{dt}\right)_{rot} = \gamma \mathbf{M} \times \mathbf{B} - \boldsymbol{\omega} \times \mathbf{M} \qquad = \gamma \mathbf{M} \times \mathbf{B} + \gamma \mathbf{M} \times \frac{\boldsymbol{\omega}}{\gamma} \qquad = \gamma \mathbf{M} \times \left(\mathbf{B} + \frac{\boldsymbol{\omega}}{\gamma}\right)$$

The term $\boldsymbol{\omega}/\gamma$ represents a fictitious magnetic field which arises because of the rotation, and thus $(\mathbf{B} + \boldsymbol{\omega}/\gamma)$ is the effective magnetic field experienced by the spins. So the motion of the magnetization in the rotating frame can be described by the same equation as in the fixed frame. This allows us to add fields due to RF pulses and predict the motion of M_0 in those conditions, if necessary using an off-resonance rotating frame. Notice that if $\mathbf{B} = B_0$ and the frame rotates at $-\boldsymbol{\omega}_0$, **M** is stationary, i.e. in the basic frame rotating clockwise around z at the Larmor frequency M_0 is static. From now on we will always use x and y for the fixed laboratory frame, and x' and y' for the rotating frame. Since z and z' are aligned, we will just use z for this axis.

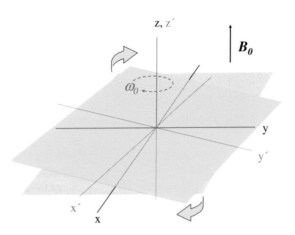

Figure 8.5 The rotating frame of reference. The coordinate system x', y', z' is considered to be rotating at the Larmor frequency in the same direction as the nuclear spins, which thus appear stationary.

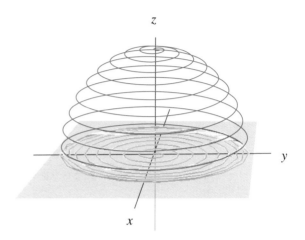

Figure 8.7 During the RF pulse M_0 spirals away from the z axis and down towards the transverse plane.

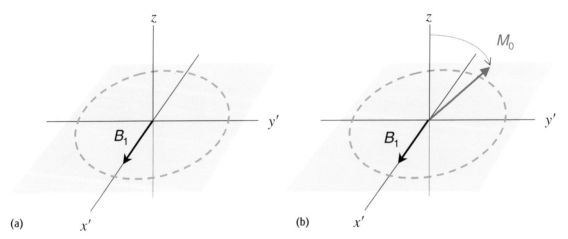

(a)

(b)

Figure 8.6 (a) The RF pulse produces a fixed magnetic field B_1 in the rotating frame. (b) M_0 precesses about B_1 until the RF is switched off.

As you can probably guess, we tip M_0 into the transverse plane using a 90° RF pulse. What exactly is going on during the pulse though? First we should note that the RF frequency used must be the Larmor frequency due to the resonance condition. The RF pulse creates a magnetic field within the transmit coil which is perpendicular to B_0 and oscillating at the Larmor frequency. In the rotating frame, this is a static field B_1 aligned along x' in the transverse plane (figure 8.6(a)). M_0 moves away from the z axis

until the RF pulse is switched off (figure 8.6(b)). In the laboratory frame the motion looks like a spiral since it is also precessing about the z axis (see figure 8.7). The maths for this isn't much fun and it is much easier to work with the rotating frame!

For a simple RF pulse switched on and then off (known as a 'hard' pulse), the flip angle (α) is given by

$$\alpha = \gamma B_1 t_p$$

In the rotating frame again

The RF wave is produced either linearly or circularly polarized (see chapter 9), and creates a fixed magnetic field $\mathbf{B_1}$ in the rotating frame (figure 8.6(a)). (A linearly polarized wave can be considered as two counter-rotating circularly polarized waves. The one which is in the clockwise direction produces $\mathbf{B_1}$, while the other is ignored.) The motion of M_0 in the rotating frame is given by

$$\left(\frac{d\mathbf{M}}{dt}\right)_{rot} = \gamma \mathbf{M} \times \left(\mathbf{B_0} + \frac{\omega}{\gamma} + \mathbf{B_1}\right) = \gamma \mathbf{M} \times \mathbf{B_1}$$

provided $\omega = -\omega_0$, i.e. the frame is rotating clockwise at ω_0. Thus the motion of M_0 will be to precess *in the rotating frame* about $\mathbf{B_1}$ (figure 8.6(b)). Note that the magnitude of B_1 is much smaller than B_0, so the precession will be much slower, typically of the order of 100 Hz (cf. 63 MHz Larmor frequency at 1.5 T). The flip angle at the end of a pulse of duration t_p will be

$$\alpha = \gamma B_1 t_p$$

To produce a 90° pulse lasting 0.25 ms for example we need a B_1 of only 23 μT.

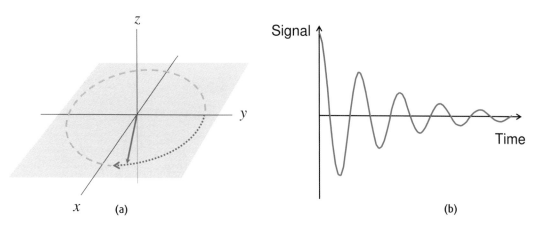

Figure 8.8 (a) Precession of the flipped magnetization in the transverse plane. (b) Signal induced in the receiver coil – the Free Induction Decay (FID).

where B_1 is the strength of the RF magnetic field and t_p is the duration of the pulse. If M_0 ends up exactly in the transverse plane, then the RF pulse is called a 90° pulse. Leaving the RF on for twice as long (or doubling its strength) would turn M_0 through exactly 180°, and the pulse would then be called a 180° pulse. Since time is always a crucial factor in MRI, we tend to just change the strength of the pulse to produce different flip angles. The RF pulse has another important effect on the spins, bringing them all into phase coherence. This means that they all point to the same position on the precession circle.

Having rotated M_0 into the transverse plane, we measure it by detecting the voltage it induces in a receiver coil which is sensitive only to magnetization perpendicular to B_0. In the laboratory frame M_0 is now precessing in the transverse plane (see figure 8.8(a)), so the coil sees an oscillating magnetic field which induces a voltage varying at the Larmor frequency. The amplitude of the signal decays exponentially to zero in only a few milliseconds (figure 8.8(b)), because the protons rapidly dephase with respect to each other. This signal is known as the **Free Induction Decay (FID)**, a rather obscure term coined by one of the original NMR researchers. We never measure the FID directly in MR imaging, instead we create echoes which are described in the next section.

8.4 Creating echoes

In MRI we use two types of echo, gradient (GE) and spin echoes (SE). In each case the sequence starts with an RF excitation pulse, 90° in the case of SE and smaller angles in GE. We will explain gradient echoes first.

In the GE sequence (figure 8.9), we apply a negative gradient lobe immediately after the excitation pulse.

This causes rapid dephasing of the transverse magnetization, much faster than the normal FID. After the negative lobe we apply a positive gradient, which simply reverses the magnetic field gradient. Spins that were precessing at a low frequency due to their position in the gradient will now precess at a higher frequency because the gradient will now add to the main field, and vice versa. Spins which were previously dephasing now begin to rephase, and after a certain time they will all come back into phase along the y' axis forming the gradient echo. However, the positive gradient only compensates for the dephasing caused by the negative gradient lobe, it does not refocus dephasing due to the

Paradoxes in QM

Some useful insights into excitation can be found by considering the quantized protons, rather than just the macroscopic magnetization. Unfortunately not all the concepts can be directly translated between QM and CM, so we will point out where the usefulness of QM stops, in our opinion at least.

When the population of protons is irradiated by an RF wave, protons can flip between energy levels. Spin-up protons can absorb energy to jump into the spin-down position, while those in the spin-down state are stimulated into giving up an equal amount of energy to drop into the spin-up state, and there is an equal probability of each transition. Since in equilibrium there are more spin-up protons than spin-down, the net effect will be absorption of energy from the RF wave, causing the temperature of the spin system to rise. The protons' temperature is considered separately from the temperature of the surrounding tissues, known as the lattice, which will eventually come into equilibrium with the spins. We will come back to this idea when we consider spin-lattice relaxation.

Taking the simple idea of population difference and absorption of RF, it can be seen that the maximum absorption will be when all the spin-down protons have flipped into the spin-up position and vice versa. This is known as population inversion, and can be easily considered as a 180° pulse which flips the magnetization from z to $-z$. The definition of a 90° pulse can then be considered to be half that amount of energy, which is thought of as equalizing the populations leaving no magnetization along the z axis. Thus far the QM concepts seem to agree with our macroscopic observations, and they can be helpful up to this point.

However, we cannot take this picture much farther, not least because pulses larger than 180° can be used and have a measurable effect on the spin system, which is difficult to reconcile with the idea that there is a maximum absorption of energy which causes population inversion. Also, from the Boltzmann distribution, we know that increasing temperature will decrease the population difference between the two states. Thus the magnetization should decrease monotonically to zero with increasing absorption of energy. It also means that population inversion would give the spins a negative temperature, which in turn places other thermodynamic constraints on the system.

This raises some strange paradoxes which are difficult to understand in everyday terms, and we would recommend that if you want to pursue these ideas you should consult some of the physics texts listed at the end of this chapter. The good news is that many people probably have rather confused internal ideas about MRI, mixing up the concepts of classical and quantum mechanics in all sorts of odd ways, but so long as you can correctly predict the effect of changing parameters such as TR, does it matter? We think probably not!

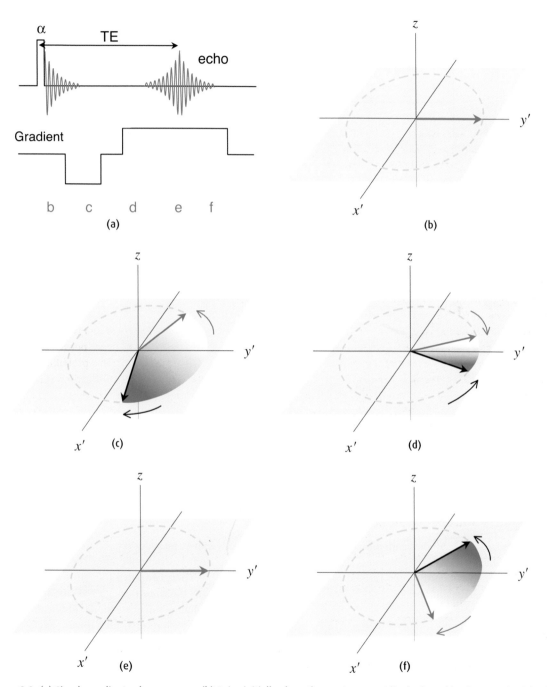

Figure 8.9 (a) Simple gradient-echo sequence. (b) Spins initially along the y axis are rapidly dephased by the negative lobe (c). When the gradient is switched positive (d), the spins begin to rephase, forming an echo (e). If the gradient is left on (f) dephasing will occur again.

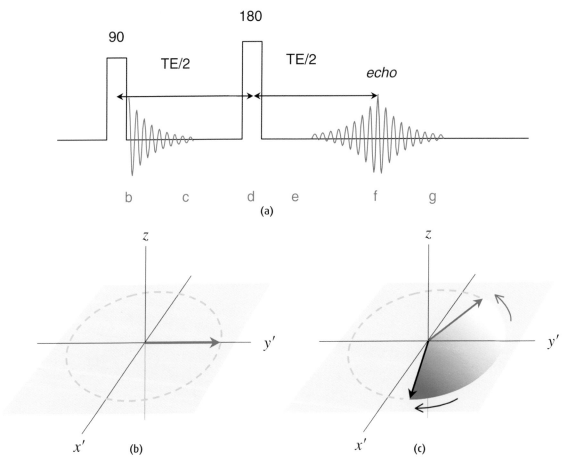

Figure 8.10 (a) Spin-echo pulse sequence. Spins initially in phase (b) dephase naturally (c) until the 180° pulse is applied. (d) Immediately after the pulse their phases are reversed, but they continue to dephase in the same direction (e) forming an echo (f) and then dephasing again (g).

main magnetic field inhomogeneities or spin-spin relaxation (which is explained in the next section). The height of the echo (S_{GE}) is thus determined by the FID decay curve which depends on T_2^*

$$S_{GE} = S_0 \exp\left(-\frac{TE}{T_2^*}\right)$$

where S_0 is the initial height of the FID. T_2^* is a composite relaxation time which includes T_2, inhomogeneities due to the main field and tissue susceptibility, and diffusion of the protons.

In the spin-echo sequence (figure 8.10) we leave the spins to dephase naturally after the 90° pulse for a certain time. Then we apply a 180° pulse on the $+y'$ axis which flips all the spins through 180° about the y' axis. It does not change the precessional frequencies of the spins, but it does reverse their phase angles. Spins which were in a lower magnetic field strength will have been dephasing anticlockwise; the 180° pulse flips them over and they now appear to have been in a higher magnetic field and have dephased clockwise. Similarly spins which were dephasing clockwise will appear to have been in a lower magnetic field and

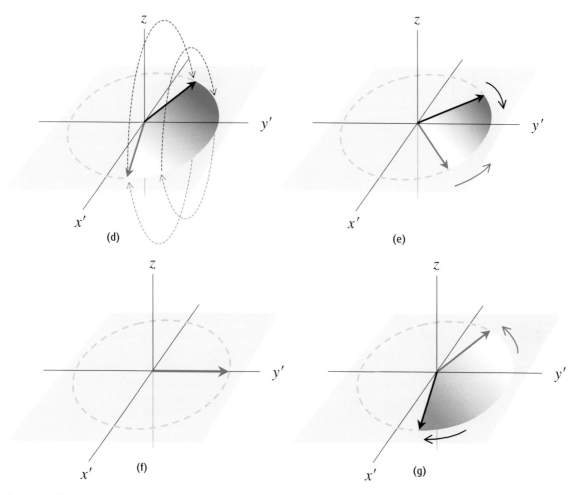

Figure 8.10 (*cont.*)

dephased anticlockwise. Assuming that the spins do not move too far within the imaging volume, they will continue to experience the same magnetic field inhomogeneities and continue to dephase in the same direction. After a time equal to the delay between the 90° and the 180° pulse, all the spins will come back into phase along the $+y'$ axis forming the spin echo. The phase-reversal trick means that the echo height will only depend on T_2 and diffusion, and not on the magnetic field inhomogeneities or tissue susceptibilities.

$$S_{SE} = S_0 \exp\left[-\frac{TE}{T_2} - \frac{2}{3}\gamma^2 \Delta B^2 D \left(\frac{TE}{2}\right)^3 \right]$$

where ΔB describes the magnetic field inhomogeneities and D is the apparent diffusion coefficient of the protons. In tissues D is typically around $10^3 \, \text{mm}^2 \, \text{s}^{-1}$, and TE is generally short compared with T_2, so the second diffusion-dependent term is very small compared with the first T_2 term. We can simplify the equation to

$$S_{SE} = S_0 \exp\left(-\frac{TE}{T_2} \right)$$

and say that the spin echo signals depend on T_2.

RF phase angles: which axis?

You may find that other texts show the 180° pulse on the $+x'$ axis so that the fan of dephasing protons is flipped a further 180° and creates a spin echo along the $-y'$ axis, i.e. a negative echo (but then of course we take the magnitude for the final image intensity). Why have we done it differently? Well partly because we have found, over many years of giving lectures, that people find the negative echo an extra complication, and we can avoid that just by putting the 180° pulse on $+y'$. Both forms create a spin echo of the same height, the only difference is in the direction of the vectors. It is also because multi-echo sequences always put the 180° pulses on $+y'$ instead of $+x'$, which partially compensates for imperfections in the RF pulse. An explanation of this can be found in the box 'Measuring T_2'.

8.4.1 The 'runners on a track' analogy (slightly reworked)

You may have come across this analogy to describe the spin echo in other textbooks or lectures. It is explained by saying that the runners all start at the same time (analogous to the 90° pulse exciting all the protons), but because they run at different speeds after a while they are spread out along the track. The 180° pulse is like turning all the runners around at this point, so that they all have to run back to the starting point. Assuming they all continue to run at the same speeds, after an equal time they will all cross the starting point together – analogous to the protons coming back into phase to create the echo.

We can modify this slightly to explain the differences between spin echo and gradient echo, and also show why the echo heights depend on T_2 and T_2^* respectively. First suppose that as well as running at different speeds, the runners get tired at different rates, so they tend to slow down. Also imagine that the track is not flat but rather lumpy, and that it is different in each lane. To explain the spin echo first, let the runners start together running in one direction; after a while they are spread out due to the differences in their running speeds and the track conditions in each lane. When the 180° pulse is applied the runners all turn around and run back towards the starting point, and magically the track conditions are reversed: the bad lanes become perfect, the good ones become difficult. So if the runners all go at the same speeds as before, the effects of the track will be evened out and they will all cross the starting point together. Since they get tired though, they don't manage to maintain their speeds, and in fact we only get some of them back at the same time.

To extend the analogy to gradient echo, the gradient reversal is the turning point instead of the 180° pulse. This time, however, the track conditions don't get fixed and the runners who had bad lanes to start with have to run back under the same conditions. As well as tiredness slowing them down, the lane conditions alter their performance. At the echo time, even fewer of the runners are back at the starting point. In this extended analogy, the runners' different tiredness rates are analogous to T_2 and the lane conditions are analogous to the magnetic field inhomogeneities.

8.5 Relaxation times

Having excited the protons in order to flip them into the transverse plane, they begin to relax back to their equilibrium position as soon as the RF pulse is switched off. There are two main features of the relaxation: a dephasing of the spins following their phase coherence after the pulse, and realignment along the z axis as they lose the energy they absorbed from the pulse.

The spins dephase because of small differences in their precessional frequencies. Thinking of the system in the rotating frame (rotating at the Larmor frequency), a slightly higher frequency will make spins dephase in the clockwise direction, while a lower frequency causes an anticlockwise phase angle. Anything that changes a spin's frequency from the Larmor frequency will add to the dephasing. For the FID, the dominant effect is the unavoidable inhomogeneity in the main magnetic field. A second effect is formed by the interactions between spins as they move around within the tissues. It is this interaction that we call spin-spin relaxation, characterized by the spin-spin relaxation time T_2, which is independent of the magnet in which it is being measured and (for practical purposes) independent of field strength.

To understand T_2, imagine a system of excited protons in a perfect magnetic field, free to move around in a random fashion. They all precess in the transverse plane, ignoring the relaxation back to the z axis for now. So long as they are evenly distributed around the volume, they are all precessing at the Larmor frequency and remain in phase in the rotating frame. However, if two protons come close together, each of them experiences a slightly higher or lower

magnetic field, as the magnetic moment of the other proton adds or subtracts from the main field (figure 8.11(a)). Their precessional frequencies change instantaneously to match the 'new' field, and each proton will dephase with respect to the Larmor frequency. When they move apart again they both return to the Larmor frequency, but the phase angles they acquire during the interaction are irreversible. Over time each proton will interact with many thousands of other protons, and the phase angles become larger and larger until all the protons are out of phase with each other. The vector sum of the magnetic moments, which is the signal we detect in the MR receiver, gradually decays from a maximum immediately after the excitation pulse down to zero (figure 8.11(b)). Since their motion is random, the dephasing is an exponential decay process, which we call spin-spin relaxation.

Measuring T_2

Since the FID includes dephasing from magnetic field inhomogeneities, how do we measure T_2? We could use a series of spin-echo sequences and measure the signal height at each TE. Plotting a graph of signal against TE allows us to measure T_2. Well it should do, but unfortunately the diffusion of protons through an inhomogeneous magnetic field adds an irreversible dephasing which messes things up! It can be shown that a series of equally spaced 180° pulses on the $+x'$ axis creates a train of spin echoes alternating negative and positive (figure 8.12) which compensates for diffusion, as well as being much more time-efficient. This is known as a Carr–Purcell T_2 measurement, and the signal at time t is given by

$$S(t) = M_0 \left[\exp\left(\frac{-t}{T_2}\right) \cdot \exp\left(\frac{-\gamma^2 \Delta B^2 D \tau^2 t}{3}\right) \right]$$

where ΔB is the magnetic field inhomogeneity, 2τ is the echo spacing, D is the diffusion coefficient and t is the overall time from the excitation to a particular echo we are measuring. Provided the echo spacing is small the second term is almost equal to 1, and we are left with an exponential decay due to T_2. A modification known as the Carr–Purcell–Meiboom–Gill (CPMG) sequence compensates for imperfections in the 180° pulses which would otherwise accumulate over the echo train. In CPMG, the initial 90° pulse is on the $+x'$ axis and the train of 180° pulses is on the $+y'$ axis and all the echoes are positive (figure 8.13). If the 180° pulse is imperfect, the first and every oddnumbered pulse will be slightly too small, but the even echoes will be the correct height, and the errors do not accumulate. To measure T_2, we should therefore use the echo height from only the even echoes. At least five echo heights should be used (implying an echo train of at least ten) with a range of echo times up to about three times T_2. Unfortunately there are other errors inherent in the imaging process; for example, imperfect slice profiles and partial volume effects, which mean that in vivo T_2 mapping is rarely accurate although it can be precise (i.e. the result isn't the true T_2 of the tissue but the measurements have good reproducibility).

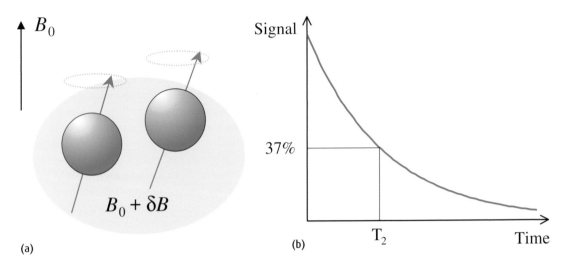

(a)

(b)

Figure 8.11 (a) As two protons come close together, they experience a change in magnetic field strength (δB) which changes their precessional frequency. (b) Because the interactions are random, the resultant transverse magnetization vector decays to zero exponentially. T_2 is the time taken for the transverse magnetization to drop to 37% of its initial size.

Measuring T_1

T_1 measurement is rather a long winded process. A series of inversion recovery sequences is used with varying TI. IR sequences start with a 180° inversion pulse (see figure 8.14a), then during the delay time TI there is T_1 recovery. When the 90° is applied some of the signals may still be negative (figure 8.14c), so a mixture of positive and negative echoes will be formed. We usually take the magnitude, giving the IR curves shown in figure 3.12; however for T_1 measurement it is better to use a 'real reconstruction' – see section 12.3.5 for details.

The TR must always be at least five times the longest T_1 present to relax after the 90° pulse (figure 8.14 d) (which presents a chicken-and-egg problem: you don't know what the T_1 is until you've measured it, and if TR is too short you won't measure it correctly!). If TR is long enough, the signal at each TI is given by

$$S(\text{TI}) = M_0\left[1 - 2\exp\left(-\frac{\text{TI}}{T_1}\right) + \exp\left(-\frac{\text{TR}}{T_1}\right)\right]$$

Assuming the longest T_1 is about 1200 ms, TR must be at least 5000 ms and, since at least five different TIs should be used, the whole process can take many minutes to do properly. A repeated 90°–TR–90°–TR– sequence can also be used, and in this case the signal is given by

$$S(TR) = M_0\left[1 - \exp\left(-\frac{TR}{T_1}\right)\right]$$

Again, to produce a reasonably accurate measure of T_1 at least five different TRs should be used, extending the total scan time required. As with T_2 measurements, there are unavoidable errors in the imaging process which mean that T_1 mapping is rarely accurate.

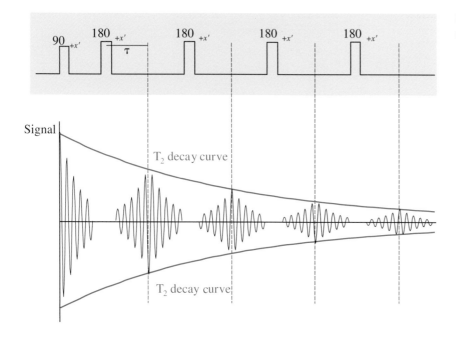

Figure 8.12 The Carr-Purcell sequence showing 4 echoes.

Although the transverse magnetization decays, there is no net loss of energy in spin-spin relaxation. To lose energy, the protons interact with the surrounding tissues (figure 8.15), known as the lattice, which can absorb the energy and disperse it via blood flow. Going back to the idea of the protons being heated up by the RF pulse, this process can be thought of as the protons getting back to thermal equilibrium with the lattice, which has a much higher heat capacity due to its larger volume. As the protons lose the extra energy from the RF pulse, they gradually return to the equilibrium populations in the spin-up and spin-down states, so that eventually the magnetization along the z axis is back to M_0. This is known as spin-lattice relaxation, characterized by the spin-lattice relaxation time T_1. Unlike T_2, T_1 changes with field strength, getting longer as the field strength increases, and in human tissues T_1 is always longer than T_2. Table 8.1 shows some approximate values at 0.5 T, 1.5 T and 3.0 T (use these with caution, remember that in vivo measurements are often inaccurate).

Since we consider the net magnetization being flipped through 90° by the RF pulse, it is tempting to think of the relaxation processes as simply being the reverse, with M_0 slowly turning through –90° back to its equilibrium position. This would explain the gradual loss of transverse magnetization and recovery of the longitudinal magnetization. However, it would also imply that T_1 and T_2 must be equal to each other, and we know that this is not the case in biological tissues. Many textbooks do not make this clear enough, showing T_1 and T_2 curves without time scales so it is difficult to see that two separate processes are at work. T_2 dephasing happens very quickly, so the transverse magnetization is zero after only a few hundred milliseconds. T_1 relaxation is much slower and it takes several seconds before M_0 is fully restored along the z axis. If we plot both curves on the same graph for a tissue with $T_1 \approx 5 \times T_2$ (figure 8.16) you can see the differences in the time scales for these two processes. Looking at table 8.1 you can see that in most tissues T_1 is several times longer than T_2.

It is better to use a more specific mental picture in which the protons rapidly dephase like a fan opening up in the transverse plane, before folding up slowly towards the z axis like an umbrella closing (see figure 8.17). If you work out the net magnetization in the laboratory frame for this model, it behaves as shown in figure 8.18, and it is important to note that the magnitude of the net magnetization is only equal to the equilibrium

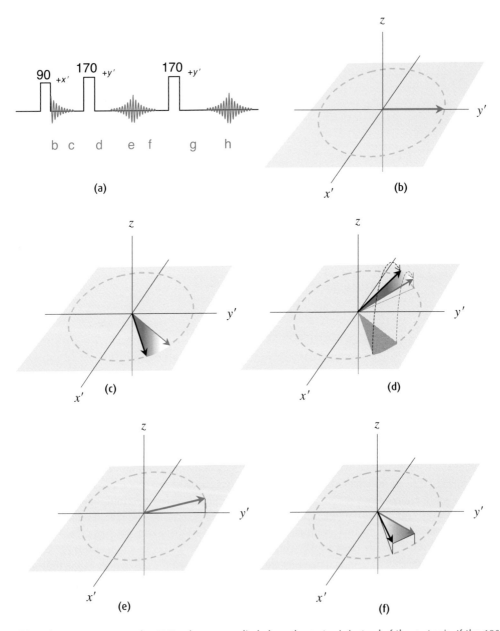

Figure 8.13 (a) In the CPMG sequence, the 180° pulses are applied along the $+y'$ axis instead of the $+x'$ axis. If the 180° pulse is imperfect, e.g. only 170° (c), the first spin echo will rephase above the transverse plane (e), giving a slightly reduced echo height. However, the second 170° brings the spins exactly back to the transverse plane (g) so that the even echoes are always correct (h).

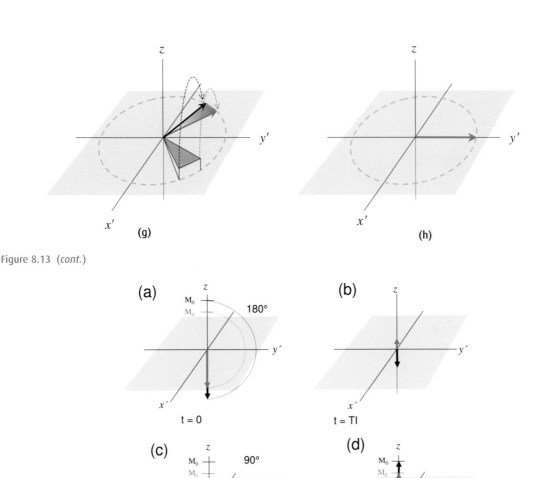

Figure 8.13 (*cont.*)

Figure 8.14 (a) The initial 180° pulse inverts the magnetization, which then starts to recover. (b) When the 90° is applied some of the signals may still be negative, so (c) a mixture of positive and negative echoes will be formed. The TR must always be at least five times the longest T_1 present to allow full relaxation (d).

magnetization immediately after the 90° pulse and after full T_1 relaxation. Compare this with the simplistic idea of M_0 rotating back and forth between the z and y axes, and you will realize that too much simplification can be seriously misleading. Although the full picture takes a bit more effort to think about, it won't let you down!

8.6 Relaxation time mechanisms

The time difference between T_1 and T_2 is extremely important in all MR imaging or spectroscopy. We always use a repeated sequence of RF and gradient pulses, with a repetition time (TR). Consider the simple case of a

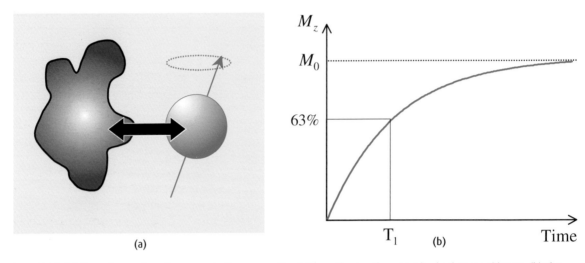

Figure 8.15 (a) The spins can transfer energy to the surrounding lattice, allowing them to relax back to equilibrium. (b) The process is random, so the recovery of M_z to M_0 is controlled by an exponential. T_1 is the time taken for the magnetization to recover to 63% of its equilibrium value.

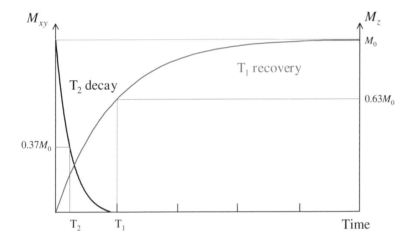

Figure 8.16 T_1 and T_2 relaxation occur simultaneously, but T_2 is much quicker than T_1.

repeated 90°-TR-90°-TR- sequence; if TR is at least five times the longest T_1 of the tissues, all tissues will be back to equilibrium before the next 90° and the signal in the transverse plane will depend only on the proton density. However, if TR is shorter, M_z will not have had sufficient time to grow back to M_0 and a smaller signal will be flipped into the xy plane. (Provided TR is still longer than five times T_2, there will be no transverse

magnetization to confuse the issue. When TR is so short that there is still M_{xy} before the next pulse, there is a more complex situation which will be discussed in chapter 12.) This loss of signal is known as saturation.

To help fix this new picture of relaxation in your mind, let us review the way TR affects T_1 contrast in spin echo images (first discussed in section 3.3), illustrated in figure 8.19. Assuming we start from full relaxation, the

Table 8.1 Selection of T_1 and T_2 values for tissues at 0.5, 1.5 T and 3.0T. All values measured in vivo from human tissues.

Tissue	T_1(ms)			T_2(ms)		
	0.5 T	1.5 T	3.0 T	0.5 T	1.5 T	3.0 T
White matter	520[f]	560[a]	832[i]	107[b]	82[c]	110[i]
Grey matter	780[f]	1100[a]	1331[i]	110[b]	92[c]	80[i]
CSF	–	2060[e]	3700	–	–	–
Muscle	560[g]	1075[d]	898[h]	34[g]	33[g]	29[h]
Fat	192[b]	200[b]	382[h]	108[b]	–	68[h]
Liver	395[b]	570[e]	809[h]	96[b]	–	34[h]
Spleen	760[b]	1025[e]	1328[h]	140[b]	–	61[h]

Notes:

[a] Steinhoff S, Zaitsev M, et al. (2001). Fast T_1 mapping with volume coverage. *Mag Reson Med* **46**: 131–40.

[b] Bottomley PA, Foster TH, et al. (1984). A review of normal tissue hydrogen NMR relaxation times and relaxation mechanisms from 1–100 MHz: dependence on tissue type, NMR frequency, temperature, species, excision and age. *Med Phys* **11**: 425–48.

[c] Pfefferbaum A, Sullivan EV, et al. (1999). Brain gray and white matter transverse relaxation time in schizophrenia. *Psychiat Res* **91**: 93–100.

[d] Venkatesan R, Lin W, et al. (1998). Accurate determination of spin-density and T_1 in the presence of RF field inhomogeneities and flip-angle miscalibration. *Mag Reson Med* **40**: 592–602

[e] Bluml S, Schad LR, et al. (1993). Spin-lattice relaxation time measurement by means of a TurboFLASH technique. *Mag Reson Med* **30**: 289–95.

[f] Imran J, Langevin F, et al. (1999). Two-point method for T_1 estimation with optimised gradient-echo sequence. *Magn Reson Imag* **17**: 1347–56.

[g] de Certaines JD, Henrikson O, et al. (1993). In vivo measurements of proton relaxation times in human brain, liver, and skeletal muscle: a multi-center MRI study. *Magn Reson Imag* **11**: 841–50.

[h] de Bazelaire CM, Duhamel GD, *et al* (2004). MR imaging relaxation times of abdominal and pelvic tissues measured in vivo at 3.0 T: preliminary results. *Radiology* **230**: 652–9.

[i] Wansapura JP, Holland SK, *et al* (1999). NMR relaxation times in the human brain at 3.0 tesla. *J Magn Reson Imaging* **9**: 531–8.

initial 90° pulse rotates all the longitudinal magnetization into the transverse plane. After the spin echo has been formed, T_2 decay continues while M_z grows in the z direction – the black vector has a longer T_1 than the blue one, so it recovers more slowly. When the second 90° pulse is applied, provided $TR > 5 \times T_2$, M_{xy} is zero, but T_1 recovery is not complete. Only the z magnetizations will be flipped into the transverse plane to create signal for the next echo. Both M_z go back to zero and begin to relax back to equilibrium again. After a further TR, both vectors have recovered to exactly the same amount, so the third and all subsequent excitations create a steady signal height which is T_1-weighted.

Strictly speaking, a dummy excitation is needed for a spin echo sequence to reach the steady state. However the normal linear phase encoding scheme means that the first echo does not affect contrast in the final image, so it is rarely done in practice. Gradient echo sequences are another matter, the number of pulses needed to reach a steady state depends on TR and the flip angle as well as the relaxation times of the tissues.

In this section we will consider the interactions between protons and their environment which cause spin-spin and spin-lattice relaxation. Much of our understanding of relaxation is based on work published in 1948 by Bloembergen, Purcell and Pound which is usually known as the BPP theory of relaxation. To understand this you must be familiar with the concept of molecular motions: every atom or molecule is rotating, vibrating and translating (i.e. moving from one position to another) in random directions. Not only that, molecules change their motion rapidly, so they will be vibrating one second and rotating the next, because they collide with each other. Actually a molecule spends only a tiny fraction of a second in a particular state of motion, as little as 10^{-12} s, before suffering a collision which changes its motion to something different. This is known as the correlation time τ_c of the molecule, and if you use the standard idea of gases, liquids and solids you will be able to imagine that solids tend to have very long correlation times (molecules are closely packed together and move slowly), while gases at the other extreme have shorter τ_c (molecules are further apart and move quicker). τ_c is also affected by

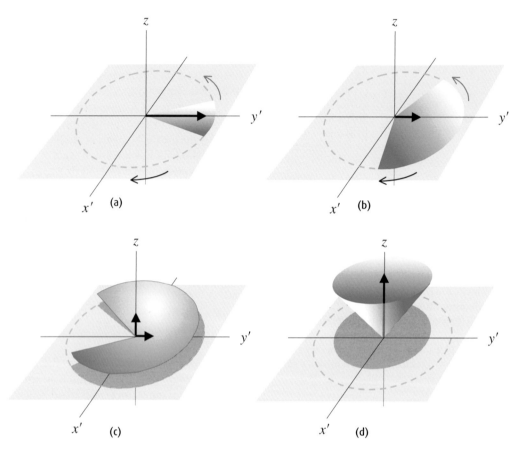

Figure 8.17 T_2 relaxation causes rapid fanning out of the protons in the transverse plane (a) and (b). T_1 is much slower, and can be thought of as an umbrella closing up (c) and (d).

temperature, with higher temperatures giving shorter correlation times.

In biological systems, water is rarely a free liquid except in CSF or blood. Large molecules such as polysaccharides and proteins form hydration layers, layers of water molecules which are closely bound to the surface of the larger molecule. There is believed to be a continuum of 'binding' from the tightly bound protons close to the surface to the 'free' protons furthest away from large molecules. In addition, protons do not stay in one place but are freely exchanged between different environments leading to a mixing of bound and free protons' properties.

8.6.1 Spin-lattice relaxation

We know that an RF pulse on average promotes protons from the low energy state to the high energy state causing a net absorption of energy. T_1 relaxation is the loss of the extra energy from the spin system to the surrounding environment, or 'lattice' (hence 'spin-lattice' relaxation time). However, the high energy state is a stable position for the proton and it does not return to the lower state spontaneously but requires an external stimulating field. Since the external B_1 field has been switched off, where does this field come from? As we have hinted in the previous section, it comes from

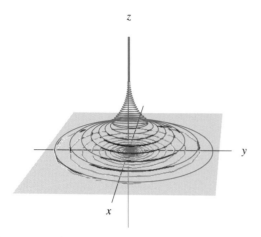

Figure 8.18 Relaxation as viewed from the laboratory (fixed) frame of reference. The vector sum of magnetization after a 90° pulse does not equal M_0 at all times.

neighbouring protons or other nuclei or molecules, which have magnetic moments. In water the nearest adjacent nucleus will be the other hydrogen atom on the same molecule. Therefore, relaxation will primarily arise through the magnetic moment that one hydrogen nucleus 'sees' as it tumbles relative to the moment of the other hydrogen nucleus. This is often called an intra-molecular dipole-dipole interaction (a dipole is simply a magnetic field with two poles, north and south – another term for a magnetic moment).

We have already seen that molecules have a range of motional frequencies, the spectral density function. So the magnetic moments of these molecules will also have a frequency distribution. In order to induce the transitions needed for T_1 relaxation the fluctuations have to be at the Larmor frequency, in the same way that the external B_1 field has to fluctuate at the Larmor

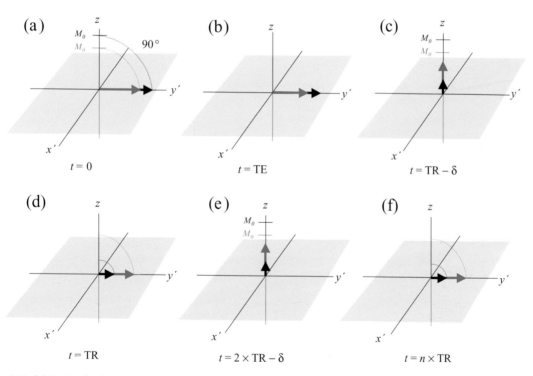

Figure 8.19 (a) During the first 90° pulse, both M_0 are rotated into the tranverse plane, producing M_{xy} (b). (c) After $5 \times T_2$, M_{xy} has decayed to zero while M_z recovers from zero with T_1 relaxation. When the second 90° pulse is applied after time TR, (d) reduced signals are rotated into the transverse plane. (e) After another TR, both M_z have recovered to the same height as before, so the third 90° pulse creates the same T_1-weighted signal in the transverse plane (f).

The Bloch equations

Bloch derived a set of differential equations which describe the changes in the magnetization during excitation and relaxation. They are sometimes called 'phenomenological' because they adequately describe what is detected in the receiver coil. Note that they are based entirely on classical mechanics. We start with

$$\frac{d\mathbf{M}}{dt} = \gamma \mathbf{M} \times \mathbf{B} = \gamma \begin{bmatrix} (M_y B_z - M_z B_y)\mathbf{i} \\ + (M_z B_x - M_x B_z)\mathbf{j} \\ + (M_x B_y - M_y B_x)\mathbf{k} \end{bmatrix}$$

We use a general expression for $\mathbf{B}$ which includes a static field along z and a second field rotating in the transverse plane

$$B_x = B_1 \cos \omega t \qquad B_y = B_1 \sin \omega t \qquad B_z = B_0$$

and add terms which account for the observed relaxations T_1 and T_2, giving

$$\frac{dM_x}{dt} = \gamma(M_y B_0 + M_z B_1 \sin \omega t) - \frac{M_x}{T_2}$$

$$\frac{dM_y}{dt} = \gamma(M_x B_1 \cos \omega t - M_x B_0) - \frac{M_y}{T_2}$$

$$\frac{dM_z}{dt} = \gamma(M_x B_1 \sin \omega t + M_y B_1 \cos \omega t) - \frac{M_z - M_0}{T_1}$$

These can then be solved with appropriate limiting conditions; for example, immediately after the RF pulse is switched off, $B_1 = 0$ and the solutions are

$$M_x(t) = [M_x(0)\cos \omega_0 t + M_y(0)\sin \omega_0 t] \cdot \exp\left(\frac{-t}{T_2}\right)$$

$$M_y(t) = [M_y(0)\cos \omega_0 t - M_x(0)\sin \omega_0 t] \cdot \exp\left(\frac{-t}{T_2}\right)$$

$$M_z(t) = M_z(0)\exp\left(\frac{-t}{T_1}\right) + M_0\left[1 - \exp\left(\frac{-t}{T_1}\right)\right]$$

If the system was initially in equilibrium and the RF pulse was a 90° pulse applied along the $+x'$ axis, $M_x(0) = M_z(0) = 0$ and $M_y(0) = M_0$, giving the results

$$M_x(t) = M_0 \sin \omega_0 t \cdot \exp\left(\frac{-t}{T_2}\right) \qquad M_y(t) = M_0 \cos \omega_0 t \cdot \exp\left(\frac{-t}{T_2}\right) \qquad M_z(t) = M_0\left[1 - \exp\left(\frac{-t}{T_1}\right)\right]$$

In complex notation this is

$$M_{xy}(t) = M_0 \exp(i\omega_0 t) \cdot \exp\left(\frac{-t}{T_2}\right) \qquad M_z(t) = M_0\left[1 - \exp\left(\frac{-t}{T_1}\right)\right]$$

This tells us that the x and y magnetizations oscillate at the Larmor frequency while decaying with time constant T_2, while the z magnetization simply grows from zero back to M_0.

The spectral density function and water binding
Statistical methods can be used to show that a collection of molecules with an average correlation time τ_c will have a range of motional frequencies described by something called the spectral density function $J(\omega)$. This simply shows the number of nuclei that tumble at each frequency. Figure 8.20 shows $J(\omega)$ for three materials with long, medium and short τ_c. Long τ_cs mean that molecules spend a relatively long time in a particular motional state before suffering a collision, and we can see that most of the motional frequencies are very low. With the shorter τ_cs molecules are highly mobile and are changing their motional states with high frequencies. Notice that the Larmor frequency of most clinical MR systems, tens of MHz, is in the middle of the frequency range. We will come back to spectral density functions in the next two sections.

frequency. So we can predict that the more protons that tumble near the Larmor frequency the more efficient the T_1 relaxation will be. For example, more protons with intermediate binding tumble at the Larmor frequency than protons in either free fluids or bound in hydration layers. Hence the T_1s of such protons are short while both bound and free protons have long T_1s. The spectral density function also predicts that T_1 is frequency dependent, since a decrease in the strength of the static magnetic field will decrease the Larmor frequency. There will be more protons tumbling at the new lower Larmor frequency so the T_1 will be shorter.

8.6.2 Spin-spin relaxation

We know that T_2 relaxation arises from the exchange of energy between spins, hence the term 'spin-spin relaxation'. No energy is actually lost from the spin system but the decay of transverse magnetization arises from the loss of phase coherence between spins, which arises from magnetic field inhomogeneities. These

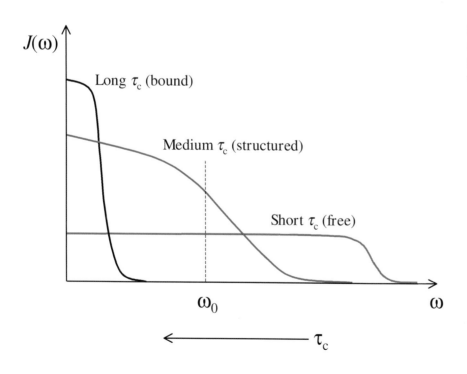

Figure 8.20 Spectral density functions $J(\omega)$ for three substances with varying correlation times τ_c

inhomogeneities may be either intrinsic or extrinsic, i.e. internal to the proton system or external in the scanner. Only the intrinsic inhomogeneities contribute to T_2.

Our description of molecular motions can also be used to describe the mechanism of T_2 relaxation. When molecules are tumbling very rapidly (i.e. free protons with short τ_c) then a particular dipole will see the local magnetic field as fluctuating very rapidly and effectively averaging out over a few milliseconds. This results in a relatively homogeneous local field and little dephasing, and is sometimes termed 'motional averaging'. Conversely a slowly tumbling molecule (bound protons close to large molecules) will see a relatively static magnetic field inhomogeneity and will be more effectively dephased with respect to other protons.

In terms of the spectral density function, we see that T_2 is affected by low-frequency motions as well as those at the Larmor frequency (for comparison T_1 is only affected by Larmor frequency fluctuations). Bound protons have very short T_2 values, so short that even at the shortest echo times we can use in MRI their signals are completely decayed to zero. Free protons in bulk fluids have the longest T_2s while those with intermediate binding have medium T_2 relaxation times.

8.6.3 BPP theory for body tissues

We can summarize the BPP relaxation theory in terms of three tissue types. Let us start with water molecules that are essentially 'free' in solution, e.g. CSF, in which there is a reasonably uniform number of protons tumbling over a wide range of frequencies. There is only a small number tumbling at the Larmor frequency so T_1 relaxation is relatively inefficient, i.e. T_1 relaxation times are long. Similarly there is only a small number tumbling at very low frequencies; therefore, T_2 relaxation is also inefficient, i.e. T_2 relaxation times are long.

If we now consider water molecules that are 'bound' to larger macromolecules through the formation of a hydration layer, e.g. myelin, then there are a large number of protons tumbling at very low frequencies because their motion is restricted by the binding. In this case T_2 relaxation is very efficient (very short T_2s) and T_1 relaxation very inefficient (long T_1s). In fact the T_2

relaxation times are so short that these molecules are 'invisible' with conventional MR imaging equipment, because by the time we collect echoes at even the shortest echo times their signals have fully decayed.

The third case to consider is when a proton is in the intermediate situation between bound and free, this is sometimes termed 'structured'. Now there are a large number of protons tumbling at the Larmor frequency and T_1 relaxation will be the most efficient. T_2 relaxation will be intermediate between bound (short T_2) and free (long T_2). Most body tissues are in the structured water category. Lipids are a special case: due to the much larger size of unbound lipid molecules, their protons intrinsically tumble at lower frequencies, i.e. more tumble at the Larmor frequency and they therefore have short T_1 relaxation times.

Exchanging protons

In describing relaxation mechanisms in this way we have ignored the fact that in reality water molecules are in fast exchange between the three states, i.e. over the time scale of an MRI scan a water proton will wander between bound, structured and free tissues. The proportion of time spent in each state will, in effect, be the same as the proportion of water in each state. The observed relaxation time is therefore a weighted-mean of the relaxation time of each fraction

$$\frac{1}{T_1^{obs}} = \frac{F^{bound}}{T_1^{bound}} + \frac{F^{struct}}{T_1^{struct}} + \frac{F^{free}}{T_1^{free}}$$

T_1^{bound} is very long, so only a small fraction of tissue water needs to be in the bound compartment to reduce the observed T_1. A similar equation can be written for observed T_2s. Whilst the bound compartment cannot be directly observed, it may however be investigated using magnetization transfer techniques (see section 8.7.4). Water binding is not the only mechanism to affect relaxation in tissues. The presence of paramagnetic material, either intrinsic (blood breakdown products) or extrinsic (exogenous contrast agents such as gadolinium), can have a profound effect on observed relaxation times as we will see in section 8.8.

8.7 Measuring relaxation times in vivo

One of the original ambitions of early MRI researchers was to characterize normal tissues and pathologies on the basis of relaxometry (the measurement of relaxation times), preferably in vivo. This has not proved possible for a number of reasons outlined below.

8.7.1 Biological variability

The basic reason is that there is substantial overlap of T_1 and T_2 values due to biological variability. For example, in the brain, grey and white matter have quite distinct T_1 and T_2 from each other and from CSF, and this makes for very good anatomical imaging. When we look at various brain lesions, e.g. astrocytomas, glioblastomas, infarction and multiple sclerosis plaques, they all have T_2 in a narrow range 170–200 ms, very distinct from white and grey matter (90–100 ms), but not uniquely distinctive from each other. The hope for MRI to be able to determine the type and grade of tumours on the basis of relaxometry is therefore unfounded. MRI is very sensitive but less specific, unless other features of the images are taken into consideration, e.g.contrast uptake, presence or absence of oedema, extent of vascularity, blood breakdown products.

8.7.2 Multi-exponential behaviour and tissue mixing

In our simplified view we have considered tissues to have a single T_1 or T_2 value. In practice the situation is usually more complex. Tissues contain a mixture of components, including the microvascular space, interstitial space and parenchymal cells. The microscopic relaxation behaviour of each of these may be distinct and thus the relaxation behaviour we observe may be a weighted average of these, as already described in the box 'Exchanging protons'. As well as the microscopic compartments, there is often a mixture of tissue types within a voxel due to the relatively low resolution of MR images, and multi-exponential behaviour may be apparent.

8.7.3 Field strength and temperature dependence

T_1 displays a marked dependence upon field strength B_0. A review of published data reveals the approximate mathematical relationship

$$T_1 \propto B_0^b$$

where the constant b lies in the range 0.3–0.4. Since there are many different field strengths commercially available, it has proved difficult to directly compare relaxation measurements from different sites. In comparison T_2 is broadly independent of B_0.

T_1 relaxation times are also strongly temperature dependent, although this should not present a major problem for in vivo measurements, as most tissues will be in the narrow temperature range 32–37 °C. However, it does make it very difficult to compare these measurements with in vitro relaxometry. The changes in T_1 with temperature can be exploited in MR thermometry; for example, in interventional MR for monitoring hyperthermia and thermal ablation therapies.

8.7.4 Magnetization transfer and J coupling

Magnetization transfer (MT) provides an additional source of contrast for certain tissues. A physical explanation is given in the box 'Getting bound up: MT explained'. MT can be exploited in imaging to reduce the intensity of certain tissues and improve the contrast in images. Table 8.2 gives examples of the degrees of attenuation achievable in this way. Fluids, including CSF and flowing blood, fat and bone marrow are unaffected. A major application for MT contrast (MTC) is for background suppression in time-of-flight angiography (see chapter 13).

Table 8.2 Magnetization transfer contrast (MTC) attenuation

Tissue	Signal reduction (%)
Muscle	50–80
Hyaline cartilage	50–75
White matter	40–70
Grey matter	40–50
Liver	40
Kidney	30

Getting bound up: MT explained

MT contrast occurs where there is fast exchange between bound and free protons. The bound or restricted protons are those associated with macro-molecules or hydration layers. This restricted pool has a very short T_2 and is invisible to direct imaging.

However, it can influence the observed MR signal through the exchange of energy (magnetization) between the two 'pools' (see figure 8.21). The bound pool has a broad resonance and therefore can be excited by an RF pulse at a frequency several kilo-hertz away from the free water frequency, which therefore has no effect on the free protons. Exchange of protons between the bound and free pools means that saturated magnetization from the (invisible) bound pool will move into the free pool, thus reduc-ing the total MR signal that can be observed.

J coupling is an interaction between the hydrogen nuclei on neighbouring atoms, which causes a splitting of the resonance peak. It is particularly important in fat molecules that contain long chains of carbon atoms. If the protons are saturated, usually by repeated RF pulses at relatively short TRs, they become decoupled and the split peak collapses to a single peak. The single peak has a higher amplitude and is narrower than the split peak, corresponding to a longer T_2. The difference between J-coupled and J-decoupled signals can be seen by com-paring fast spin echo (FSE) T_2-weighted images to conventional spin-echo (SE) T_2-weighted images. The FSE images have brighter fat signals than they should because the protons are decoupled and their T_2 is apparently lengthened. In the conventional SE images, J coupling in the lipids reduces their T_2 and they have a darker appearance.

8.7.5 Sources of error in in vivo relaxometry

Apart from all these problems, there are still others which introduce significant errors in in vivo relaxome-try. These include poor sequence parameter choice, particularly too short a TR for the PD-weighted image, inhomogeneous RF pulses, unwelcome MTC effects in multiple-slice acquisitions arising from selective

(therefore off-resonance) pulses intended for other slices, and slice profile distortions. Some can be cor-rected by acquiring only a single slice, but all in all there are too many problems to make the routine measure-ment of T_1 and T_2 a useful clinical tool.

8.8 Contrast agent theory

Now that you have a good idea of the relaxation mech-anisms in MR, it is time to look more closely at the effect of exogenous contrast agents such as gadolinium and iron oxides. You should already know that gadolinium is a paramagnetic element, while the iron oxides are known as superparamagnetic. Both of them become quite strongly magnetized when placed in a magnetic field, whereas most body tissues are diamagnetic and only become weakly magnetized.

8.8.1 Gadolinium contrast agents

Gadolinium has seven unpaired electrons in its elec-tronic structure and consequently has strong paramag-netic properties. It is toxic in its elemental state, but it can be chelated to a ligand such as diethylene-triamine penta-acetic acid (DTPA, as in Magnevist® by Schering). You can think of these complexes as safe chemical 'wrappers' around the gadolinium atom which elimi-nate toxicity but preserve its paramagnetic properties. When a gadolinium contrast agent is injected into the body, it is distributed via the vasculature to all perfused tissues. Although it is too large a molecule to cross the blood–brain barrier quickly, it does slowly leak out into the brain tissues, and rapidly accumulates in lesions where the blood–brain barrier is disrupted. In most other organs it passes from the vasculature into the interstitial space relatively quickly. After the initial redistribution into the extracellular fluid space with a half-life of about 11 min, gadolinium is gradually excreted via the kidneys with a biological half-life of approximately 90 min, so in most patients it is not detectable in tissues after about 6 h although it may linger in the urine and bladder for a day.

The effect of the strongly paramagnetic gadolinium is to decrease T_2 and T_1 relaxation times of protons in the

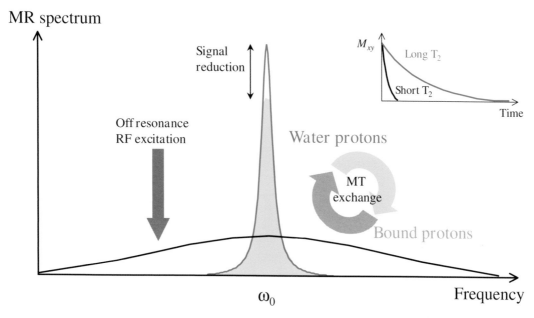

Figure 8.21 Magnetization transfer between bound and free protons. The free protons have long T_2 and the bound protons have a short T_2, as shown in the inset. The bound protons are not normally 'visible' in the image.

immediate vicinity of the molecule. In this respect gadolinium behaves just like any magnetic field inhomogeneity but acting over a very small distance not much larger than the complex itself. As these protons exchange with other protons (see section 8.6) further away from the gadolinium complex there is an overall reduction of T_1 and T_2. At low concentrations such as those used in normal clinical practice the major effect is the T_1 shortening (see figure 8.22), and tissues which take up the agent have an enhanced signal intensity on T_1-weighted images. Many studies have been performed to find the optimum dose for various conditions, but most clinical sites use a standard dose of 10 or 15 ml for adult patients, which approximates to 0.1 mmol Gd per kilogram of body weight (known as single dose). Doses for children should always be adjusted based on the child's weight. Double and even triple dose injections are routinely used for MR angiography, viability and perfusion imaging and have been shown to improve the conspicuity of lesions in multiple sclerosis and metastatic disease. At concentrations higher than about 1 mmol Gd kg⁻¹, ten times the standard dose, the

effect on T_2 begins to dominate and a loss of signal occurs (see figure 8.22).

There are several different formulations available commercially with various osmolalities and safety profiles. In general gadolinium is a safe drug well tolerated by subjects, with only a handful of serious adverse effects noted in the literature. The only absolute contraindication to using gadolinium is in pregnant patients. This is because the gadolinium crosses the placenta into the fetal circulation and gets excreted into the amniotic fluid where it will linger for the entire remaining duration of the pregnancy. Gadolinium also crosses into breast milk, so lactating mothers are also contraindicated, or should not breastfeed for 24 h following gadolinium administration. Full details of contraindications and clinical applications can be found on the information insert in any preparation of gadolinium.

8.8.2 Iron oxide contrast agents

Iron oxides have much stronger paramagnetism than gadolinium, and are injected as carbohydrate-coated

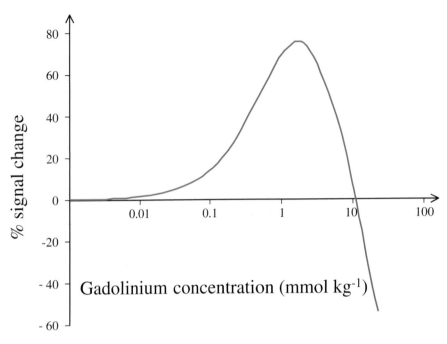

Figure 8.22 Signal intensity versus concentration of gadolinium, calculated using a T_1-weighted SE sequence (TR = 400 ms, TE = 15 ms) and a tissue with T_1 = 800 ms and T_2 = 75 ms.

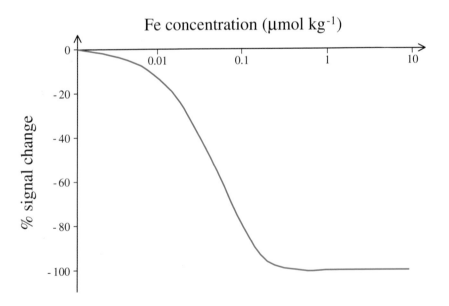

Figure 8.23 Signal intensity versus concentration of Fe, calculated using a T_2-weighted spin-echo sequence (TR = 10000 ms, TE = 100 ms) and a tissue with T_1 = 800 ms and T_2 = 75 ms.

particles in a solution such as mannitol. They are usually known by the acronym SPIO (**S**uper**P**aramagnetic **I**ron **O**xide). Like gadolinium agents they are distributed by the circulation and are

taken up preferentially by Kupffer cells in the liver and spleen. They tend to be rather less well tolerated than gadolinium contrast agents and licensing of the drugs was initially rather slow due to reports of serious

Contrast agent relaxivity

The effect of contrast agents on tissue relaxation times is best described using relaxation rates rather than times. The relaxation rate is simply the inverse of the relaxation time, so we can define

$$R_1 = \frac{1}{T_1} \qquad R_2 = \frac{1}{T_2} \qquad R_2^* = \frac{1}{T_2^*}$$

Relaxation rates are additive, so for example we can redefine the effective transverse relaxation rate as

$$R_2^* = R_2 + \frac{1}{2}\gamma\Delta B_0$$

For contrast agents we can define a specific relaxivity, which describes how much they change relaxation rates per molar concentration. Multiplying the specific relaxivity by the concentration in a particular tissue gives the increase in relaxation rate caused by the contrast agent, so the new relaxation rate will be

$$R' = R + rC$$

The relaxivity r may be different for longitudinal and transverse relaxation rates (usually denoted r_1 and r_2 respectively), but in the case of gadolinium they are approximately the same, 4 and 5 $\text{mmol}^{-1}\,\text{s}^{-1}$ respectively. Thus at a concentration of 0.1 mmol kg^{-1} in a tissue with a T_1 of 700 ms and T_2 of 75 ms, we can calculate the new relaxation times

$$R_1' = R_1 + r_1 C = \frac{1}{0.700} + 4 \cdot 0.1 = 1.828 \Rightarrow T_1' = \frac{1}{1.828} = 0.547$$

$$R_2' = R_2 + r_2 C = \frac{1}{0.075} + 5 \cdot 0.1 = 13.833 \Rightarrow T_2' = \frac{1}{13.833} = 0.072$$

As you can see, at this concentration the biggest effect is the reduction of T_1 from 700 ms to 547 ms, whereas T_2 only changes from 75 to 72 ms. We say that the relaxation rate due to the gadolinium dominates the T_1, while for transverse relaxation the normal T_2 is the dominant relaxation rate.

The relaxivity of iron oxides is much higher and quite different for R_1 and R_2; for example, 25 $\text{mmol}^{-1}\,\text{s}^{-1}$ and 165 $\text{mmol}^{-1}\,\text{s}^{-1}$ respectively (Resovist®, Schering). A concentration of 0.1 mmol kg^{-1} in tissue causes a significant drop in both T_1 and T_2

$$R_1' = R_1 + r_1 C = \frac{1}{0.700} + 25 \cdot 0.1 = 3.929 \Rightarrow T_1' = \frac{1}{3.929} = 0.255$$

$$R_2' = R_2 + r_2 C = \frac{1}{0.075} + 165 \cdot 0.1 = 29.833 \Rightarrow T_2' = \frac{1}{29.833} = 0.034$$

However, for a given TR and TE, the transverse relaxation effect dominates (see figure 8.23) and therefore signals are reduced. Notice that although SPIOs are injected at low concentrations of about 10 $\mu\text{mol Fe kg}^{-1}$, the concentration in the liver and spleen is much higher because the Kupffer cells take up the iron preferentially. Abnormalities are left relatively enhanced, making them easier to detect. Unlike gadolinium, different SPIO formulations vary considerably in their uptake and relaxivities, depending on the size of the particles.

adverse effects. Most of these problems have now been resolved and iron oxides are recommended for clinical applications including focal and diffuse liver disease and to evaluate lymph nodes.

The iron particles are many times bigger than gadolinium complexes, typically between 50 and 150 nm in diameter. The magnetic field from such a particle is significant and creates a large inhomogeneity when the agent is injected into the body. Like any inhomogeneity they increase the dephasing rate of protons, reducing T_2^* as well as T_2 and T_1. The effect of the inhomogeneity extends over a volume many times larger than the particle size, in contrast to gadolinium which has a very localized effect on protons. Thus very low concentrations are sufficient to cause a reduction of intensity in tissues which take up the agent on either T_2- or T_2^*-weighted images. Increased doses are not useful, as T_2 gets too short to provide a signal, and the optimum dose is 8–16 µmol Fe kg^{-1} body weight. The T_1 effect can also be seen but is rather less useful in liver scanning. This is because normal tissues take up the agent, so abnormalities become relatively enhanced only in T_2 or T_2^*-weighted scans. (It is generally easier to spot a bright object on a dark background than the other way round.)

See also:

- Image contrast: chapter 3
- Quality control: chapter 11
- In vivo spectroscopy: chapter 15

FURTHER READING

Abragam A (1983) *The Principles of Nuclear Magnetism.* Oxford: Clarendon Press (ISBN: 019852014X), Chapters I, II & III.

Bernstein MA, King KF and Zhou XJ (2004) *Handbook of MRI Pulse Sequences.* London: Elsevier Academic Press (ISBN: 0120928612), Chapters 4 & 6.

Elster AD and Burdette J (2001) *Questions and Answers in Magnetic Resonance Imaging,* 2nd edn. London: Mosby-Yearbook (ISBN: 0323011845), Chapter 2.

Farrar TC and Becker ED (1971) *Pulse and Fourier Transform NMR: Introduction to Theory and Methods.* New York: Academic Press (ISBN: 0122496507), Chapters 1, 2 & 4.

Haacke EM, Brown RW, Thompson MR and Venkatesan R (1999) *Magnetic Resonance Imaging: Physical Principles and Sequence Design.* London: Wiley-Liss (ISBN: 0471351288), Chapters 2–6 & 8.

Kuperman V (2000) *Magnetic Resonance Imaging: Physical Principles and Applications.* New York: Academic Press (ISBN: 0124291503), Chapters 1 & 4.

Let's talk technical: MR equipment

9.1 Introduction

At the start of this book we said that you do not need to understand the workings of the internal combustion engine to be able to drive a car. However, if you're curious, this chapter provides an opportunity to get down and dirty with the innards of the equipment. The basic components of an MRI scanner were introduced in chapter 2. By now you will be familiar with many aspects of MR hardware, especially the use of various coils. In this chapter we provide more technical information. A lot of the detail is in the advanced topics boxes, as many of you will not be especially interested in the engineering and only need a basic understanding. In particular we will see that:

- Magnets for clinical MRI are available with field strengths from approximately 0.2 T to 3 T with even higher field magnets constructed for research purposes. In general higher field strengths give a better signal-to-noise ratio (SNR). Magnets can be classified as either open or closed systems depending on the ease of patient access.
- Four major types of magnets are used in MRI: air-cored resistive magnets, iron-cored electromagnets, permanent magnets and superconducting magnets. Each has advantages and disadvantages in terms of cost, ease of siting, patient and physician friendliness and image quality.
- The main design criteria for the magnetic field gradients are the maximum amplitude and rise time together with good linearity over the imaging field of view. The gradient system should also minimize the

effects of eddy currents that can be induced in the magnet.
- The radiofrequency transmission system needs to produce a uniform excitation within the patient. Techniques such as quadrature excitation can reduce the specific absorption rate (SAR) of the radiofrequency energy.
- For signal reception, coils that closely match the anatomy of interest maximize sensitivity and minimize noise. Phased array coils enable high SNR for large fields of view. Digital signal processing can also improve SNR and help avoid image artefacts.
- Multiple computers within the MRI system synchronize the operation of the various sub-systems and perform the necessary mathematical operations required for image reconstruction.

Figure 9.1 shows the basic architecture of a typical MR system.

9.2 Magnets

The magnet is the main component of the MR system. Due to design constraints the static magnetic field is inherently nonuniform and its homogeneity is optimized by a process known as shimming whereby pieces of steel and/or electrical coils are incorporated into the magnet to improve the uniformity over a given volume. This process is usually performed at system installation; however, many systems give the user limited ability to improve the homogeneity on a per-patient basis during scan set-up. This is particularly important

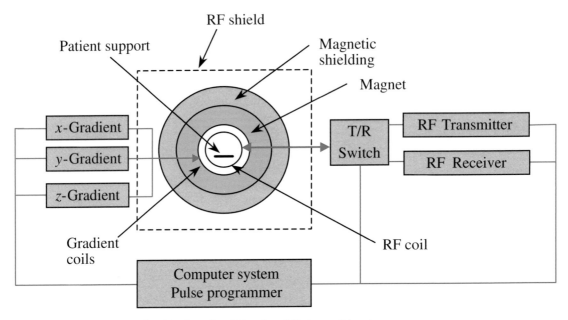

Figure 9.1 Basic components and architecture of an MR system. T/R, transmit/receive.

for techniques such as fat suppression, steady state imaging or spectroscopy. A magnet will also generate a magnetic field outside of the patient aperture. Considerable effort is invested in designing magnets whereby the extent of this fringe field is minimized. However, for some sites additional magnetic field shielding may be required either for safety reasons or to avoid interference with nearby sensitive electronic components.

9.2.1 Field strength

Magnetic field strength (or flux density) is measured in tesla (T). Whole-body magnets have been constructed with field strengths of 0.02–8 T. Typical clinical systems operate in the range of 0.2–3.0 T. Spectroscopy is generally performed at 1.5 T and above. The advantages of higher field strengths are a better SNR (see chapter 11) and increased chemical shift effects, improving spectral fat suppression and spectroscopy. The improvement in SNR with increasing field strength may be traded for increased spatial resolution, or decreased imaging time.

9.2.2 Homogeneity

The homogeneity of a magnetic field is usually expressed in parts per million within a given spherical volume. The size of this volume is given as the diameter of a spherical volume (DSV). For example, a 1.5-T magnet with a maximum variation of 7.5 μT (0.0000075 T) over a 40-cm DSV has an inhomogeneity given by

Inhomogeneity (ppm)

$$= \left(\frac{\text{variation (T)}}{\text{nominal field strength (T)}} \right) \times 10^6$$

$$= \left(\frac{0.000\,0075}{1.5} \right) \times 10^6$$

$$= 5 \text{ ppm}$$

Manufacturers' technical sheets often quote inhomogeneity over a range of different DSVs. Care is required in their interpretation, as these figures may represent only the mean or average inhomogeneity, typically called the root mean square (RMS) value, and not the maximum (peak-to-peak) value which may be considerably more.

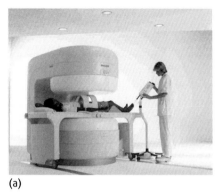
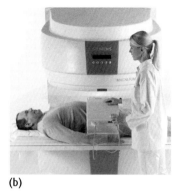
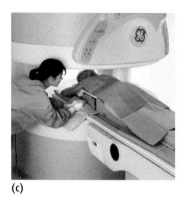

(a)   (b)   (c)

Figure 9.2 Commercial examples of resistive, permanent and superconducting magnets. (a) 0.23 T Philips Panorama, (b) 0.23 T Siemens Magnetom C, (c) 0.7 T General Electric OpenSpeed. All three systems are "open" and have vertical main fields B_0.

9.2.3 Magnet types

There are four main types of MR magnet:
- air-cored resistive magnets;
- iron-cored electromagnets;
- permanent magnets;
- superconducting magnets.

Air-cored resistive magnets were used for the first generation of MRI systems and are now most likely to be found in science museums. An air-cored resistive magnet typically comprises four large coils wound with either copper wire or aluminium bands. An electric current passed through the windings generates a magnetic field up to about 0.2 T. The electrical power (typically 40–100 kW) required to generate the field is dissipated as heat in the windings necessitating water-cooling. The homogeneity is moderate (50–200 ppm over a 50-cm DSV) and stability is largely determined by the thermal properties of the magnet. The magnet may have to be turned off completely or left in stand-by mode to maintain thermal equilibrium. Figure 1.4 shows a very early 0.15 T air-cored resistive magnet.

Iron-cored electromagnets use coils wound around soft iron pole pieces. When an electric current flows through the coils the iron becomes a magnet. The use of iron means that higher magnetic fields can be achieved, e.g. 0.6 T, compared with air-cored magnets. Homogeneity is typically <5 ppm over a 20-cm DSV. These systems tend to be quite heavy due to the large mass of iron required.

Permanent magnets use materials in which large magnetic fields are induced during manufacture. They have maximum field strengths around 0.2–0.3 T and, like electromagnet designs, the field is often orientated vertically (figure 9.2). Installation and running costs are low. It should be remembered that permanent magnets cannot be 'switched off'. A modern commercial permanent magnet system typically has a field strength of 0.2 T with a homogeneity of 40 ppm over a 36-cm DSV and weighs around 9500 kg.

Superconducting magnets use the special properties of certain materials, which at temperatures approaching absolute zero (−273.16°C, 0 K) have zero electrical resistance. An electric current established in a loop of superconducting wire, held below its transition temperature, will therefore continue to circulate indefinitely. Superconducting magnets have the advantages of higher fields, up to approximately 8 T whole-body and considerably higher for smaller bores, together with excellent field uniformity, e.g. 5 ppm over 50 cm DSV at 1.5 T, and stability, e.g. <0.1 ppm h^{-1} and <1000 ppm year^{-1}. A modern superconducting magnet typically weighs 3000–4000 kg inclusive of the cryogens.

Superconducting magnets are usually cylindrical in shape with the patient being placed inside the bore. Although both ends are open, patients may experience claustrophobia from being inside this 'tunnel'. Since the anatomy of interest must be positioned at the centre of the magnet these feelings can be worse for

Design matters 1: permanent and iron-cored electromagnets

Permanent magnets and electromagnets booth utilize magnetic materials to induce the magnetic field. The former is constructed from magnetic materials such as high-carbon iron, in which a large intrinsic magnetic field is induced at the time of manufacture. Permanent magnet designs for MRI typically include a yoke of soft iron, either C-shaped (figure 9.3(a)) or H-shaped (figure 9.3(b)), which is easily magnetizable with a pair of permanent magnets configured as the pole pieces. This generates a homogeneous magnetic field between the pole pieces with most of the magnetic flux carried within the yoke. This design means that the magnetic field is vertical and that stray fields are considerably reduced.

The first whole-body permanent magnets were exceedingly heavy, weighing up to 100 tonnes. More recently permanent magnets that produce higher fields with lower mass (10–16 tonnes) have been constructed using rare-earth alloys such as samarium cobalt ($SmCo_5$) and neodymium-iron-boron (Nd-Fe-B). Permanent magnets obviously have no running costs but have poor thermal stability requiring siting in temperature-controlled rooms. The magnetic field strength of neodymium iron, for example, decreases 1000 ppm for a 1 °C temperature rise. The large mass of the magnet, however, tends to even out fluctuations in the ambient temperature.

Electromagnets are very similar except that they use coils wound around the soft iron pole pieces of the yoke to establish the magnetic field; these obviously require electric current to generate the field between the poles. Since the flux lines are confined within the iron yoke, comparatively small currents can produce relatively high and homogeneous magnetic fields.

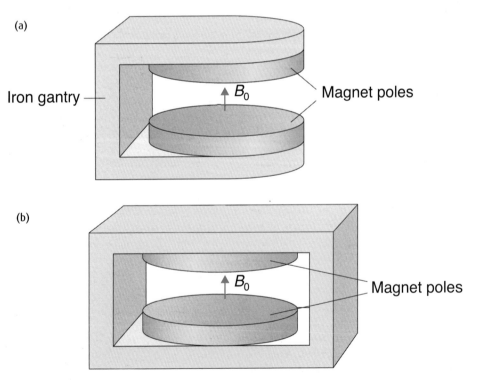

Figure 9.3 Resistive magnet using (a) a C-shaped or (b) an H-shaped core design.

patients having their head scanned compared with, for example, a knee. This has led manufacturers to invest considerable effort in the design of more patient-friendly shorter superconducting magnets. However, these shorter designs tend to compromise field homogeneity.

Whilst electrical power is not required to maintain the field in routine operation it should be noted that the liquid helium coolant slowly boils off, requiring a refill every 3 to 18 months depending on the magnet design and how effectively evaporating helium is recondensed. A cross-section through a typical superconducting magnet is shown in figure 9.4.

9.2.4 Quench

If any part of the windings ceases to be superconducting some of the stored electrical energy will be dissipated as heat. This warms up neighbouring parts of the windings, taking them above their critical temperature, which will in turn dissipate more heat and propagate the effect throughout the magnet. This is known as a 'quench' and results in the collapse of the magnetic field together with very rapid boiling-off of the helium. Magnets incorporate bursting-disks that blow out under high pressure permitting the large volume of gaseous helium to leave the cryostat. Exhaust or quench pipes vent the gas outside the imaging room to prevent asphyxia and cold burns. Oxygen level monitors are sometimes installed in the magnet or technical rooms to alert the users to a dangerous depletion of oxygen should any helium gas leak from the quench pipe. Spontaneous quenches are extremely rare occurrences, but there may be occasions when it is necessary to 'ramp down' the magnet through a controlled quench. In this situation the electrical energy is deposited in a dummy load to avoid damaging the magnet. In either case re-energizing the magnet can be a costly procedure.

9.2.5 Shimming

All magnets suffer from some degree of inhomogeneity as a consequence of design limitations and compromises. Fixed shimming is used to improve the magnet homogeneity and to correct for field distortions

Design matters 2: super cool magnets

Superconducting magnets are constructed from a number of coils, usually from four to eight depending on the required homogeneity. The coils are usually wound from niobium-titanium (NbTi) filaments embedded in a copper matrix. The copper matrix protects the superconducting windings in the event of a quench. The NbTi filaments have a superconducting transition temperature of 7.7 K and become superconducting when immersed in liquid helium (boiling point 4.2 K). A typical superconducting magnet consists of a cryostat, i.e. a large chamber of liquid helium, in which the magnet coils are immersed, surrounded by further vacuum chambers. In early magnets this was followed by a further chamber of liquid nitrogen (77 K) to help reduce the continual boil-off of the expensive helium caused by external thermal energy entering the cryostat.

Modern MRI magnets use cryogenic coolers to reduce boil-off and do not need liquid nitrogen cryostats. Compressed helium gas is circulated around a two-stage 'cold head' mounted on the magnet. Controlled gas expansion is used to cool two thin circumferential aluminium heat-interception shields within the cryostat operating at typically 70 K and 20 K. When the cooling cycle is completed the helium gas is returned to a water-cooled compressor. Depending on their design modern cryo-cooled 1.5-T magnets boil-off helium at a rate of $<0.02\%$ h^{-1} and typically have a capacity of 1200–2000 litres of liquid helium.

Whilst not requiring any external electrical power during normal operation, an external power supply is used when the magnet is first energized or 'ramped' up to the required field strength. A superconducting switch is used to short-circuit the magnet once the desired magnetic field has been established.

The latest development in superconducting magnet technology uses novel materials that have higher transition temperatures and consequently do not require cryogens. The required cooling is provided by a version of the cryo-cooler described above. These magnets however are currently more expensive than conventional superconducting systems, and have not found widespread acceptance.

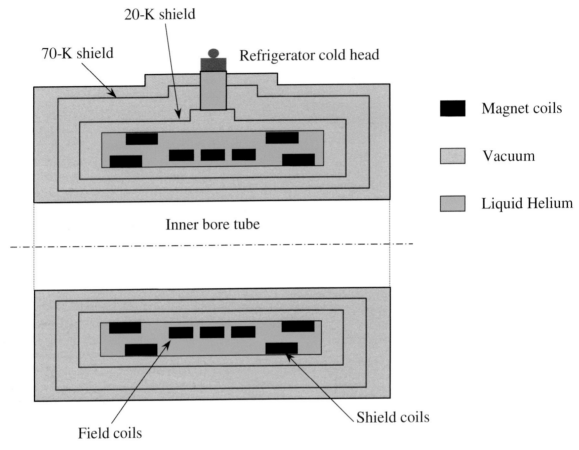

Figure 9.4 Cross-section through a superconducting magnet.

induced by nearby ferromagnetic structures and may be performed either passively, actively, or as a combination of both. The homogeneity achievable using these fixed shims is usually adequate for the purposes of imaging over relatively large volumes. The homogeneity may be further adjusted on a per-patient basis using dynamic shimming.

9.2.6 Shielding

The fringe field from the magnet, especially high-field superconducting systems, extends beyond the magnet in all three directions. Magnetic field shielding reduces this. Self-shielding uses iron plates, either attached to the outside of the cryostat on-site or incorporated into the magnet design. A considerable mass of iron is required to shield the magnet satisfactorily (e.g. 32 000 kg of iron for a 1.5 T magnet). Alternatively the magnet may be positioned inside a free-standing framework to which iron plates are bolted. This framework distributes the weight of the shield over a larger area, but requires more space. Most modern magnets are actively shielded. With active shielding, the superconducting coil winding is continued in the opposite direction outside the inner main magnet winding. This partially cancels the field outside the main magnet coils thereby reducing the stray field strength.

Fixed shimming

Passive shimming involves the positioning of pieces of steel around the magnet, with the amount and position of the steel usually determined by a computer program. Active shimming involves the use of additional coils in which currents of accurately determined magnitude are running. The shim coils in superconducting magnets may also be positioned inside the cryostat, i.e. they are also superconducting. The required currents are determined during system installation and remain fixed until the service engineers re-shim the magnet.

Dynamic shimming

Dynamic shimming may be performed by the user to optimize the homogeneity over a given volume on a per-patient basis. Simple dynamic shimming involves the use of the gradient coils to produce the necessary static magnetic fields to optimize the uniformity. The required gradient magnetic fields are calculated either manually or automatically. In spectroscopy where <0.1 ppm over a 10 ml volume is desirable, the manufacturer may offer an additional set of resistive (i.e. nonsuperconducting) shim coils, which may be manually or automatically adjusted. The usual optimizing techniques are to minimize the line-width of a Fourier-transformed free induction decay (FID) or to analyse phase-difference images.

9.3 Gradients

As we saw in chapter 7 spatial localization of the MR signal requires the use of three orthogonal linear magnetic field gradients. These are generated by gradient coils mounted on a cylindrical former just inside the bore of the magnet. In a standard cylindrical magnet, such as a superconducting system, the direction along the bore is termed the z axis, the left–right direction is termed the x axis and the top–bottom direction is termed the y axis. Although the gradients are oriented in the three orthogonal directions, the gradient magnetic fields themselves are parallel to the main magnetic field B_0. The null point at the centre of the gradient coils, and also the centre of the magnet, is called the isocentre. Gradient pulses in conventional pulse sequences are trapezoidal in shape with a sloping rise, followed by a flat plateau and a sloping fall (figure 9.5). The strength of

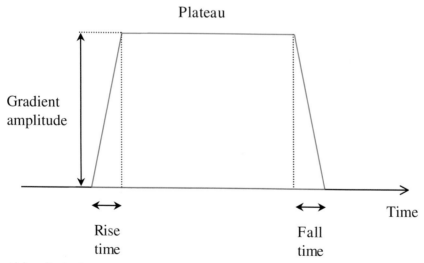

Figure 9.5 Trapezoidal gradient pulse.

the gradient, or how rapidly the field changes over distance, is expressed in millitesla per metre ($mT\,m^{-1}$), with maximum values being in the range of 10–50 $mT\,m^{-1}$. Increasing the maximum gradient amplitude permits images to be acquired with smaller fields of view and thinner slice widths. Large peak gradient amplitudes are also required for some specialist scanning techniques, e.g. diffusion imaging. The gradient rise time, or how rapidly the field changes with time from zero to the peak amplitude, is usually expressed in microseconds (μs), with typical values from 1000 μs down to 200 μs. The gradient slew rate is calculated by dividing the peak gradient amplitude by the rise-time (see 'High slew rates'). Typical slew rates are in the range of 20 to 150 $T\,m^{-1}\,s^{-1}$. High performance gradient coils with high peak amplitudes and short rise times may require cooling, either by forced airflow across the coils or by circulating water or other coolant within the coil assembly.

Gradient amplifiers generate the electrical currents and voltages that need to be applied to the coils to produce the pulsed-gradient magnetic fields. These pulses may also induce *eddy currents* in the surround-

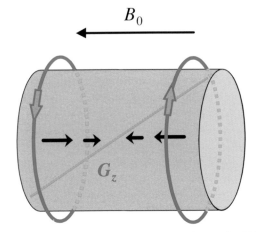

Figure 9.6 Maxwell pair configuration for a longitudinal (z) gradient field.

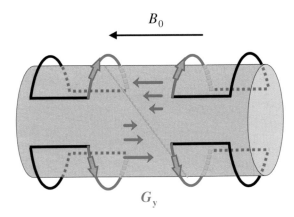

Figure 9.7 Golay coil configuration for transverse (x and y) gradient fields. Only the blue arcs contribute usefully to forming the gradient, which is linear only for a fraction of the length of the coil system.

Z axis gradient

The *z* gradient (G_z) can be generated through the use of a single pair of coils with counter-rotating currents known as a Maxwell pair shown in figure 9.6. The optimum gradient linearity occurs when the coils are separated by $r\sqrt{3}$, where *r* is the coil radius. Other designs can generate *z* gradients with much better radial linearity, e.g. spiral windings with variable pitch along the *z* axis.

X axis and Y axis gradients

G_y can be generated using the Golay configuration shown in figure 9.7 comprising four coils on the surface of the cylindrical former with the currents producing a quadrupolar magnetic field (i.e. one having two North and two South poles). Only the innermost arcs contribute usefully to producing a transverse gradient with the field parallel to B_0. The G_x gradient can be generated using an identical set of Golay coils rotated through $90°$.

ing metallic structures of the magnet, e.g. the metal walls of the cryostat in a superconducting magnet, which can cause artefacts in images unless they are properly controlled.

9.3.1 Gradient linearity

A fundamental specification for a gradient is its linearity. Linear variation in the gradient field is required for

Eddy currents

The rapid switching of the gradients induces eddy currents in nearby conducting components of the magnet cryostat. These persist for varying durations depending on the resistivity of the metal involved. The field generated by the eddy currents combines with the intended gradient field to create waveform distortions, which can result in image artefacts and signal loss.

Eddy current effects can be reduced by deliberately pre-emphasizing the gradient waveforms so that, when combined with the eddy current field, the resultant is close to the ideal gradient waveform (figure 9.8). Pre-emphasis requires extra electronic circuits that add additional voltages, with adjustable amplitudes and time constants, to the gradient driving waveform. Although this method significantly reduces eddy currents it is not totally effective because, in general, the spatial distribution of the eddy current field is not the same as the gradient field.

A better approach is to use active shielding where additional coils surround the gradient coils and are driven with the opposite gradient waveform. This cancels the gradient field outside the shield coils, magnetically isolating the gradients from the cryostat so that eddy currents cannot be induced. However, the shield coils make the entire gradient assembly larger, reducing the free space available inside the bore, and also require more power to generate a given gradient amplitude.

Actively shielded gradients also contribute to reduced superconducting magnet cryostat costs, since there is no longer a need for the large separation between the gradient coils and the first metal wall of the cryostat.

accurate spatial encoding. Linearity is typically 1–2% over a 50-cm DSV. Linearity usually decreases fairly rapidly towards the edge of the imaging volume. The consequence of nonlinearity on an image is misplaced signal and geometric distortion. Figure 9.9(a) shows how the nonlinearity of the gradients can result in geometric distortion of an object. The true edge of the image should be encoded at x_1 but because the actual gradient is non-linear this point gets effectively encoded at x_2, resulting in the object being artificially contracted. Some manufacturers make use of computer algorithms that warp the images after reconstruction to compensate for the gradient nonlinearities. Figure 9.9(b) shows an image with a gradient warp applied; note how the image is stretched at the top and bottom of the field of view.

9.3.2 Gradient amplifiers

High-power audiofrequency amplifiers (similar to those used for high-quality concert sound systems) supply the current required to produce the gradient fields. The requirement for high-peak-gradient amplitudes means that the amplifier must be capable of generating large electrical currents through the coils.

Furthermore, the requirement for short rise and fall times means that this current must be rapidly increased from zero to the maximum and then back down. However, whenever you attempt to change the current flowing through a coil a 'back-emf' is generated. The amplifier therefore needs to generate a sufficient driving voltage to overcome this back-emf. The capacity of the gradient amplifier to generate this voltage limits the slew rate. Since the electrical power required to set up a gradient is proportional to the fifth power of the radius (r^5) of the volume over which the gradient acts, obtaining short rise times with whole-body-sized coils necessitates substantial amplifier capabilities.

9.4 Radiofrequency system

The radiofrequency (RF) system comprises a transmitter, coil and receiver. The purpose of the transmitter is to generate suitably shaped pulses of current at the Larmor frequency. When this current is applied to the coil an alternating B field is produced. The coil will also detect the MR signal from the patient. The frequency-encoding

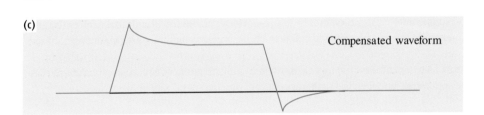

(a)   Ideal gradient waveform

(b)   Actual response due to eddy currents

(c)   Compensated waveform

Figure 9.8 Gradient pulses. (a) Ideal gradient waveform, (b) actual response due to eddy currents and (c) compensated waveform.

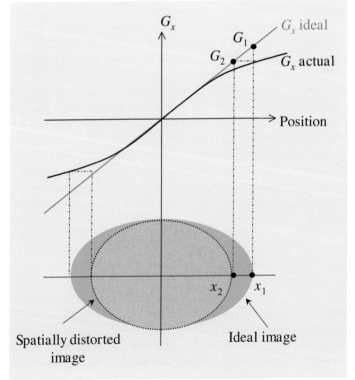

(a)

Spatially distorted image

Ideal image

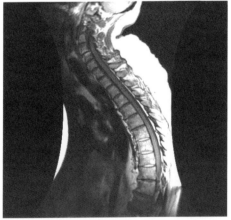

(b)

Figure 9.9 (a) Gradient field nonlinearity and (b) the effects of gradient warping to correct nonlinearities.

High slew rates

High slew rates have not, until relatively recently, been routinely available. This limited the abilities of commercial MRI systems to perform very fast imaging techniques, in particular echo planar imaging (EPI), that require the gradients to be switched very rapidly. In order to overcome this hardware limitation a number of unique approaches have been taken. The first generation of high-performance gradients was based on the principle of resonance. A resonant gradient system makes the gradient coils and their power supply behave as a tuned electrical circuit. The gradient waveforms could therefore be made to oscillate at a very rapid but fixed frequency, e.g. 1 kHz (figure 9.10(a)). Since the frequency and amplitude of the gradient were fixed the spatial resolution was also fixed.

   This limitation drove further research into the development of more flexible technology. The next development, albeit rather short-lived, was the catch-and-hold principle. A catch-and-hold gradient system can momentarily interrupt its resonating and hold a fixed gradient amplitude (plateau) for some period of time (figure 9.10(b)). Modern systems have non-resonant gradient power supplies using conventional gradient amplifiers in combination with unique 'pulse width modulated' (PWM) voltage supplies (figure 9.10(c)). The PWM voltage supply is capable of producing the high voltages required for fast slew rates, whilst a conventional gradient amplifier is used to supply the electric current needed to maintain the flat plateau of the gradient. A typical amplifier could have an efficiency of approximately $10\ \mathrm{mT\ m^{-1}}$ for every 100 A. Therefore, a whole-body gradient coil of 1 m diameter with an inductance of 1 mH switched to its maximum amplitude of $40\ \mathrm{mT\ m^{-1}}$ in a rise-time of 200 μs, would require an amplifier capable of delivering 2000 V at 400 A or 800 kW.

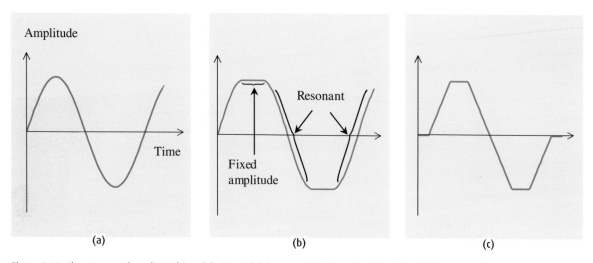

Figure 9.10 Three types of gradient drive: (a) sinusoidal (resonant), (b) catch-and-hold and (c) trapezoidal.

process will result in a narrow range of useful frequencies, e.g. ±16 kHz, centred at the Larmor frequency. It is the function of the receiver to remove, or more correctly demodulate, this ±16 kHz range of interest from the much higher (Larmor frequency) carrier signal.

9.4.1 Transmitter

The transmitter has to generate RF pulses with appropriate centre frequencies, bandwidths, amplitudes and phases in order to excite nuclei within the desired slices

On the air: transmitter theory

As we saw in chapter 7, the slice-selective RF pulse is amplitude modulated by a function $S(t)$ to create a slice. It has a frequency slightly offset from Larmor in order to select the required slice position and may also have a phase angle. The required output is

$$S(t)\cos(\omega_{ss}t+\phi)$$

where

$$\omega_{ss}=\omega_0 \pm \Delta\omega$$

To avoid the possibility of stray RF reaching the receiver coil from the transmitter (and completely bypassing the patient!), its internal frequency source does not operate at the Larmor frequency but at a fixed frequency ω_{fix}. For that reason ω_{ss} is only generated when the RF pulse is about to be applied, by combining a variable offset frequency ω_{off} with the fixed frequency ω_{fix}:

$$\omega_{ss}=\omega_{fix}-\omega_{off}$$
$$\Rightarrow \omega_{off}=\omega_{fix}-\omega_0-\Delta\omega$$

This combination is performed in an electronic 'mixer' that multiplies the two frequencies and generates the sum and difference frequencies, known as side-bands, using the trigonometric identity

$$2\cos(\omega_{fix}t)\cos(\omega_{off}t)=\cos((\omega_{fix}+\omega_{off})t)+\cos((\omega_{fix}-\omega_{off})t)$$

We want the lower side-band at $(\omega_{fix}-\omega_{off})$, and the unwanted side-band at the higher frequency $(\omega_{fix}+\omega_{off})$ is filtered out.

To generate the RF pulse, the transmitter (figure 9.11) takes the digitally generated amplitude-modulation function $S(t)$ and mixes it with the offset frequency ω_{off} and phase ϕ. This waveform is then passed to a digital-to-analogue converter (DAC). The power of this analogue RF pulse coming from the transmitter will only be about 0.1 mW. In order to perturb the spins in a patient this will need to be amplified with high linearity using an RF power amplifier.

or slabs. The slice position and the strength of the slice select gradient at that location determine the centre frequency of the pulse. The bandwidth, or the range of frequencies within the pulse, controls the thickness of the excited slice. The shape and duration of the RF pulse envelope determines the bandwidth. The amplitude of the RF pulse controls how much the magnetization is flipped by the pulse, whilst the phase controls along which axis the magnetization is flipped (in the rotating frame of reference). In modern MRI systems the RF pulse envelope is generated digitally.

9.4.2 Transmit coils

The coils used to excite the MR signal must produce a uniform field B_1 at right angles to the static magnetic field. Transmit coils are usually large to optimize their uniformity, and encompass a significant volume of tissue. A transmit coil may also be used to detect or receive MR signals, provided an appropriate transmit/receive (T/R) switch is used. This protects the receiver circuitry from the very high voltages applied during transmit and also prevents the small NMR signal from being lost in the

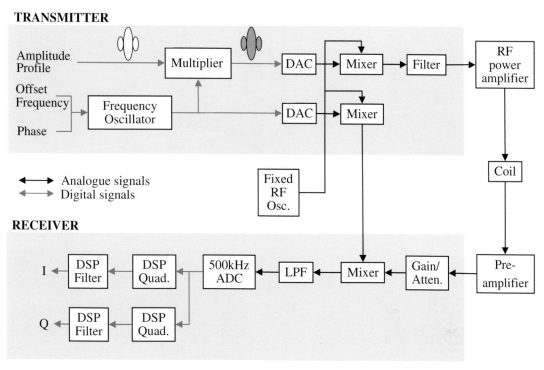

Figure 9.11 Digital radio frequency transceiver. DAC denotes digital-to-analogue converter, ADC, analogue-to-digital converter; LPF, low-pass filter, DSP, digital signal processor. See text for details on the theory of operation. Figure redrawn from Holland GN & MacFall JR (1992) *J Magn Reson Imaging* 2: 241–246.

electronic noise generated by the transmitter even in its off state.

The main transmitting coil is usually the body coil, which surrounds the entire patient. This is usually built into the scanner bore and is not generally visible. Since this coil is large it has a very uniform transmission field, but this also means that it is not particularly sensitive if used as a receiver coil. In some systems other coils, e.g. head or knee, may also be used for transmission, in which case less power is required to flip the magnetization, but excitation uniformity may be sacrificed.

In horizontal bore MR systems, cylindrical transmit coils may be of a saddle or birdcage design. Theoretically, to obtain a perfectly homogeneous B_1 field within a cylindrical coil requires the current around the surface of the cylinder to vary sinusoidally.

In a saddle coil this arrangement can be approximated by six wires arranged at 60° intervals (figure 9.12). In practice only four conductors are required, each carrying the same current (the conductors at 0° and 180° are unnecessary since they would carry zero current). The birdcage coil (figure 9.13) improves homogeneity over the saddle coil by increasing the number of conductors and improving the approximation to the theoretical ideal of a sinusoidal distribution of current around the circumference. For a vertically oriented B_0 field the most homogeneous B_1 field is achieved through the use of a solenoidal coil (figure 9.14).

9.4.3 Radiofrequency polarization

A simple saddle or solenoidal coil generates linearly polarized RF (figure 9.17(a)). Since a linear alternating

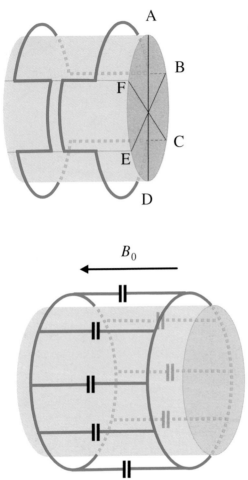

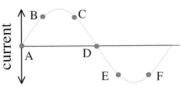

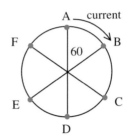

Figure 9.12 Saddle coil for use with a horizontal magnetic field. This figure shows the azimuthal current distribution around the coil.

B_0

Figure 9.13 Low -pass birdcage coil.

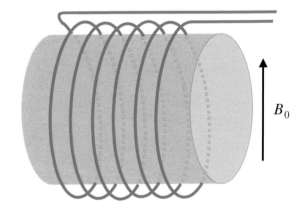

Figure 9.14 Solenoidal coil for use with a vertical static magnetic field. The B_1 field is horizontal.

field can be decomposed into two counter-rotating components, each of half the amplitude, only one of these will be rotating in the same sense as the magnetization and will contribute to B_1. The other one is ineffective and wastes power, which is deposited within the patient increasing the specific absorption rate (SAR).

Circularly polarized (CP) or quadrature coils consist of two orthogonal coils fed alternating currents 90° out of phase, so that there is only one rotating component of magnetization that rotates in the same sense as the nuclear magnetization (figure 9.17(b)). This results in more efficient excitation, since now half the B_1 power

is not wasted. Quadrature transmission therefore reduces patient RF exposure.

9.4.4 Receiver coils

The function of a receiver coil (or simply 'coil') is to maximize signal detection, whilst minimizing the noise. Usually the major source of noise is from the patient's tissue (from the Brownian motion of electrolytes). To minimize the noise, and maximize the SNR, it is necessary to minimize the coil dimensions, i.e. the coil's volume should be filled as much as possible by the sample. A compromise needs to be made between adequate RF homogeneity and high SNR. There are two types

Play that tune

An RF coil is essentially a tuned electrical circuit that comprises an inductor (the actual coil wires) and a capacitor connected in parallel (figure 9.15(a)). The inductor has an electrical reactance $X_L = i\omega L$, where $i = \omega - 1$ and L is the inductance in henrys. The capacitor has a reactance $X_C = -i/\omega C$, where C is the capacitance (farads). The parallel tuned circuit gives a sharp frequency response (figure 9.15(b)), peaking when the reactances cancel, at a resonant frequency of

$$f_0 = \frac{1}{2\pi\sqrt{LC}}$$

At this frequency the impedance of the tuned circuit is a pure resistance

$$Z_p = \frac{LR}{C}$$

RF signals are usually piped around circuits using transmission lines, a typical example being coaxial cable. The transmission line will have a characteristic impedance of typically 50 Ω; therefore, for efficient power transfer the RF circuits should also have an input and output impedance of 50 Ω. Therefore, in order to match the tuned circuit to the 50 Ω output of the power amplifier, the impedance of the coil needs to be matched to 50 Ω. At some frequency off-resonance the coil will have a resistance of 50 Ω in series with an inductive reactance. The addition of a series (matching) capacitor will cancel this inductive reactance resulting in a pure 50 Ω resistance at this frequency (figure 9.16(a)). The parallel tuning capacitor may then be adjusted to make this frequency the desired Larmor frequency. A measure of the tuned circuit (coil) performance is the Q or quality factor, which is the ratio of stored energy to dissipated energy. It may also be written as

$$Q = \frac{\omega L}{R}$$

Q is also a measure of the current or voltage magnification achieved by the tuned circuit. Q can be measured by dividing the centre frequency by the frequency difference at the half power points, or the –3 dB bandwidth (for voltage) (figure 9.15(b)).

Coils should have reasonably high Qs, typically 200 when empty, but not too high since the circuit will continue to oscillate after the RF pulse. A good Q means that the frequency response is quite narrow and the coil is behaving like a band-pass filter, eliminating noise from outside the bandwidth of interest.

When a conducting sample, such as a human body, is placed inside the coil the Q (the loaded Q) decreases. The coil inductance also changes due to mutual inductance between the coil and the conducting tissues, changing its resonant frequency and impedance. In some systems the unloaded Q is deliberately decreased so that the coil has a fixed tuning for more operational convenience.

of receiver coil: volume and surface. Volume coils completely encompass the anatomy of interest and are often combined transmit/receive coils. Surface coils are generally receive only, due to their inhomogeneous reception field. They are however, as their name suggests, good for detecting signal near the surface of the patient.

Receiver coils can also operate in quadrature. During reception the signals from the two-quadrature modes add constructively, whilst the noise from each is uncorrelated, i.e. it 'averages out', resulting in a $\sqrt{2}$ improvement in SNR over a comparable linear coil. Further consideration of SNR is given in chapter 11. Note that

(a)

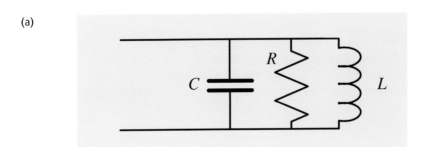

Figure 9.15 Tuned circuit (a) and typical frequency response (b).

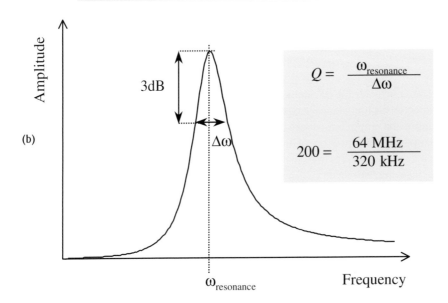

(b)

$$Q = \frac{\omega_{resonance}}{\Delta\omega}$$

$$200 = \frac{64\ \text{MHz}}{320\ \text{kHz}}$$

Birdcage coils

In a birdcage coil the necessary sinusoidal variation in current is generated by the components acting to delay the current around the conductors. The birdcage coil physically consists of two circular end rings connected by N equally spaced straight conductors. The straight conductors and segments of end rings connecting adjacent conductors can be treated as inductors. In the low-pass configuration each of the straight conductors includes a capacitance C, whilst in the high-pass configuration the capacitance is placed on the end rings. Breaking the two end rings and unrolling the coil results in an equivalent circuit of N elements each introducing a phase shift of $\Delta\phi(\omega)$. The requirement for a sinusoidal current distribution is that the total phase shift around the coil must equal a multiple of 2π

$$N\Delta\phi(\omega) = 2\pi M$$

where M is the resonant mode number and $1 \le M \le N/2$. A standing wave in the $M = 1$ mode produces the most homogeneous B_1 field.

The birdcage design also naturally lends itself to CP techniques. Driving the coil with two alternating currents 90° out of phase with each other results in circularly polarized RF.

(a)

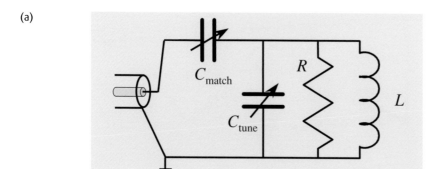

(b)

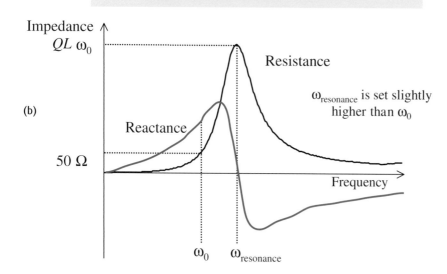

Figure 9.16 Tuned and matched circuit. (a) A matching capacitor is added to cancel the inductive reactance at ω_0 and make the impedance of the circuit appear as a pure 50 Ω resistance (b).

receiver coils also require tuning and matching in the same way as transmitter coils.

9.4.5 Surface coils

Surface coils are placed directly over the anatomical region of interest. A typical example is a small rectangular coil, sometimes known as a licence-plate coil, for imaging the spine. This coil is positioned against the subject's back and produces images with a high SNR because of its limited size, but with the obvious tradeoff of reduced penetration depth and field of view (FOV). The signal response of a surface coil is nonlinear with depth, resulting in an intensity fall-off into the patient. Surface coils are therefore only useful for imaging structures that lie relatively close to the surface of the patient.

Flexible surface coils are very useful since they can be wrapped around the region of interest. Surface coils can function in quadrature by utilizing partially overlapping loops and suitable phase-changing circuitry, but act in quadrature only over a limited spatial extent. Care must be taken to ensure that the surface coil is orientated perpendicular to B_0 otherwise no signal will be detected. Decoupling, i.e. detuning, during RF transmission is required to avoid damaging or saturating the preamplifier or distorting the transmitted RF field. Because of their nonuniform response surface coils are generally unsuitable for transmission.

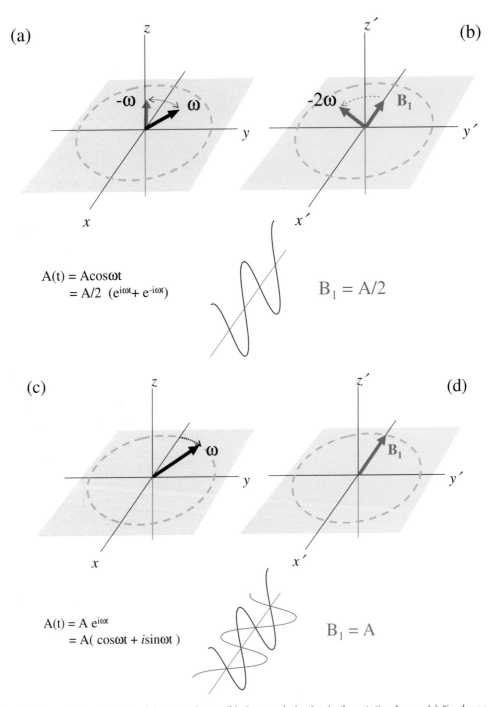

(a)

$$A(t) = A\cos\omega t$$
$$= A/2 \ (e^{i\omega t} + e^{-i\omega t})$$

(b)

$$B_1 = A/2$$

(c)

$$A(t) = A \ e^{i\omega t}$$
$$= A(\cos\omega t + i\sin\omega t)$$

(d)

$$B_1 = A$$

Figure 9.17 (a) Linear polarization in the laboratory frame. (b) Linear polarization in the rotating frame. (c) Circular polarization in the laboratory frame and (d) in the rotating frame.

Beauty is only skin deep

Coils are physically constructed from either wide copper tape or tubing. Due to the skin effect, RF currents only flow near the surface of a conductor. Solid conductors offer no advantage; circumference and net cross-sectional area are key factors in determining the electrical resistance R. The RF resistance of a coil is several times its DC resistance. A measure of how rapidly electromagnetic waves are attenuated is called the skin depth δ given by

$$\partial = \sqrt{\frac{2}{\mu\omega\sigma}}$$

where μ is the magnetic permeability and σ is the material conductivity. The skin depth in copper is about 10 μm at 64 MHz. A further increase in RF resistance arises from the proximity effect when the wire is bent into a coil.

At lower field strengths, the resistance of the coil windings is important in maximizing SNR, but less so at higher field strengths. This is also true when the coil dimension is much larger than the sample, i.e. it has a small 'filling factor'.

9.4.6 Phased array coils

The problem of the limited FOV of surface coils can be solved by using a number of coils simultaneously, known as an array. On modern systems array coils will be available to image most areas, e.g. a spine array coil or a torso array coil. These coils need to be constructed very carefully so that the individual coils (also known as elements) do not interact with each other, a phenomenon known as coupling which reduces SNR in the images. One way of effectively 'decoupling' one element from its neighbours is to geometrically overlap the coils in a particular way. Each element is connected to an entirely separate preamplifier and receiver (see sections 9.4.8 and 9.4.9) which has the advantage that the noise in each receiver is completely different, i.e. uncorrelated, resulting in a higher SNR in the final image.

Images can be produced from the individual elements, but generally they are combined together to produce an image with the large FOV advantage of the array but with the SNR advantage of the small individual elements. A commonly-used method for combining the signals is the 'sum-of-squares' technique, where the signal in a voxel of the final image is the sum of the squared signals intensities for that voxel measured by each element of the coil. Figure 9.18 shows the individual images from a four-element phased array coil for spine imaging.

Phased array coil imaging generates more data than single receive coils, and reconstruction times may be longer due to the additional processing required. A key advantage of multi-element coils is the possibility of using parallel imaging techniques such as SMASH or SENSE (see chapter 17 for full details). Parallel imaging has become very important particularly for techniques like 3D CE-MRA, steady state imaging and for high field (3.0T) imaging since it offers another way to reduce SAR. 8-element coils are quite common. 16, 32 and even higher channel systems are the latest 'big thing' in MRI. It is useful to be able to connect two or more array coils simultaneously, particularly for whole body screening where the patient is imaged from head to toe using several stations. With this technique, a particular FOV is scanned (e.g. the head and neck), then the patient is automatically moved into the magnet by a fixed distance and the next station is scanned (e.g. the upper thorax). This is repeated up to six times to provide complete coverage without having to change coils.

9.4.7 Radiofrequency shields

It should be remembered that gradient and room temperature shim coils can cause losses in the RF coil and cause spurious resonances. Therefore, coil designers usually include an RF shield around the coil that acts to decrease the coupling between the coil and it surroundings. The shield can also affect the performance of the coil and should be taken into account during the design process.

9.4.8 Preamplifier

The small MR signal detected by the coil needs to be boosted by an extremely low-noise preamplifier before being fed to the receiver. Preamplifiers are often

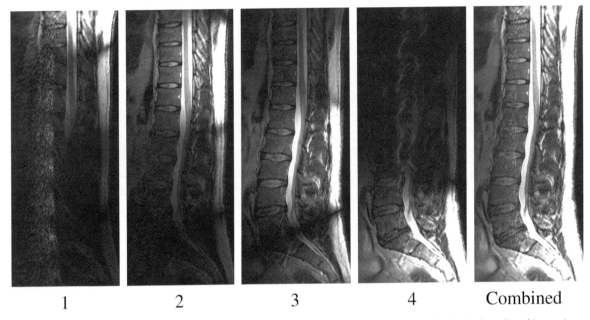

1   2   3   4   Combined

Figure 9.18 Separate images from each of the four channels of a lumbar spine phased array coil. The final combined image is also shown.

Noise figure

The noise figure (NF) is measured in decibels (dB) and is defined as

$$NF = \frac{SNR\ at\ output}{SNR\ at\ input}$$

and is a measure of how much additional noise the amplifier adds. Noise figures are less than 1 dB typically. The noise figure of the preamplifier depends upon the source impedance, in this case the parallel impedance of the tuned circuit Z_p.

mounted on the coil assembly to avoid degradation of the signal by the leads. The quality of an amplifier is given by its *noise figure*.

9.4.9 Receiver

The MR signal only contains a narrow frequency range of interest, typically ± 16 kHz, but is embedded in or carried by the Larmor frequency. The function of the receiver is to retrieve or demodulate this signal, i.e. eliminate the high-frequency carrier. In all modern MR systems this is performed digitally to minimize image artefacts due to drift in the earlier analogue receiver circuitry. Although the chosen receiver bandwidth may only be ± 16 kHz, if the anatomy of interest extends outside the chosen field of view then signals with frequencies outside of this range will also be present. These signals will be effectively undersampled in the reception process and will appear as aliasing or image wrap artefacts in the frequency-encoding direction. Therefore, the detected signals must be strongly filtered (usually digitally) to suppress these unwanted frequencies.

9.4.10 Prescan

Usually each imaging sequence is preceded by a prescan or preparation phase, in which the characteristics of the transmitter and receiver are optimized. Since the presence of the patient within the magnet may alter the precessional frequency very slightly the first step

Digital demodulation

The MR signal is at a high frequency close to ω_0, but offset slightly due to the frequency encoding and with a bandwidth $\Delta\omega$. Mathematically this is shown as

$$\cos(\omega_0 + \omega_{FE} \pm \Delta\omega)$$

It is necessary to digitise the signal and measure the real and imaginary components of the magnetization. The latter process is known as "quadrature detection" and involves splitting the incoming signal and creating a 90° phase shift between the two components. Demodulation to a lower frequency is also desirable, to reduce the sample frequency required in the analogue-to-digital converter (ADC). In early MR systems this was done with analogue components, multiplying the signal by sine and cosine waves at the Larmor frequency:

$$\cos(\omega_0 + \omega_{FE} \pm \Delta\omega) \cdot \sin(\omega_0) = \frac{1}{2}\sin(\omega_0 + \omega_{FE} \pm \Delta\omega + \omega_0) + \frac{1}{2}\sin(\omega_0 + \omega_{FE} \pm \Delta\omega - \omega_0)$$

$$= \underbrace{\frac{1}{2}\sin(2\omega_0 + \omega_{FE} \pm \Delta\omega)}_{\text{unwanted high frequency side band}} + \underbrace{\frac{1}{2}\sin(\omega_{FE} \pm \Delta\omega)}_{\text{Real component}}$$

$$\cos(\omega_0 + \omega_{FE} \pm \Delta\omega) \cdot \cos(\omega_0) = \frac{1}{2}\cos(\omega_0 + \omega_{FE} \pm \Delta\omega + \omega_0) - \frac{1}{2}\cos(\omega_0 + \omega_{FE} \pm \Delta\omega - \omega_0)$$

$$= \underbrace{\frac{1}{2}\cos(2\omega_0 + \omega_{FE} \pm \Delta\omega)}_{\text{unwanted high frequency side band}} - \underbrace{\frac{1}{2}\cos(\omega_{FE} \pm \Delta\omega)}_{\text{Imaginary component}}$$

Numerous artefacts could arise from this process, including quadrature ghosts if the sine and cosine waves were not exactly 90° out of phase and DC artefacts from subtracting the Larmor frequency. The latter can be avoided by demodulating the signal to an intermediate frequency ω_{if} e.g. 125 kHz instead of subtracting exactly ω_0. By digitising the signal at $4 \times \omega_{if}$ (500 kHz) it is possible to create the two digital components and add the phase delay in a single step. Alternate digital samples are sent to the real and imaginary channels, and then every other point on each side is inverted. In effect the real channel is the input signal multiplied by {0, 1, 0, −1}, the imaginary by {1, 0, −1, 0}, which corresponds to a sine and cosine respectively at the intermediate frequency, with perfect 90° phase difference between them.

Advances in ADC technology mean that it is now possible to digitise at much higher frequencies, up to tens of MHz, and most modern scanners now have a completely digital receiver. In general they are operated at something less than Larmor frequency, which means they measure a series of alias frequencies ω_A of the true signal,

$$\omega_A = (\omega_0 + \omega_{FE} \pm \Delta\omega) - n \cdot \omega_s$$

where ω_s is the sample frequency of the ADC, and n is an integer. Provided that ω_s and n are chosen such that the bandwidth of the received MR signal is well within the sampled bandwidth, i.e. $\Delta\omega \ll \omega_s$, the MR signal is accurately measured.

involves determining the exact Larmor frequency so that the appropriate slice offsets can be calculated. The second stage involves the scanner determining how much RF power is required to generate a known flip angle. Remember that the required power will be dependent upon the type of transmitter coil and the weight of the patient. The desired RF power is achieved by adjusting the output of the RF power amplifier. Finally the gain of the receiver circuitry is adjusted so that the signal coming back from the patient matches, as closely as possible, the input voltage range of the analogue-to-digital converter. The prescan phase may also be used for optimizing the frequency and amplitude of chemical shift selective fat saturation pulses and also for locally shimming the magnet to improve the fat saturation uniformity. Most scanners also offer the user the capability to manually adjust all these parameters.

9.5 Computer systems

The multi-tasking nature of MR means that it is impractical to control the many processes requiring accurate timing directly from the main or host computer, so many subsystems will have their own microprocessors whose commands can be downloaded from the host. A typical MRI system will have a host computer on which the operator will prescribe the scan in terms of the pulse sequence, its timing and various geometry factors, etc. These parameters will then be converted into commands that are transferred to another microproces-

Pulse programmer

The pulse programmer (PP) normally performs the complex timing control of sequences. The PP is usually a separate, microprocessor-controlled, highly flexible array of sequencers and memory. The user, via the host computer interface, enters the required scan prescription, e.g. pulse sequence, echo time, repetition time, etc. The host computer checks that the values entered are within any hardware limits, e.g. maximum gradient strength, or software constraints, e.g. maximum number of slices, before passing the values to the PP, which converts the sequence parameters into digital representations of the desired gradient or RF pulses. The PP can also communicate with the data-acquisition software sending information about the data to be collected. Once a scan is initiated the sequencers play out their waveforms to the transmitter and the gradient controllers. Whilst the sequence is playing out the PP will queue up any updates to the sequencers, e.g. new phase-encoding gradient, required the next time the sequence is played out. The PP must also be capable of responding to environmental inputs, e.g. patient ECG for cardiac-triggered scans.

Array processor

An array processor (AP) is a specialized computer capable of executing instructions in which the operands may be arrays rather than individual data elements. They are therefore very e fficient at performing operations such as the fast Fourier transform (FFT) on MRI raw data matrices. MRI systems often have multiple array processors so that the raw data matrix may be shared between APs resulting in even faster reconstruction times. The FFT algorithm is inherently linear allowing this natural division between processors.

sor system, known as the pulse programmer (PP), that controls the hardware. The PP ensures that the RF, gradients and data acquisition are all properly synchronized. Once the data have been acquired, a separate computer system known as the array processor carries out the image reconstruction. The host computer then manages the image display, processing, for example, windowing, hardcopy production, archiving and networking.

9.6 Open MRI systems

Open MRI systems are much more patient friendly than the restricted tunnels of superconducting systems. Such systems offer the possibility of MRI-guided interventional procedures, since the physician now has access to the patient during scanning. Open MRI systems based on either permanent or iron-cored electromagnet designs operate primarily between 0.06 T and 0.3 T. Open superconducting systems are available in the range 0.5–1.0 T. Examples of high field open systems are GE Healthcare's 0.7 T OpenSpeed and Philips 1.0 T Panorama. These systems have vertically oriented magnetic fields and have specially designed flat planar gradient coils and efficient solenoidal RF coils. In addition to the open environment for patients, most of these systems also have the capability of moving the patient sideways in the field so that areas such as the shoulder that would normally be off-centre in a cylindrical superconducting magnet can be positioned at the centre of the field. Systems have also been developed that allow

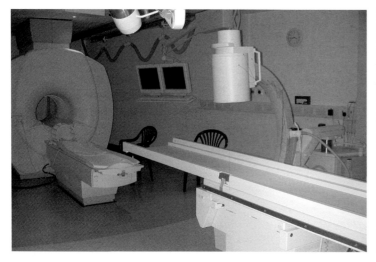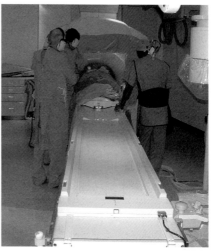

Figure 9.19 Interventional MRI system with integral C-arm X-ray tube over an extended patient couch. This system is used for pediatric cardiac endovascular procedures (courtesy of Dr S Keevil, Guys' Hospital, London).

for imaging during weight bearing, e.g. the Easote G-scan 0.25 T permanent magnet system that can tilt.

9.6.1 Interventional systems

There is continuing interest in the use of MRI for image guided interventional procedures. Although there have been a number of attempts to develop dedicated systems for intervention, including open surgery, they haven't generally developed into mainstream products. Therefore most interventional procedures are now carried out using conventional or open systems (see figure 9.19). The major advantage of performing interventional procedures under MRI guidance is its ability to monitor the progress of a procedure. An example is MR guided focused ultrasound (FUS) in which MRI is used to monitor the thermal ablation of tissue, e.g. uterine fibroids, using temperature sensitive pulse sequences. Fast dynamic MR imaging is also being used to track catheters for cardiac or vascular interventions.

9.6.2 Dedicated systems

In addition to the whole-body open magnets there is also growing interest in niche magnet designs for particular applications. Systems have been developed for imaging the extremities, head and breast. These have the advantage of potentially significantly reduced cost and installation requirements.. High field head-only systems (e.g. at 3 T and above) have been available for neuro-imaging research applications such as fMRI, however now that whole-body 3 T systems are commercially available, the market for head only systems is diminishing (see section 16.5).

9.7 Siting and installation

When purchasing an MRI system there are a number of considerations with respect to the siting and installation of the system that need to be addressed.

9.7.1 Fringe field

Depending on the field strength and the design of the magnet a stray field can extend for a considerable distance in all three directions as noted in chapter 2. Containment of the 0.5 mT fringe field contour away from public access, to avoid potential heart pacemaker malfunction, may require additional magnetic shielding. Figure 9.20 shows various field contours for a typical 1.5 T clinical system.

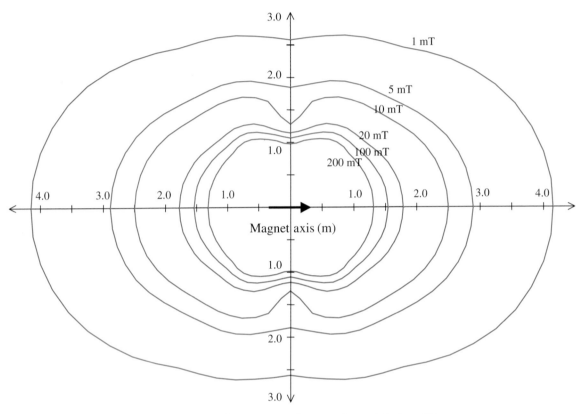

Figure 9.20 Fringe field plots for a 1.5 T system. Figure courtesy of Magnex Research Systems Ltd.

9.7.2 Radiofrequency shielding

To avoid any extraneous sources of RF from interfering with the MR signals most scanners are placed in an RF-shielded enclosure, or Faraday cage. Typically this consists of a room lined on all six sides with copper, aluminium or steel sheeting. All electrical connections between the magnet system and the system's electronics cabinets are connected via electrical filters through a 'penetration panel' in the RF shield. Special wire-embedded glass is used for windows, and any doors need to make a proper electromagnetic seal with their frame. It is possible to allow tubes or fibre-optic through the screen via the use of waveguides (metal pipes of a specific length and diameter through which unwanted RF signals below a certain frequency cannot pass).

Conducting wires, including power cables, should not be passed through waveguides since they may act as aerials, picking up unwanted RF interference outside the room and radiating it inside.

9.7.3 Siting and environment

Every iron or steel object in the stray field of the magnet will have a temporary magnetization induced into it. The stray fields from these items will in turn affect the homogeneity of the magnet. Providing they are static then the effect can be counteracted, up to a limit, by shimming of the magnet. Proximity to moving objects such as elevators or trucks can make siting even more complex.

MRI systems also have quite significant environmental requirements, particularly with respect to adequate cooling of the equipment racks and reliable electric power. Adequate air conditioning must be installed to maintain temperature and humidity within the equipment room. The air conditioning unit should also provide the chilled water required by the cryo-cooler. A good quality electrical supply is required since the sensitive electronic components do not react well to sudden losses of power, particularly if one phase of the three-phase supply fails. If necessary, additional transient suppression devices, line conditioners or even uninterruptible power supplies (UPS) may be required. In the event of power failure, a superconducting magnet will remain functioning but the absence of a cryocooler will result in increased helium boil-off. Fluorescent lights should not be used in the magnet room since they produce RF interference. Standard alternating current (AC) lighting should not be used either, since the bulb filaments oscillate in the magnetic field, significantly reducing the lifetime of the bulb. Ideally low-voltage direct current (DC) incandescent lighting should be used.

See also:

- Chapter 2: Early daze: your first week in MR
- Chapter 10: But is it safe? Bio-effects

FURTHER READING

Chen C-N and Hoult DI (1989) *Biomedical Magnetic Resonance Technology*. Bristol: IOP Publishing (ISBN: 0852741189), Chapters 3–6.

Haacke EM, Brown RW, Thompson MR and Venkatesan R (1999) *Magnetic Resonance Imaging: Physical Principles and Sequence Design*. New York: Wiley-Liss (ISBN: 0471351288), Chapter 27.

Holland GN and MacFall JR (1992) An overview of digital spectrometers for MR Imaging. *J Magn Reson Imaging* **2**: 241–6.

But is it safe? Bio-effects

10.1 Introduction

For centuries magnets have been attributed with alleged healing and hypnotic powers despite a lack of any scientific evidence or hypotheses on mechanisms. Magnets certainly don't make you better, but are they harmful? In the course of undergoing a clinical MR examination, the patient will be exposed to a static field, time-varying gradient fields and RF fields. Staff normally will only be exposed to the fringe field from B_0. In 25 years of MR, there have been ten documented fatalities related to magnet safety, seven of these involving persons with cardiac pacemakers, one involving displacement of an aneurysm clip and one involving a projectile and the other from an unknown cause. You must thoroughly know your institution's safety practices and patient screening procedures, as outlined in chapter 2. Carrying out a metal check on yourself and others will be second nature to you by now, but you can never be too vigilant. The purpose of this chapter is to provide background on the underlying potential biological effects of magnetic fields. In particular we show that:

- The main effect of RF exposure is tissue heating. This is restricted to less than 1 °C by monitoring and limiting the SAR (specific absorption rate). Care is required to avoid the heating of leads used for physiological monitoring.
- Peripheral nerve stimulation (PNS) is the main bioeffect of the time-varying magnetic fields generated by the gradients. It may cause discomfort but it is not harmful. Modern scanners have a stimulation monitor to alert the user to the likelihood of causing PNS.

- At very high B_0 (i.e. greater than 1.5 T) mild sensory effects may be experienced associated with movement in the field. These are not harmful.
- Care is required for staff and patients who are pregnant, although there is no evidence of deleterious effect on the foetus.
- Potential displacement and heating must be considered when metallic implants are present.

10.2 Radiofrequency effects

RF effects arguably give the greatest cause for concern in terms of potential bio-effects, partly because they are under the operator's control. The principal physical effect is deposition of energy, leading to tissue heating with possible physiological effects including changes in cardiac output and decreased mental function. Of particular concern are heat-sensitive organs such as the eyes and testes, although there is no evidence of any deleterious effect of MR on either. Other so-called nonthermal RF bio-effects are contentious but there is much interest in the effect of RF encountered in mobile phone use. (Mobile phones operate in the frequency range 900–1800 MHz, very different from clinical MR.) One case that requires some caution is where the patient has a metallic (but nonferromagnetic) implant that may result in greater heating. The use of inappropriate physiological monitoring leads can also result in heating of the electrodes and the possibility of skin burns.

SAR maths

For a uniform conducting medium of conductivity σ the SAR can be calculated as follows. The energy deposition is given by the product of induced current density $\mathbf{J}$ and induced electric field $\mathbf{E}$ (this is just 'power = voltage times current', but for a volume conductor)

$$P = \mathbf{J} \cdot \mathbf{E} = \sigma E^2$$

and then

$$SAR = 0.5\sigma \frac{E^2}{\rho}$$

where ρ is the density of tissue and the factor 0.5 comes from time-averaging the alternating electric field (just as in AC power calculations). Thus SAR has units of $W\,kg^{-1}$.

From Faraday's law (section 10.3) and allowing for a sinusoidal B_1 (and for simplicity assuming rectangular pulses) we get an average SAR

$$SAR = 0.5\sigma \frac{\pi^2 r^2 f^2 B_1^2 D}{\rho}$$

where D, the duty cycle, is the fraction of total scan time for which the RF is present. This tells us the following relationships:

- SAR increases with the square of Larmor frequency or B_0;
- SAR increases with the square of flip angle;
- SAR increases with the patient size;
- SAR increases with the number of RF pulses in a given time.

Of course, this calculation is a huge simplification. The details of anatomical geometry can change the power levels. The possibility of local hotspots has led to the development of localized SAR limits for partial body exposure.

10.2.1 Specific absorption ratio

The RF exposure is measured in terms of the SAR defined as the total power in watts (W) per kilogram of tissue. This is why you need to enter the patient's mass when registering them. The scanner monitors its RF transmitter output then computes an average SAR (see also 'SAR maths'). Normally two levels of RF exposure are permitted. The lower level can be applied without restriction. Exposure to the upper level requires positive confirmation from the operator.

10.2.2 Staying cool – reducing SAR

SAR is under the control of the MR operator. Some factors that help to reduce the SAR are:

- the use of quadrature rather than linear coils for transmission;
- avoiding the use of the body coil for certain examinations, i.e. when you have a head, knee or other coils that can transmit as well as receive;
- increasing TR;
- using fewer slices;
- reducing echo train length (ETL, turbo factor) in fast or turbo spin echo (FSE/TSE) sequences;
- reducing the refocusing pulse flip angle, especially in FSE sequences.

10.2.3 RF exposure standards

The IEC 60601-2-33 standard is based upon limiting RF induced core temperature rises to 0.7 °C or 1 °C for normal and first-level controlled operations, respectively. This translates into SAR terms as 2 and 4 W kg^{-1} averaged over 6 min. Further details are given in 'Normal and controlled RF limits'.

In the USA, the FDA currently recommends that the RF exposure should be limited to producing less than a 1 °C core body temperature rise. Furthermore, it currently defines a significant risk criteria for SAR values of:

- 4 W kg^{-1} whole body for 15 min;
- 3 W kg^{-1} averaged over the head for 10 min;
- 8 W kg^{-1} in any gram of tissue in the head or torso for 15 min, or;
- 12 W kg^{-1} in any gram of tissue in the extremities for 15 min.

The IEC 60601-2-33 standard gives the following limits for the temperature rise (table 10.1) and SAR limits (table 10.2) for the first and second-level controlled modes.

Table 10.1 RF temperature limits

Operating mode	Core temperature rise (°C)	Spatially localized temperature limits (°C)		
		Head	Torso	Extremities
Normal	0.7	38	39	40
First-level controlled	1	38	39	40
Second-level controlled	>1	>38	>39	>40

Table 10.2 SAR limits

Operating mode	SAR (W kg^{-1})					
	Whole body	Partial body		Localized region		
		Any	Head	Head	Trunk	Extremities
Normal	2	2–10	3.2	10	10	20
First-level controlled	4	4–10	3.2	10	10	20
Second-level controlled	>4	>4	>3.2	>10	>10	>20
Short-term SAR	The SAR limits over any 10-s period should not exceed three times the stated SAR average					

Note: The averaging time is 6 min.

10.3 Gradient effects

The time-varying fields generated by the gradients fall in a part of the frequency spectrum known as extremely low frequency (ELF). There is much controversy about the effect of chronic exposure to ELF fields from high-voltage power lines and household appliances. However, in MRI we are concerned with acute effects. There is no evidence of MR switched gradient fields causing terato-genic (literally, the production of monsters!) effects.

10.3.1 Stimulation effects

The switching of the gradients induces electrical currents in conducting tissues according to Faraday's law (see 'Faraday induction'). In modern EPI-capable MR systems, the rapidly changing magnetic field associated with the switching of the magnetic field gradients is able to generate currents in tissue, which may exceed the nerve depolarization threshold and cause peripheral nerve stimulation (PNS). The possibility also exists, at least theoretically, of stimulating cardiac muscle, thus

presenting a hazard. Stimulation of motor nerves and skeletal muscle may be disconcerting to the patient (discomfort being reported for levels 50% to 100% greater than the sensation threshold) but is not itself hazardous and will not normally occur in routine clinical scans. Animal research (with dogs) has shown that respiratory stimulation occurs at exposure levels of the order of three times that required for PNS, whilst cardiac stimulation requires 80 times the PNS threshold.

PNS is most likely to occur in EPI. In particular we have to be careful of two scenarios:

(a) When oblique slices are used and it is possible to have a greater slew rate by summing the contributions from two or three sets of gradient coils (indeed some manufacturers use this trick in their technical specifications to make their systems look better than they are).

(b) For coronal or sagittal EPI where the possible current loops in the torso are greatest when the read gradient is in the head–foot direction. Normally the scanner will monitor dB/dt and advise on the likelihood of stimulation.

Mental stimulation

Neurostimulation is used diagnostically and therapeutically in trans-cranial magnetic stimulation (TMS), which is used in the diagnosis of certain neurological conditions and is claimed to alleviate severe depression. It is not thought to be harmful (although I wouldn't fancy it myself). Whilst the underlying physical mechanism for stimulation is Faraday induction (see below) there is still debate within the neurological community about the detailed electrophysiology of magnetic stimulation and the effect of different stimulus waveforms. The view expressed within the MR community, namely that biphasic stimuli (as generated by a gradient ramp up and down) are less effective for stimulation than monophasic stimuli, has not been shown in TMS.

Another well-documented effect is magnetophosphenes, or experiencing the harmless sensation of flashes of light. This is thought to originate from retinal stimulation by induced currents. The same effect has been reported for sudden head movements within strong static fields.

10.3.2 Gradient noise

The characteristic knocking or drilling noise heard when an MRI sequence is in progress can be considered simply the result of the Lorentz force generated by the coils when a current is pulsed through them in the presence of the static magnetic field. The noise is caused by the movement of the coils against their mountings, and can be in excess of 100 dB for some manufacturer's sequences. This is why hearing protection is recommended for patients during MRI scanning. The reduction of gradient noise is an active area of development for system manufacturers, with various approaches including vacuum packing under investigation.

10.3.3 Gradient exposure standards

The principle behind the IEC 60601-2-33 standard is to prevent cardiac stimulation and minimize PNS at any

Faraday induction

Faraday's law gives the EMF (or voltage) induced in a conducting loop of area A from a uniform time-varying field as

$$EMF = A\frac{dB}{dt} = \pi r^2 \frac{dB}{dt}$$

for a circle (see figure 10.1).

The induced electric field round a circular loop is given by volts/distance (strictly $\int \mathbf{E}.\mathbf{dl}$ for the mathematically unchallenged) or

$$E = \frac{1}{2}r\frac{dB}{dt}$$

around the circumference of the circle.

Electrical current flowing in wires is measured in amps. When considering electrical conduction in volumes (rather than in wires), we speak of a current density measured in amps per square meter, $A\,m^{-2}$. For a uniform conductor with a conductivity $\sigma\,S\,m^{-1}$ (siemens per metre) the current density flowing in a circular path or loop of radius r is

$$J = \frac{1}{2}\sigma \cdot r \cdot \frac{dB}{dt}$$

We can work out the likely current density by assuming a tissue conductivity in muscle of $0.4\,S\,m^{-1}$ and a maximum loop radius of 0.3 m (along the length of the trunk). We also have to calculate it at the point of peak value of the gradient, where the field generated by the gradient is highest. If we consider that to be the maximum tissue radius, then the current density is

$$J = 0.018 \times \text{max slew rate in T}\,m^{-1}\,s^{-1}.$$

A slew rate of $55\,T\,m^{-1}\,s^{-1}$ (or $mT\,m^{-1}\,ms^{-1}$) is required to give a current density of the order of $1\,A\,m^{-2}$, the lower limit for stimulation. This is well within the capabilities of modern gradients.

operating mode. IEC standard thresholds for normal and the first-level controlled operating mode for PNS and for cardiac stimulation are shown in figure 10.2. Further details are considered in 'Crossing the

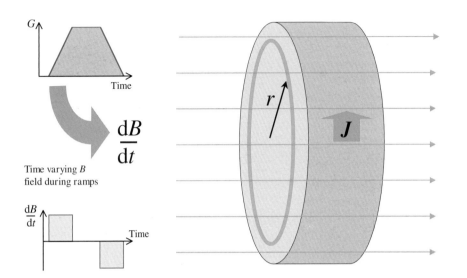

Figure 10.1 Faraday induction in a time-varying magnetic field. With a trapezoidal gradient waveform dB/dt only exists during the ramp up and ramp down periods. In a uniform conductor a current density J flows in loops.

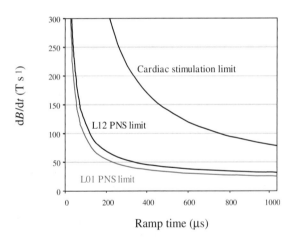

Figure 10.2 Derived hyperbolic strength–duration (SD) curves for the IEC 60601-2-33 limits for cardiac stimulation and the normal (L01) and first-level controlled (L12) operating modes for peripheral nerve stimulation (PNS).

threshold'. The FDA takes a more pragmatic approach in that it limits dB/dt to that 'sufficient to produce severe discomfort or painful stimulation'.

The risk to hearing is also addressed by the IEC, which states that the system manufacturer must issue a warning on the system console if a particular pulse sequence is likely to exceed 99 dB(A). The FDA advice is effectively the same. Note that the threshold for

Crossing the threshold

In IEC 60601-2-33, cardiac stimulation is assumed to be avoided when the combined gradient output of all gradient units of the gradient system satisfies

$$\frac{dB}{dt} < 20 \cdot \left(1 + \frac{3}{ts}\right)$$

where dB/dt is in T s^{-1} and ts is the duration of the gradient field change (i.e. the time to ramp from maximum negative to maximum positive) in ms.

PNS limits for the normal operating mode (L01) and the first-level controlled operating mode (L12) are

$$L01 = 0.8 \cdot rb \cdot \left(1 + \frac{0.4}{ts}\right)$$

$$L12 = 1.0 \cdot rb \cdot \left(1 + \frac{0.4}{ts}\right)$$

where again ts is the effective stimulus duration and rb is the rheobase, the threshold below which no further excitation is possible, independent of the stimulus duration.

The IEC 60601-2-33 rheobase values are given in table 10.3 below and may be expressed either as the electric field E (V m^{-1}) induced in the patient or as the time rate of change of the magnetic field in the patient dB/dt (T s^{-1}).

The strength–duration curve

Both the gradients and the RF are examples of time-varying magnetic fields and both induce electrical currents in tissue. So why are their associated bioeffects so different? The reason lies in the strength–duration (SD) curve. The form of the SD curve for electrical stimulation (via electrodes) has been known for a long time. It is a plot of the threshold for stimulation plotted against the duration of the pulse. In MRI terms, the duration of the pulse refers to the duration of the leading and trailing slopes of the gradient pulses, the part during which tissue currents are produced (figure 10.1).

Each type of muscle fibre or nerve may have a different time constant that determines the shape of the SD curve. For MRI the following hyperbolic relationship is considered to apply

$$\left(\frac{dB}{dt}\right)_{threshold} = C \cdot rb \cdot \left[1 + \frac{\tau_{chron}}{\tau}\right]$$

where (dB/dt)threshold is the threshold for peripheral nerve stimulation, τ is the duration of the gradient field change (i.e. the time to ramp from maximum negative to maximum positive) and τ_{chron} (the chronaxie) is a type of tissue electrical time constant. Typical values for τ_{chron} are 0.4 ms for a peripheral nerve and 3.0 ms for cardiac muscle. rb is known as the 'rheobase', the threshold below which no further excitation is possible, independent of the stimulus duration. C is a constant taking into account the tissue radius and the gradient orientation. Theoretical hyperbolic SD curves for cardiac stimulation and the PNS limits for the IEC L01 and L12 operating modes are illustrated in figure 10.2. Interestingly we see that the lowest thresholds occur for the longest ramp times and therefore gradients that switch faster, i.e. have very short rise times, actually allow much greater amplitude changes as well. Cardiac stimulation, which would be very dangerous, requires a lengthy duration of switching, and is therefore difficult to envisage in an MR system (it has never been reported as happening). In any event, owing to the different likely conduction paths or loops, one would almost always experience peripheral muscular stimulation first, which would serve as adequate warning.

Table 10.3 Rheobase values for different types of gradient system

Type of gradient system	rb expressed as dB/dt	rb expressed as E
Whole-body gradient system (cylindrical magnet)	(not applicable)	$22.8\,T\,s^{-1}$
Special purpose gradient system	$3.65\,V\,m^{-1}$	(not applicable)

instantaneous acoustic trauma is 140 dB and that properly fitting ear-plugs offer about 20 dB(A) attenuation. dB(A) is a unit of sound pressure level which takes into account the normal hearing curve for most people.

10.4 Static field effects

There is evidence for some mild sensory effects of static magnetic fields, including vertigo, nausea and taste sensations, with the suggestion of a dose–effect relationship for 1.5 T and 4 T whole-body magnets. However, some subjects reported sensations in cases when the magnet was switched off! Other effects, namely headache, tinnitus, vomiting and numbness, have not been substantiated. At very high fields the possibilities exist of altering nerve conduction characteristics at least theoretically (e.g. for a field of 450 T!), of changing the rate of ion transport across cell membranes, and of altering chemical reactivities.

Published animal-based experiments have been beset by contradictory evidence, failure to be replicated, poor control and lack of exposure details. For example, prolonged exposure to 9.4 T fields had no effect on numbers of offspring, growth rates, feeding patterns, blood and urine biochemistry and behavioural development for male and female adult and fetal rats. In another study on mice at 4 T (although with combined RF and switched fields and ultrasound) small changes in fetal weight, birth rates, delayed motor skill learning and adult sperm production rates were reported. At 10 T some behavioural changes in laboratory animals have been noted.

Magneto-hydrodynamic effect

The one static field mechanism that is not negligible in vivo is the magneto-hydrodynamic effect (figure 10.3). A charged particle moving at velocity v within and at an angle θ to a magnetic field B generates an electric field E

$$E = vB \sin \theta$$

Flow along the field direction will produce no effect, the maximum occurring for flow perpendicular to the field. In an idealized case the voltage across a vessel of diameter d containing conducting fluid (e.g. blood) will be

$$V = dvB \sin \theta$$

The above expression estimated for aortic flow gives a voltage of about 40 mV at 2.5 T. Although these voltages have been demonstrated in vivo, there is no evidence of any consequent ill-effects.

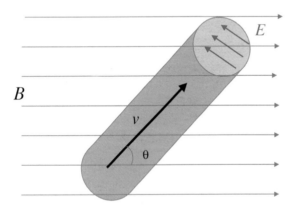

Figure 10.3 Magneto-hydrodynamic effect. An electric field E is induced across the moving conducting fluid, giving an EMF (voltage) across the vessel. v is velocity.

It needs to be remembered that the exposure of human subjects in MRI is for short periods only and that these effects cease with the exposure. Epidemiological studies on female magnet workers have shown no deleterious effects on fertility, pregnancies or children. A cautious approach should nevertheless be adopted for both patients and staff who are pregnant.

So what about 'mag lag', the idea that cognitive function or memory is affected by exposure to fringe fields? There is no evidence for it. It simply doesn't exist. (That loss of short-term memory you are experiencing is simply old age!)

10.4.1 Flow effects

One well-established bio-effect is the generation of electric potentials in moving, conducting tissue, e.g. across blood flowing in vessels, particularly the aorta (the magneto-hydrodynamic effect). Although this is not known to be hazardous, the possibility exists, at least theoretically, of the induced potential exceeding the threshold for depolarization of cardiac muscle (about 40 mV). This has led to the current field limits of 2 T as a lower uncontrolled level and 4 T for the firstlevel controlled mode level.

10.4.2 Force fields

Static fields also pose hazards through the displacement of ferro-magnetic implants (clips, coils, stents, etc.). The field will exert both a translational force and a torque (twisting force) on magnetic objects (see 'Of frogs and forces'). The field may disrupt the function of cardiac pacemakers. Of the ten reported deaths in MR incidents, seven resulted from the inadvertent scanning of persons with pacemakers. In specialist centres, under strict protocols, it has become possible to scan patients with certain newer kinds of pacemakers. However we strongly recommend that you don't do this, unless you happen to be working in one of those centres.

10.4.3 Static field exposure standards

The IEC 60601-2-33 standard gives the following static magnetic field limits:
- Normal operating mode: equal or lower than 2 T;
- First-level controlled operating mode: higher than 2 T and equal to or lower than 4 T;
- Second-level controlled operating mode: higher than 4 T.

Of frogs and forces

Biological tissue is diamagnetic, which means it is essentially, but not entirely, nonmagnetic. A diamagnetic material responds to an applied magnetic field by generating fields that oppose the applied field, i.e. generating a repulsive force. This effect has been demonstrated dramatically by magnetically levitating frogs in a 16 T field (I always thought frogs were repulsive).

Forces and torques were examined in section 2.3.1. Aside from floating frogs, the theoretical effect of these forces on biological tissues in vivo is negligible compared with the normal mechanical and haemodynamic forces involved with life. Although red blood cells in sickle cell anaemia have shown displacement in vitro in a 0.5 T field, this has not been replicated in patients, or for normal blood cells.

Occupational exposure

In some countries legislation may exist covering occupational limits for exposure to static magnetic fields and time-varying magnetic fields (table 10.4). However, it should be noted that no evidence exists to support cumulative effects with time of exposure to static magnetic fields.

Assuming these limits apply to an 8-h day, then at 0.5 T, only 1 h per day could be spent in the field using the 60 mT level. In the European Union, whilst no static field limit applies, an 'action level' of 200mT for occupational exposure has been established. Special protective measures are required for occupational exposures which exceed this action level.

Table 10.4 Static field occupational limits

Source	Whole-body time average (8 h) (mT)	Whole-body maximum	Extremities time average (8 h) (mT)	Extremities maximum (T)
ICNIRP[a]	200	2	–	5
NRPB[b]	200	2	200	4
ACGIH[c]	60	2	600	2
LLNL[d]	60	2	600	2
ARL[e]	60	5	200	10
EU[f] action level (no time average)	200			

Notes:

[a] International Commission on Non-Ionizing Radiation Protection (1994) Guidelines on limits of exposure to static magnetic fields. *Health Physics* **66**: 100–6.

[b] National Radiological Protection Board (2004) Advice on Limiting Exposure to Electromagnetic Fields (0-300 GHz) Documents of the NRPB Vol 15 No 2 Available direct from the Health Protection Agency at http://www.hpa.org.uk/radiation/publications/documents_of_nrpb/index.htm [accessed 12th April 2005]

[c] American Congress of Government Industrial Hygienists (1993–1994) Threshold limit values for chemical substances and physical agents. Cincinnati, OH: American Conference of Governmental Industrial Hygienists.

[d] Miller G (1987) Lawrence Livermore National Laboratory 'Exposure guidelines for magnetic fields'. *Am Ind Hyg Assoc Jour* **48**: 957–68.

[e] Australian Radiation Laboratory (1991) *Safety Guidelines for Magnetic Resonance Diagnostic Facilities*. Melbourne, Australia: Australian Radiation Laboratory.

[f] European Union (2004) Directive 2004/40/EC of the European Parliament and of the council of 29 April 2004 on the minimum health and safety requirements regarding the exposure of workers to the risks arising from physical agents (electromagnetic fields), *Official Journal of the European Union* **L 184** p 1-9 24.5.2005. Available direct from http://europa.eu.int/eur-lex/lex/LexUriServ/site/en/oj/2004/l_184/l_18420040524en00010009.pdf [accessed 12th April 2005]

The Food and Drug Administration (FDA) Center for Devices and Radiological Health (CDRH) advice on static fields is that a field of greater than 4 T constitutes significant risk investigation.

See also:

- Safety first: section 2.3

FURTHER READING

Food and Drug Administration (2003) *Criteria for Significant Risk Investigations of Magnetic Resonance Diagnostic Devices*. http://www.fda.gov/cdrh/ode/ guidance/793.pdf [accessed 12th April 2005]

InternationalElectro-Technical Commission (1995) *Medical Electrical Equipment – Part 2: Particular Requirements for the Safety of Magnetic Resonance Equipment for Medical Diagnosis Edition 2.0*. IEC 60601–2–33. Available direct from IEC at http://www.iec.ch/webstore/ [accessed 23rd October 2004]

International Commission on Non-Ionizing Radiation Protection (2004) *Medical Magnetic Resonance (MR) Procedures: Protection of Patients*. Health Physics **87**:197–216. Available direct from ICNIRP at http://www.icnirp.de/documents/MR2004.pdf [accessed 12th April 2004]

National Radiological Protection Board (1991) *Principles for the Protection of Patients and Volunteers During Clinical Magnetic Resonance Procedures*. Documents of the NRPB Vol 2 No 1 (ISBN 0859513394). Available direct from the Health Protection Agency at http://www.hpa.org.uk/radiation/publications/documents_of_nrpb/index.htm [accessed 12th April 2005]

Ordidge RJ, Kanal E and Shellock FG (eds) (2000) *Journal of Magnetic Resonance Imaging* special issue: MR safety. *J Magn Reson Imaging*, **12**.

Shellock FG (2003) *Reference manual for Magnetic Resonance Safety 2003*. Salt Lake City: Amirsys Inc (ISBN: 1931884048).

Part B

The specialist stuff

11

Ghosts in the machine: quality control

11.1 Introduction

Quality control (QC) or assurance (QA) often raises many questions. How do you do it? Who should do it and how often? (Do I have to do it – can't someone else?) Quality has become more and more a part of service provision and professional practice in many sectors of work. QA has long been established in the imaging modalities that utilize ionizing radiation, in response to regulatory pressure. No such pressure exists for MR, nevertheless 'best practice' dictates that quality programmes should be implemented. With all QA activity, the importance is to achieve a balance between spending too much time and resources checking everything, and getting on with clinical work. This chapter will look at the aspects best covered by a QA programme, with other elements covered in the boxes.

MR QA is largely concerned with image quality. This is normally quantified through the measurement of particular image quality parameters using specially designed phantoms or test objects (figure 11.1). Most MR manufacturers produce their own phantoms and use them in installation and routine preventative maintenance. In this chapter we will see that:

- Signal-to-noise ratio (SNR) is the most useful (and fundamental) image quality parameter and should be measured and monitored both regularly and frequently.
- At field strengths above 0.5 T SNR is fundamentally related linearly to B_0
- Geometric parameters, e.g. spatial resolution and distortion, including slice-related quantities are

essential measurements for the initial commissioning of a system or after a re-shim, and more routinely for geometry-critical clinical applications such as radiotherapy treatment planning.
- Spatial resolution is normally 'pixel-limited', except for highly segmented sequences or where excessive signal filtering is applied.

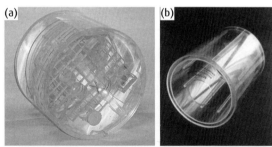
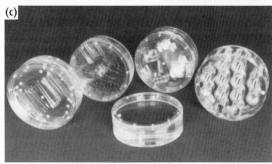

Figure 11.1 Phantoms for quality assurance (QA). (a) ACR multipurpose phantom, courtesy of the American College of Radiologists. (b) Loading ring, courtesy of MagNET, Imperial College, London. (c) Eurospin test object set, courtesy of Diagnostic Sonar Ltd., Livingston, UK.

- Relaxation parameters, particularly contrast and contrast-to-noise ratio (CNR) are important for protocol development and sequence and evaluation.
- Ghost artefacts and problems with fat saturation or water selection may give an indication of underlying technical problems with the scanner.
- National and international QA standards have been developed.
- Specialized QA procedures are required for specific applications such as spectroscopy and fMRI.

We will underpin this chapter with physics theory relating to SNR and resolution.

11.2 The quality cycle

The quality cycle for an item of radiological equipment begins with the drawing up of specifications, i.e. before purchase. On installation of a new or upgraded MR system, acceptance procedures should be carried out by an appropriately qualified MR physicist or engineer with any noncompliance receiving corrective action from the manufacturer. The acceptance report can then form the baseline for routine QA. This sort of QA is concerned with equipment aspects of the scanner. Human aspects (working practice, safety procedures, training, skill, etc.), which are much more likely to be problematical, are best addressed through clinical audit or quality management systems such as ISO9001 or equivalent. One such scheme, organized by the American College of Radiology (ACR), consists of an initial accreditation and the development of a QA programme for all MRI facilities. All QA should be subject to audit, review and corrective action. At each point in the cycle reference to local, manufacturer or national/international standards can be made. Further details are in the box 'National and international standards'.

11.3 Signal parameters

Signal parameters include SNR, uniformity and centre frequency. SNR is without doubt a key parameter. Equipment-related factors that affect SNR include field strength, choice of coil, coil loading (see 'Theoretical field dependence of SNR') and bandwidth. Sequence-related factors include voxel size, sequence choice and timings. For SNR measurement it is important to use standard set-up arrangements and sequence parameters. Saving these into a user-defined QA protocol is highly recommended.

Signal parameters are normally measured using a uniform or 'flood field' phantom filled with a material with appropriate relaxation times (see box 'Filling factors'). A crucial issue is whether to load the coil or not. Loading means using a slightly conductive solution (i.e. saline) to mimic the reduction of coil quality factor and to generate realistic patient noise. For head and body coils a loading ring is often used (see figure 11.1(b)). For other coils saline can be added to the paramagnetic solution to obtain the desired effect (see box 'A loaded question').

Measurement of the centre (Larmor) frequency may also be carried out using the uniform phantom. This value is normally available through the manufacturer's prescanning software.

11.3.1 SNR

SNR measurements are very useful and should be carried out daily or weekly. Two methods are common for measuring SNR. In the signal-background method, the signal is given by the mean pixel value from a region of interest (ROI) within the phantom. For head and body coils it is recommended that the ROI should include at least 75% of the phantom area (see figure 11.2). Alternatively, the AAPM suggests a small ROI of at least 100 pixels although the mean value obtained can then be dependent upon the exact position. The noise is measured from the standard deviation of the pixel values from small ROIs (between one and four) placed within ghost-free regions of background outside the phantom. You must take care to avoid using areas with filter roll-off, which may have atypical standard deviations. The average of the standard deviations from these noise regions is used in the calculation of SNR

$$SNR = \frac{0.66 \times \text{mean signal}}{\text{average of noise region standard deviations}}$$

The factor of 0.66 is the Rayleigh distribution correction factor (see box 'What's in the noise?').

The second (NEMA) method involves acquiring two identical images consecutively and subtracting them. An ROI covering 75% of the phantom area is used to measure the signal as before. Noise is measured from the standard deviation of pixel values within this ROI placed in the subtraction image. The SNR is

$$SNR = \sqrt{2} \cdot \frac{\text{mean signal in image ROI}}{\text{standard deviation in subtraction image ROI}}$$

The factor of $\sqrt{2}$ is required to compensate for the greater standard deviation from the subtraction of images. The Rayleigh correction factor is not required.

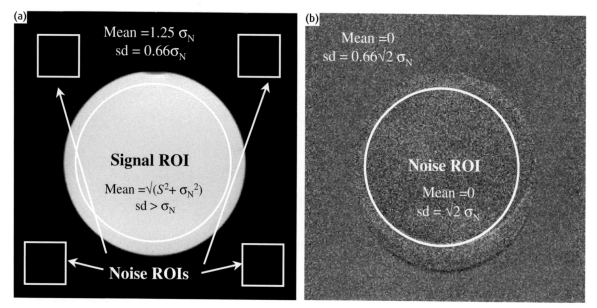

Figure 11.2 Signal-background and National Electrical Manufacturers Association (NEMA) SNR methods: (a) Magnitude image. (b) Subtraction of two consecutive magnitude images. In this example the subtraction was affected by scan-to-scan inconsistencies. σ_N is the standard deviation of the normal (Gaussian) noise distribution. S is the mean MR signal intensity of a region of interest (ROI).

National and international standards (NEMA, AAPM, IPEM, Eurospin and ACR)

The National Electrical Manufacturers Association (NEMA) has published a series of standards for the methodology of image quality parameter measurement and phantom design principles. NEMA has stopped short of defining specific performance expectations or 'action criteria'. A similar approach has been taken by the American Association of Physicists in Medicine (AAPM) and includes action criteria. By contrast, the Eurospin Test System developed by a European Community Concerted Action programme in the 1980s is a set of five test objects for image quality evaluation, with a particular emphasis on the measurement and characterization of relaxation times in vivo (figure 11.1(c)). Because of this emphasis on T_1 and T_2 measurement, the Eurospin phantoms are not especially suited to the QA requirements of modern MR systems. The same group has published protocols, phantom designs and results of a multi-centre trial for spectroscopic QA.

The American College of Radiology (ACR) has developed a standard for performance monitoring of MRI equipment, and its accreditation and quality control scheme uses a custom-designed phantom (figure 11.1(a)) and protocol. The ACR also has defined clinical standards for performing and interpreting MRI and specialist standards for neurovascular MR angiography and cardiovascular MRI. ACR standards include a summary of techniques, indications and contraindications, education, training and experience of personnel, staff responsibilities, examination specifications, documentation, equipment specifications, safety guidelines, quality control and patient education. The ACR states that its standards 'are not rules but are guidelines that attempt to define principles of practice which should generally produce high-quality radiological care.'

The International Electotechnical Commission (IEC) is working on a standard for test methodologies and reporting of results in a uniform format. At the time of writing it is only in draft form and is unavailable to the MR community.

These standards can be found in:

American Association of Physicists in Medicine

Price RR, Axel L, Morgan T et al. (1990) Quality assurance methods and phantoms for magnetic resonance imaging: report of AAPM Nuclear Magnetic Resonance Task Group No 1a. *Med Phys* **17**:287–95.

The American College of Radiology

The following documents are available to download or purchase from http://www.acr.org/frames/fpublications.html [accessed 4th November 2001]

ACR standard for performing and interpreting magnetic resonance imaging (MRI) (2000).

ACR standard for diagnostic medical physics: performance monitoring of magnetic resonance imaging equipment (2000).

ACR standard for the performance of cardiovascular MRI (2000).

ACR standard for the performance of pediatric and adult neurovascular magnetic resonance angiography (MRA) (2000).

Phantom Test Guidance for the ACR MRI Accreditation program (2000). ACR MRI Quality Control Manual (2001) ISBN 1–55903–144–1.

European Concerted Action Research Project

European Communities Research Project (COMAC BME II 2.3) (1988) Protocols and test objects for the assessment of MRI equipment. *Magn Reson Imaging* **6**:195–9.

European Communities Research Project (1995) Quality assessment in in-vivo NMR spectroscopy: results of a concerted research project for the European Economic Community I–IV. *Magn Reson Imaging* **13**: 117–58.

Lerski RA, de Wilde J, Boyce D and Ridgway J (1998) Quality control in magnetic resonance imaging. *IPEM Report no 80.* (ISBN: 0904181901).

International Electrotechnical Commission

Medical Electrical Equipment – Magnetic resonance equipment for diagnostic imaging Part 1 determination of characteristics (Draft only)

National Electrical Manufacturers Association

The following documents can be purchased via http://www.nema.org/index_nema.cfm/703 [accessed 4th November 2001].

MS1 Determination of the signal-to-noise ratio (SNR) in diagnostic magnetic resonance images (1988).

MS2 Determination of two dimensional geometric distortion in diagnostic magnetic resonance images (1989).

MS3 Determination of image uniformity in diagnostic magnetic resonance images (1989).

MS5 Determination of slice thickness in diagnostic magnetic resonance images (1992).

MS6 Characterization of special purpose coils for diagnostic magnetic resonance images (1991).

See also 'Further reading' at the end of the chapter.

Filling factors

The choice of filling materials for phantoms usually involves aqueous paramagnetic solutions. Common substances include nickel, sodium and manganese used in ionic compounds as chlorides or sulphates. Alternatively one can simply dilute leftover gadolinium or super-paramagnetic iron oxide (SPIO) contrast. It is important to understand the MR properties of the solution. These include the ratio of T_1 and T_2, field dependence, magnetic susceptibility and temperature coefficient, and are summarized in table 11.1. The AAPM recommends having T_1 between 100 and 1200 ms and T_2 between 50 and 400 ms. NEMA recommends only the upper limit for T_1 and the lower for T_2. We favour keeping both T_1 and T_2 quite short, e.g. both about 200 ms, as this means that the QA can be completed more quickly by using a shorter TR, and that transverse coherence artefacts can be avoided.

Table 11.1 MR Properties of paramagnetic ions

Ion	T_1/T_2 ratio	Relaxivity R_1 $(s^{-1}\,mmol^{-1})$ 3 MHz (0.07 T)	60 MHz (1.4 T)	Temperature coefficient dR/dT	Comments
Cu^{2+}	1.1	1.7	0.5	0.038	Varies with B_0 and temperature
Gd^{3+}	1.1	22.1	10	0.28	Varies with B_0 and temperature
Mn^{2+}	2–10*	13	7		* T_1/T_2 ratio varies with B_0 but can get more 'tissue-like' T_2
Ni^{2+}	1.1	0.6	0.65	−0.006	B_0-independent up to 1.5 T; fairly independent of temperature

The relaxation time is calculated as follows:

$$\frac{1}{T_1} = \frac{1}{T_{1,0}} + R_1 C$$

where $T_{1,0}$ is the T_1 of pure water (distilled and de-ionized – about 3000 ms for all B_0) and C is the molar concentration of ions. For example a 7 mM solution of $NiCl_2$ gives T_1 and T_2 approximately equal to 200 ms. The ACR phantom uses 10 mM nickel chloride plus 75 mM sodium chloride for loading, giving it a T_1 and T_2 of approximately 150 ms independent of B_0 for most clinical systems. However beware of significant relaxation time shortening for 3 T systems if using nickel-based solutions.

A loaded question

Should you load the coils or not? NEMA recommends loading only for SNR measurements, either by a loading phantom or electrically. The AAPM recommends not loading for any parameter (to determine system performance independently of the patient). Our advice is to load for signal parameter measurements in the head and body coils. For other parameters, loading is generally unnecessary but, if used, does not adversely affect the tests provided SNR is good enough. If a loading ring is used it must be aligned with its axis along the main z axis of the scanner to work properly.

Theoretical field dependence of SNR

In a uniform static magnetic field of strength B_0 the equilibrium magnetization M_0 is given by the Langevin equation

$$M_0 = \frac{\gamma^2 h^2 B_0 \rho}{4kT}$$

where k is Boltzmann's constant, T is the absolute temperature in kelvin (K), ρ is the number of nuclei per unit volume and γ is equal to 42 MHz T^{-1} for proton imaging.

The signal induced in the receiver coil is proportional to the rate of change of the magnetization, i.e. the Larmor frequency ω_0, the coil efficiency (field per unit current) B_1 and M_0

$$S \propto \omega_0 \cdot B_1 \cdot B_0$$

Since both the Larmor frequency and M_0 are proportional to B_0, the signal (S) can be written as

$$S \propto B_1 \cdot B_0^2$$

Random noise arises from the Brownian motion of electrons within a conductor. The thermally induced random noise or Johnson noise is given by

$$V_{\text{noise (rms)}} = \sqrt{4 \cdot k \cdot T \cdot R \cdot \text{BW}}$$

where R is the effective resistance and BW is the bandwidth of the measuring equipment. The overall noise variance is the sum of the noise variances due to the patient, receiver coil and receiver electronics. Effectively the resistance R is the sum of the coil resistance R_c and the resistance induced by the conductive losses in the patient R_p. Therefore $R = R_c + R_p$. In high-field imaging the dominant source of noise is the patient, whereas at low field the coil can be the dominant noise source.

If we consider the coil noise first then we need to take account of the fact that at radiofrequencies the resistance of the coil increases with the square-root of the frequency due to the phenomenon of skin effect described in chapter 9 ('Beauty is skin deep'). Therefore

$$V_{\text{noise(rms)}} \propto \omega_0^{1/4} \propto B_0^{1/4}$$

and for low-field systems

$$\text{SNR} \propto \frac{B_1 \cdot B_0^2}{B_0^{1/4}} \propto B_1 \cdot B_0^{7/4}$$

At low B_0 then SNR depends upon B_0 to the power of 7/4 and the coil efficiency is crucial.

However, at high field strengths (≥ 0.5 T) the effective patient resistance should dominate over the coil resistance. For the simplified case of a saline sphere of radius r with conductivity , for a uniform B field (i.e. a coil with a perfectly uniform sensitivity), R_p is given by

$$R_p = \frac{2\pi\sigma\omega_0^2 B_1^2 r^5}{15}$$

Therefore

$$V_{\text{noise(rms)}} \propto \sqrt{B_1^2 \cdot \omega_0^2} \propto B_1 \cdot B_0$$

and

$$\text{SNR} \propto \frac{B_1 \cdot B_0^2}{B_1 \cdot B_0} \propto B_0$$

So at high field strengths the theoretical SNR is only proportional to B_0. In practice other factors, e.g. signal bandwidth and gradient strength, may reduce this dependence further. Notice that although SNR is independent of the coil efficiency, noise and SNR are highly dependent upon the amount of tissue the coil 'sees' (to the fifth power). This is the underlying reason for the greater SNR of surface and array coils.

What's in the noise?

The measurement of background noise in MRI is quite instructive. For an ROI in the background noise of a magnitude-reconstructed image, the ratio of the mean pixel value to the standard deviation should be very close to a fixed number

$$\frac{\text{mean}}{\text{standard deviation}} = 1.8$$

This is because the background noise follows a Rayleigh distribution rather than a normal (or Gaussian) one. In a normal distribution the mean of the background would be zero. But because we use magnitude images, all the negative numbers are made positive and the mean is greater than zero. This results in the standard deviation being smaller and is the reason for the 0.66 factor used in the signal-to-background method. The constant value of 1.8 for the ratio of mean to standard deviation in the background breaks down for some fast imaging sequences or when phased array coils are used, and in parallel imaging.

Noise of course pervades the whole image, and in a high signal region or in the subtracted images of the NEMA SNR method the variance of the signal, i.e. the noise, does have a normal distribution. These noise relationships apply for 'white noise' only, where the noise has a flat frequency spectrum, i.e. the same noise power per unit bandwidth. White noise gives a Gaussian distribution of pixel values with zero mean. These noise relationships are illustrated in figure 11.2.

Absolutely fabulous SNR

The absolute SNR provides a calculation of the fundamental signal-to-noise performance of the system when measured under appropriate loading conditions and with minimal signal saturation and T_2 decay, i.e. a long enough TR and short enough TE. Absolute SNR (ASNR) can be directly related to the magnetic field strength. It is defined for two-dimensional Fourier transform (2D FT) as

$$\text{ASNR} = \text{SNR} \cdot \frac{\sqrt{\text{pixel bandwidth}}}{\Delta x \cdot \Delta y \cdot \Delta z \cdot \sqrt{\text{NSA} \cdot N_{\text{PE}}}}$$

where the pixel bandwidth is measured in Hz and SNR is measured by any suitable method. As before NSA is the number of signal acquisitions and N_{PE} is the phase-encode matrix size. ASNR has units of $\text{Hz}^{1/2}\,\text{mm}^{-3}$. As a rule of thumb we expect ASNR to be at least 10 per tesla for an appropriately loaded head coil. So for a 1.5 T scanner with pixel dimensions of 1 mm by 1 mm and a 5 mm slice with a pixel bandwidth of 100 Hz and 256^2 matrix expect an image SNR of $10 \times 5 \times \sqrt{256} \, / \, \sqrt{100} = 80$ assuming minimal T_1 saturation and minimal T_2 decay.

Ideally both SNR methods should yield the same result. Performance criteria are not normally quoted, being dependent upon fundamental and equipment-related factors (see box 'Theoretical field dependence of SNR'). For a practical approach refer to 'Absolutely fabulous SNR'. SNR is usually measured on a daily or weekly basis for either head or body coils.

These methods can be applied to surface and special purpose coils only with a great deal of care on the exact positioning and choice of ROI. NEMA has attempted to define a standard method for such coils. The ACR recommends measuring the 'maximum SNR' for surface coils using small ROIs for both signal and background noise.

11.3.2 Uniformity

Uniformity is particularly important for RF coils which transmit and receive, as any RF inhomogeneity will affect the flip angles and hence the contrast. Nonuniformity in receive-only surface coils is a feature of their design and is usually quite well tolerated by the observer. Homogenizing (image intensity correction) filters may be provided in the system. For this reason uniformity is usually only measured for head and body coils using a uniform phantom.

Integral uniformity I is defined as

$$I = 1 - \frac{M - m}{M + m} \cdot 100\%$$

where M is the maximum pixel value and m is the minimum pixel value within an ROI of 75% of the phantom area. A value of 100% represents perfect uniformity. (NEMA uses a nonuniformity parameter U = (1 − I) with a value of zero representing perfect uniformity.) To overcome inaccuracies arising from a low SNR, NEMA recommends an image smoothing stage. In practice we have found this achieves little, and for systems with low SNR it is better to increase the number of acquisitions, NSA. Performance criteria have been defined for head coils, and these are shown in table 11.2. Uniformity

Table 11.2 Action criteria and expected performance for head coil

Parameter	ACR[a]	AAPM
SNR	Not specified	Not specified
Uniformity	≥ 87.5%	≥ 80%
Linearity/distortion	≤ ±2 mm in 190 mm on diameterof phantom	≤ 5% over 25 cm or greater
Spatial resolution	±1 mm using ACR specified sequence	Pixel size, e.g. 1 mm for 256×256, 256 mm FOV
Slice thickness	≤ 0.7 mm for 5-mm slice	±1 mm for ≥ 5 mm
Slice position accuracy	Bar length difference should be ≤5 mm[b] (see figure 11.3)	≤ ±2mm
Slice separation	Not defined	±1 mm or 20% of slice width, whichever is greater
Low contrast object Detectability	Specific to phantom	Not specified
Ghosting	≤ 2.5%	≤ 5%
Centre frequency	Not specified	≤ ±50 ppm

Notes:
[a] American College of Radiology (ACR) action criteria are dependent upon using the ACR phantom and test guidance and are somewhat stricter than those used by the ACR for accreditation, but in all cases are indicative of a minimum level of performance one can reasonably expect from a well-functioning MRI system. On the other hand, being minimum levels of performance, these criteria are not to be construed as indicators of typical or normal levels of performance.
[b] This is equivalent to an error of ±2.5 mm.

measurements are important for accepting new coils. They can usually be incorporated with scans performed for SNR measurements. At higher field strengths (1.5 T and above) there is a possibility of nonuniformity arising through standing wave effects caused by the dielectric properties of water. In this case an oil-based filling substance may be used.

11.4 Geometric parameters

Geometric parameters are mainly concerned with the accuracy of the spatial encoding, and reflect various technical factors, e.g. field uniformity, gradient linearity and eddy current compensation. Examples of specific action criteria are contained in table 11.2. Appropriate phantoms may afford the measurement of different parameters in particular slice positions or throughout an extended volume. These are illustrated in figure 11.3.

11.4.1 Linearity and distortion

Linearity refers to the accuracy of distances within the image, and is usually associated with gradient ampli-

tude calibration. Nonlinearity indices L_{FE} and L_{PE} can be defined with respect to the frequency and phase axes as

$$L_{FE} = \frac{x - l}{l} \cdot 100\%$$

$$L_{PE} = \frac{y - l}{l} \cdot 100\%$$

where x is the measured distance in the frequency-encode direction, y is the measured distance in the phase direction and l is the true length in the test object. NEMA and the AAPM do not distinguish between linearity and distortion, using similar definitions to those above (AAPM actually use the negative). The ACR uses the term 'geometric accuracy'. In Europe distortion is calculated as the precision of linearity from several distance measurements, usually between a regular array of points spaced throughout an image. Indices for distortion include the maximum deviation of a location from its true position or the standard deviation of the measured distances. These tests are essential at commissioning and after a field ramp or re-shim. The measurement of linearity can indicate gradient amplifier problems and is useful in routine QA. Some distortion phantom images are shown in figure 11.4.

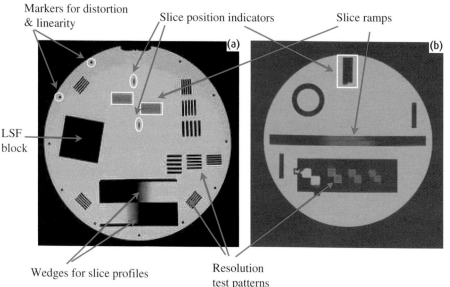

Markers for distortion & linearity

Slice position indicators

Slice ramps

(a)

(b)

LSF block

Wedges for slice profiles

Resolution test patterns

Figure 11.3 General purpose geometric phantoms. (a) Volume phantom for which all parameters are measurable on every slice, courtesy of Charing Cross Hospital, London. (b) Slice from ACR phantom showing insert for measuring spatial resolution, slice width and slice position accuracy. LSF denotes line spread function. Courtesy of the American College of Radiologists.

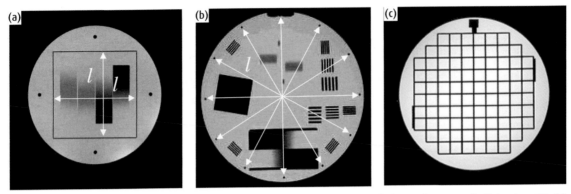

Figure 11.4 Distortion measurement phantom images: (a) Eurospin TO2, courtesy of Diagnostic Sonar Ltd., Livingston, UK. (b) Charing Cross TO2A, courtesy of Charing Cross Hospital, London. (c) ACR geometric accuracy insert, courtesy of the American College of Radiologists. l is the true length in the test object.

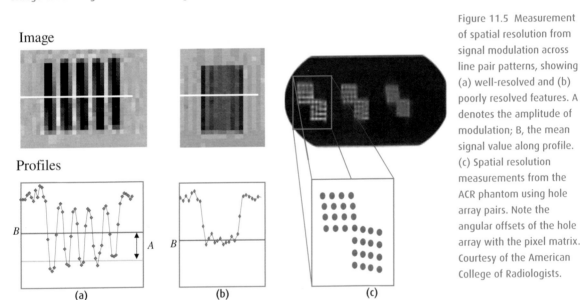

Figure 11.5 Measurement of spatial resolution from signal modulation across line pair patterns, showing (a) well-resolved and (b) poorly resolved features. A denotes the amplitude of modulation; B, the mean signal value along profile. (c) Spatial resolution measurements from the ACR phantom using hole array pairs. Note the angular offsets of the hole array with the pixel matrix. Courtesy of the American College of Radiologists.

11.4.2 Resolution

Spatial resolution is often pixel limited in MRI, except for certain highly segmented sequences such as single-shot fast spin echo (FSE) and echo planar imaging (EPI) and when heavy signal filtering is applied. It is therefore of minimal use in QA but may be helpful in evaluating new sequences. Quantitatively it can be assessed using bar patterns or line pairs (figures 11.3 and 11.5). These can be assessed visually or by measuring the modulation, defined (for a 100% contrast pattern) as

$$\text{modulation (line pairs)} = \frac{\text{amplitude of pattern}}{\text{mean signal across pattern}}$$
$$= \frac{A}{B}$$

Care is required with alignment of the patterns with the pixel matrix. Aliasing of the patterns can occur and excessive Gibbs' ringing may also render the measurement void. Both effects are apparent in figure 11.3(a).

Modulation transfer function

In X-ray CT we would measure the modulation transfer function (MTF) of the scanner. This is not commonplace in MRI because of its Fourier pixel-limited nature, and also because an accurate method of MTF measurement is difficult. Where it has been attempted, Judy's method of scanning a high-contrast edge at a slight angle θ (e.g. 10°) to the pixel matrix (figure 11.6) is used. For a square ROI centred on the edge, the centre of each pixel will be at a slightly different distance (as the crow flies) from the edge. The difference in distance of neighbouring pixels to the edge will be less than the pixel dimension (Δx). Hence from this ROI a magnified or over-sampled edge response function (ERF) may be reconstituted. In a simpler variant of the Judy method, a line profile obliquely crossing the edge yields a similar result.

In either method the effective sampling interval is given by

$$\delta = \Delta x \times \sin \theta$$

Differentiation of the ERF produces a line spread function (LSF). In CT one could take the normalized Fourier transform of this to obtain an MTF. However, in MRI, unless real-valued inversion recovery (with positive and negative signals) is used the LSF will be distorted and asymmetric and does not yield a true MTF. In this case a measurement of the full width at half maximum (FWHM) of the LSF will give a good indication of the spatial resolution. It is vital to remember that the axis in which you are measuring the resolution is the one nearly perpendicular to the edge, i.e. the horizontal axis in figure 11.6.

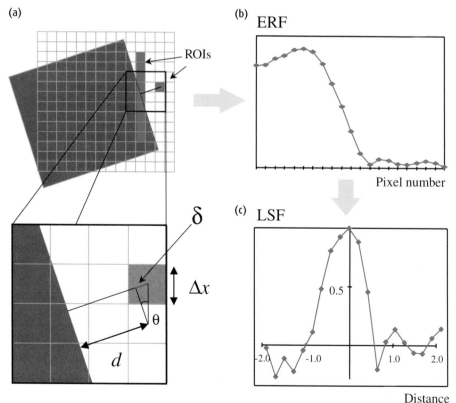

(a)

(b) ERF

Pixel number

(c) LSF

δ

Δx

θ

d

0.5

-2.0   -1.0   1.0   2.0

Distance

Figure 11.6 Derivation of the line spread function from an angled edge. (a) The edge response function (ERF) can be obtained from either a square region of interest (ROI) or a linear profile. In the latter case, the resolution measured is that perpendicular to the profile. (b) Example of an ERF. (c) The line spread function (LSF) is the normalized derivative of the ERF.

Resolution limits

The spatial resolution of an imaging method is defined as the smallest resolvable distance between two different objects. In MRI it is easy to think of the pixel size as the intrinsic spatial resolution of the image; however, this is not necessarily the case.

The pixel-limited resolution was given in section 7.5.6. For the frequency-encode (FE) axis this was

$$\Delta x = \frac{1}{\gamma G_x M \Delta t} = \frac{1}{\gamma G_x T_{acq}}$$

where T_{acq} is the data acquisition time $= M\Delta t$. We could in principle increase G_x, M or Δt to achieve any desired resolution, although in practice both gradient strength and acquisition time are subject to physical limits.

The frequency spread across a pixel from the spatial-encoding gradient is

$$\Delta f = \gamma G_x \Delta x$$

However, if the signal from a point source decays over the readout period with time constant T_2^* then, following Fourier transformation, this results in the point spreading out to give a characteristic line width of $\Delta \omega = 2 \div T_2^*$, i.e. the point would be blurred by this amount. The line-width broadened frequency Δf^* is therefore given by

$$\Delta f^* = \frac{1}{\pi T_2^*}$$

To avoid T_2^* blurring we require that

$$\Delta f \gg \Delta f^*$$

i.e.

$$G_x \gg \frac{2}{\gamma \Delta x T_2^*}$$

This also implies an ultimate limit on the spatial resolution determined by T_2^* of $2/(\gamma G_x T_2^*)$.

An alternative method uses arrays of small holes of varying diameters. The ACR phantom (figure 11.5(c)) has hole diameters of 0.9, 1.0 and 1.1 mm to allow visual assessment of spatial resolution for a nominal pixel size of 1 mm. These are slightly offset with regard to the main gradient axes to avoid aliasing problems with the pixel matrix.

11.4.3 Slice parameters

Slice parameters include slice position, slice width and slice profile (see 'In profile'). Slice position can be measured from a phantom containing a pair of crossed rods or ramps inclined at θ to the slice plane (figure 11.7). The slice position p is then given by

$$p = \frac{d}{2\tan\theta}$$

where d is the measured distance in the image plane. In figure 11.7 θ is 45°. Slice separation is the distance between adjacent slice positions.

Slice width measurements can be obtained by two methods: ramps and wedges (figure 11.3 and 11.8). Ramps may be either 'hot' or 'cold' depending upon whether they produce signal or lack of signal, e.g. a glass plate immersed in water would constitute a cold ramp. Figure 11.3 shows examples of both hot and cold ramps. The effect of the ramp is to project a magnified image or shadow of the signal in the z axis (the slice profile) onto one of the in-plane axes. A line profile drawn across this is related to the slice shape. If the ramp makes an angle θ with the slice plane the slice thickness can be determined, defined as the full width half maximum (FHWM) as

Slice width = in-plane FHWM $\cdot \tan \theta$

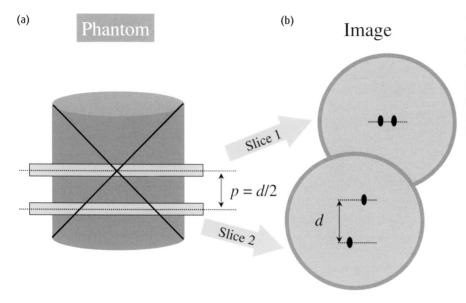

Figure 11.7 Slice position measurements from a pair of rods crossed at 45°: (a) view of phantom perpendicular to the slice-select axis showing slice positions. (b) schematic of images produced from (a).

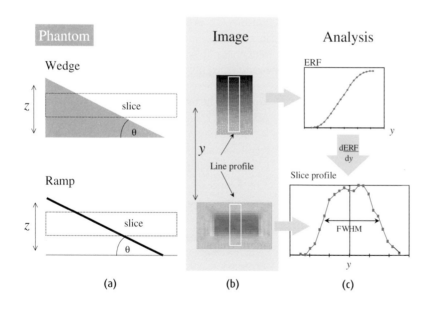

Figure 11.8 Slice width and profile measurement from a wedge and cold ramp. (a) View of phantom perpendicular to the slice-select axis showing slice position. (b) images resulting from (a). (c) Line profiles from (b). ERF denotes edge response function and FWHM full width at half maximum.

Using a different angle for the ramp or wedge changes the 'stretch factor' or degree of magnification, e.g. 26.6° gives a magnification of two whilst 11.3° magnifies by five. This method is adequate for slice widths down to about one-third of the ramp thickness. Below this you get an overestimation of slice thickness caused by the convolution of the ramp thickness with the slice profile (and also the in-plane pixel dimension).

Wedges can be used to measure very thin slices. An edge response function (ERF) is obtained from a line profile drawn along the wedge. The derivative of this represents the scaled slice profile, again according to

In profile
The slice profile P is a plot of the transverse magnetization (or signal) in the slice-select axis and is related to flip angle α by

$$P(z) = \rho(z)\sin \alpha(z)$$

Slice profiles are sensitive to relaxation effects, particularly T_1 for short TR in gradient-echo sequences. When TR/T_1 becomes less than 1, significant broadening and other distortions to the slice profile can occur in the regions where the flip angle is varying most, i.e. at the edges of the slice. These can be minimized by the use of a suitably low flip angle. For a perfectly rectangular profile, these would not occur. The need for short duration RF pulses means that, in practice, profiles are never perfect. Once again, it's a case of the Fourier 'less-is-more' principle. Slice profile distortions can lead to changes in image contrast and unexpected partial volume effects (see section 7.4).

the stretch factor above. This method requires a high SNR.

In both methods, using pairs of opposed ramps or wedges allows one to correct for geometric misalignment with respect to the slice plane. Whilst an exact correction is possible, it is usually sufficient to take the geometric mean of measurements across both features.

$$\text{True slice width} = \sqrt{\text{slice width 1} \cdot \text{slice width 2}}$$

Manufacturers often specify a tolerance of 10% of the slice width. These tests are important at acceptance and for sequence evaluation, especially where selective inversion pulses are used, but may not be useful in routine QA. Ramps or wedges may also be used for slice position measurements as in the ACR phantom.

11.5 Relaxation parameters

Relaxation parameters include contrast, contrast-to-noise ratio (CNR) and T_1 and T_2 measurement accuracy and precision. Contrast is probably the most important feature of MRI; however, because it is so sequence dependent, standard QA methodologies are not common. Nevertheless contrast can be measured for pairs of samples with differing relaxation times from the mean pixel values S_1 and S_2 in ROIs placed in each sample as

$$\text{Contrast} = \frac{S_1 - S_2}{|S_1| + |S_2|}$$

where $S_1 > S_2$. The moduli on the denominator are required for inversion recovery sequences where negative signals may be encountered. This gives a contrast range of 0–1 for all sequences.

CNR may be defined as

$$\text{CNR} = \frac{S_1 - S_2}{\text{Noise}}$$

for a suitable measurement of noise (e.g. standard deviation of background).

These tests would not commonly form part of a routine QA programme, but may be very helpful in protocol optimization and for evaluating new sequences. To be useful, one needs to know the appropriate relaxation times for the tissues of interest and have a suitable material that mimics them. Physical properties of tissue, such as proton density, heterogeneity, T_1/T_2 ratio, magnetization transfer and partial volumes, may not be adequately modelled by simple test materials. The Eurospin TO5 (figure 11.1(c)) contains a set of doped polysaccharide gels with a range of T_1 and T_2.

Contrast-detail detectability
A test that is very important in X-ray-based imaging methodologies is low-contrast-detail detectability. This is a test of the resolving power of the system for low values of contrast. A typical phantom is shown in figure 11.9 where differing diameters of disk details have a different signal contrast. The image is evaluated subjectively by counting the number of disks clearly seen for each diameter group. Constructional difficulties with contrast phantoms limits this test to proton density contrast evaluation. It can also provide a subjective assessment of SNR.

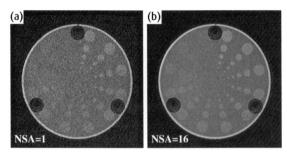

Figure 11.9 Examples of contrast-detail detectability phantom with a different number of signal acquisitions. (a) NSA = 1. (b) NSA = 16. Phantom by Philips Medical Systems.

11.6 Artefacts

Artefacts tend to occur sporadically and would not be subject to a routine QA test, except for ghosting.

11.6.1 Ghosting

Ghosting is best measured using a small phantom offset diagonally in the field of view (FOV). Phase ghosts will then be apparent in the phase-encode (PE) direction. Additionally, 'quadrature ghosts' (which are extremely rare these days) appear as a reflection of the primary image through the origin. The fourth quadrant (figure 11.10) should contain only random noise. A ghost-to-signal ratio (GSR) can be defined as

$$GSR = \frac{\text{mean SI of ghost ROI} - \text{mean SI of background ROI}}{\text{mean SI of primary image ROI}}$$

where SI is signal intensity. You may have to manipulate the display window and level to extreme values to visualize the ghosts, but they will always be in there somewhere. The AAPM action level is set at 5%. In practice we would recommend a more stringent 2% for most sequences (except EPI). Owing to the sensitivity of 2D FT to ghosting, this is a very useful test, although care needs to be taken to ensure that ghosts are not induced by mechanical vibration caused by the gradients. The presence of ghosting should be routinely investigated on a daily or weekly basis.

Evaluation of clinical images: ACR standard

The ACR accreditation process includes an image quality evaluation for clinical images, carried out by an independent radiologist. Images required include:

(a) Routine brain examination (for headache)
- sagittal short TR/short TE with dark cerebrospinal fluid (CSF)
- axial or coronal long TR/short TE (or FLAIR)
- and long TR/long TE (e.g. long TR double echo)

(b) Routine cervical spine examination (for radiculopathy)
- sagittal short TR/short TE with dark CSF
- sagittal long TR/long TE or T_2^*-weighted with bright CSF
- axial long TR/long TE or T_2^*-weighted with bright CSF

(c) Routine lumbar spine examination (for back pain)
- sagittal short TR/short TE with dark CSF
- sagittal long TR/long TE or T_2^*-weighted with bright CSF
- axial short TR/short TE with dark CSF and/or long TR/long TE with bright CSF

(d) Complete routine knee examination (for internal derangement)
- to include sagittal(s) and coronal(s) with at least one sequence with bright fluid

The images are evaluated subjectively for choice of pulse sequence and image contrast, filming technique, anatomical coverage and imaging planes, spatial resolution, artefacts and examination annotation.

Items (a)–(d) are reprinted with permission of the American College of Radiology, Reston, VA, USA. No other representation of this material is authorized without express, written permission from the American College of Radiology.

11.6.2 Chemical shift and fat suppression

Chemical shift, as an artefact, is not worth measuring as we can determine the pixel shift if we know the bandwidth (section 6.5.1). However, it is very worthwhile to measure the effectiveness of fat suppression or

(a) Original image

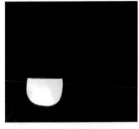

Windowed image

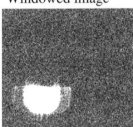

(b) Measurement ROIs

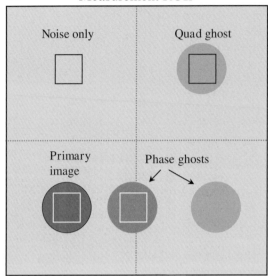

Figure 11.10 Ghosting. (a) Extreme windowing is usually required to see the ghosts. (b) Schematic diagram of ROI positions for signal–ghost ratio measurement.

water-only excitation methods as these critically depend upon the shimming of the magnet and can have a major effect upon the diagnostic value of certain examinations, especially musculo-skeletal and any use of echo planar imaging (EPI).

This can be done simply using a water-based and a fat-based phantom (e.g. cooking oil) and taking the ratio of mean pixel values in images acquired with and

Other specialist QA

Certain clinical situations may require a more specialized QA program. Examples of these include the use of MRI for radiotherapy treatment planning and stereotactic surgery where geometric distortion may need to receive special attention. The same may be true for interventional MRI, certainly when new instruments are introduced. Functional MRI (fMRI) places high demands upon the short-term stability of the MR system and may require additional QA based upon stability of the MR signal, SNR and artefact level in EPI sequences.

In addition to image quality, the ACR recommends weekly sensitometric QA for hard copy devices used in MRI.

QA for high field systems

The principles of QA are exactly the same for high field systems (e.g. 3 T), however certain practical considerations need to be made. The relaxation times of the test materials need to be considered. The electrical conductivity of the test object may result in an unrealistic RF deposition : always use an oil phantom for uniformity measurements. Expect increased susceptibility problems: these may be related to the phantom design and construction rather than to the scanner.

without fat-suppression enabled. The effect of frequency-selective fat suppression on the water signal should also be tested to ensure that unwanted water signal saturation is not occurring. Care needs to be taken over shimming and the shape and positioning of the phantoms.

11.7 Spectroscopic QA

Centres using spectroscopy should also perform QA regularly with an appropriate MR spectroscopy

Phantom problems

Care has to be taken with phantom measurements to avoid obtaining misleading results. Phantoms generally contain higher signals than humans and have a different distribution of spatial frequencies, often with many high-contrast edges. The phantom geometry and materials may result in spurious susceptibility effects and the automatic shim may have trouble obtaining convergence. The filling materials may have atypical relaxation times with various consequences: greater occurrence of coherence and stimulated echoes due to long T_2, and greater high spatial frequency signals in segmented sequences. There are simple practical considerations to remember:

- allow the phantom fluid to settle
- let the phantom fluid reach thermal equilibrium with the environment, if temperature-dependent
- avoid bubble formation
- minimize mechanical vibration

It's also important to remember that patients breathe, pulsate and fidget (the usual cause of image quality problems) but that phantoms do not.

phantom which will be provided by the manufacturer. At the very least phantom spectra should be acquired weekly using the clinical protocols (PRESS and/or STEAM at appropriate echo times; see sections 15.3.1 and 15.3.2). The SNR of the main peaks (creatine, N-acetyl-aspartate and choline) should be examined and ideally their linewidths should also be measured.

If quantification of metabolite ratios is being used, a calibration scan is usually necessary and this should be performed weekly. The same phantom may be used, but it may be better to use a single metabolite phantom such as N-acetyl-aspartate at a precise concentration in de-ionized water. When such a phantom is made up, it must include a buffer to regulate the pH to approximately 7 and 0.1% sodium azide as a fungicide and bactericide. Peak area (i.e. absolute metabolite concen-

tration) is extremely sensitive to RF coil characteristics, so care must be taken to ensure that the phantom can be placed in exactly the same location each time to produce the same coil loading. It is also sensitive to temperature, and if the ambient room temperature fluctuates by more than 2 °C it will be necessary to store the phantom in a fridge. In this way although the phantom begins to warm up as soon as it is placed in the scanner, it will be at the same temperature when the MRS scan is done provided the QA is performed in the same way each time – which of course is the whole point!

As well as the weekly QA, spectroscopy results should be checked immediately after each service and especially after software upgrades. If the eddy current compensation is changed in any way, spectroscopy results will be affected and the QA should be performed. In these situations a good working relationship with the service engineers is essential, so that they tell you what they've actually done to the system.

See also:
- Image optimization: chapter 5
- MR safety standards: chapter 2
- Equipment-related artefacts: chapter 6

FURTHER READING

Edelstein WA, Bottomley PA and Pfeifer LM (1984) A signal to noise calibration procedure for NMR imaging systems. *Med Phys* **11**: 180–5.

Judy PF (1976) The line spread function and modulation transfer function of a computed tomography scanner. *Med Phys* **3**: 233–6.

Lerski RA, McRobbie DW, Straughan K et al. (1988) Multi-center trial with protocols and prototype test objects for the assessment of MRI equipment. *Magn Reson Imaging* **6**: 201–14.

McRobbie DW (1996) The absolute signal-to-noise ratio in MRI acceptance testing. *Br J Radiol* **69**:1045–8.

Och JG, Clarke GD, Sobol WT, et al. (1992) Acceptance testing of magnetic resonance imaging systems: report of AAPM Nuclear Magnetic Resonance Task Group No 6a. *Med Phys* **19**: 217–29.

Acronyms anonymous: a guide to the pulse sequence jungle

12.1 Introduction

In previous chapters we have seen how the image appearance can be manipulated by altering the sequence parameters such as TR, TE, TI and flip angle to give T_1-weighted or T_2-weighted contrast. We have examined the practical aspects of image acquisition: choosing the matrix size, field of view and slice thickness, the relationship between resolution and signal-to-noise ratio, and how, in practice, to avoid artefacts. Hopefully by now, you have got your head round spatial frequencies and spatial encoding. You will also have noticed by now that there are literally hundreds of pulse sequences. Every year at MR conferences around the world scores of new pulse sequences are launched and, in the tradition of the MR scientific community, all sporting stylish acronyms.

The trouble with acronyms is that despite sounding memorable and snappy (e.g. FLASH, HASTE, DRESS, SLIT-DRESS, DIET, PEPSI, etc.) it's virtually impossible to remember what they stand for, and therefore what they do. Moreover, MR manufacturers have the annoying tendency to use different names for the same things (a manufacturer conversion chart is given at the end of the chapter). Whilst the end-point of an acquisition can be expressed in terms of T_1 or T_2 weighting, there are numerous ways of achieving this – few destinations but many routes. So if you are lost in the pulse sequence jungle with a bewildering variety of sequence species, and cannot see the wood for the trees, this chapter is for you.

You will see that:
- there are two major pulse sequence families: spin echo (SE) and gradient echo (GE);

- segmented k-space acquisition schemes dramatically speed up SE-based acquisitions whilst retaining SE-like contrast, but with possibly a reduced number of slices and increased specific absorption rate (SAR);
- single-shot fast spin echo and echo planar imaging (EPI) offer the ultimate speed for T_2-weighted images but with image quality compromises;
- speed enhancement in GE is achieved by a combination of low flip angle and short TR, which minimizes the T_1 recovery required between successive TR periods;
- spoiled GE sequences produce T_1, proton density (PD) or $T_2{}^*$ contrast;
- rewound GE sequences give mixed contrast depending upon the ratio of T_2 and T_1 but higher SNR than spoiled GE, and are also subject to $T_2{}^*$ decay;
- time-reversed GE sequences have 'spin echo' type properties giving T_2 weighting;
- k-space segmentation applied to GE results in ultra-fast sequences such as turbo-FLASH and GE-EPI.

To understand this chapter you need to be familiar with the material from chapters 7 and 8 and have some grasp of the concept of k-space. For each sequence examined we will answer the following questions: how fast is it, how does it localize signal, what contrast does it produce and how does it avoid artefacts?

12.2 Getting above the trees: a sequences overview

Before venturing into the pulse sequence jungle, it is useful to find our bearings and remind ourselves of the

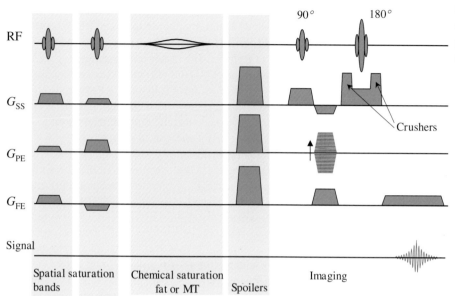

RF

90°   180°

G_{SS}

Crushers

G_{PE}

G_{FE}

Signal

Spatial saturation   Chemical saturation   Imaging
bands   fat or MT   Spoilers

Figure 12.1 Generic spin-echo sequence showing pulse sequence options in shading.

purposes and functions of pulse sequences, and also to survey the wider view of the terrain or (with a slightly alarming mixing of metaphors) the pulse sequence family tree.

12.2.1 Physiology of a pulse sequence

It can be helpful to list the purposes of MR imaging pulse sequences. They include generating contrast between different tissues and especially between healthy tissue and pathology, producing spatial localization, being sensitive or insensitive to flow or to some dynamic parameter, e.g. contrast uptake or blood perfusion, and the avoidance of artefacts. Additionally a sequence must achieve the desired anatomical coverage within a particular time frame, for example within a breath-hold.

Every imaging sequence must contain a means of exciting and localizing an MR signal. Therefore, there will always be RF pulses and gradients, one of which will always be a read or frequency-encode (FE) gradient. There will almost always be one or two sets of phase encode (PE) gradient pulses and some form of slice or slab selection. Additionally various other features may be added to ensure that scans are diagnostic. These are

shown in the context of a generic spin-echo sequence in figure 12.1 and include:

- Spatial saturation, to remove unwanted artefact-producing signals (e.g. from breathing). Usually there will be a choice of several saturation bands, all freely selectable in space.
- Fat suppression or saturation.
- Magnetization transfer saturation to improve contrast, or reduce background signal intensity in cerebral angiography.

These are repeated within every TR period and thus reduce the time available for each slice and also the number of slices possible.

12.2.2 The pulse sequence family tree

A great deal of the variety of MR sequences arises from the need to speed up MR acquisitions. Section 7.7 outlined a few Fourier transform tricks to speed things up, each offering at best a 50% reduction in scan time. The basic reasons for the slowness of conventional spin echo arose from the need to acquire each phase-encode line of the k-space raw data matrix from separate MR excitations, and the need to allow time for the magnetization to recover sufficiently between successive excitations.

The latter is fundamentally determined by the bio-physical properties of tissue and therefore not particu-larly negotiable. Addressing both these problems, ways of speeding up an acquisition are therefore:

- To acquire more than one line of data at once – this is called segmentation. It is done by fast or turbo spin echo – basically any sequence with the word 'fast' or 'turbo' in it.
- To only partially excite the MR signal with a low RF flip angle, achieving a 'steady state' and getting round the relaxation problem, as in gradient-echo tech-niques.

Despite the enormous variety of sequences and the bewildering jungle of names, there are just two basic underlying contrast mechanisms (three if you include PD weighting) and sequence character can be broadly divided into T_1-weighted or T_2-weighted or, more accu-rately, will exploit either T_1 or T_2 relaxation behaviour. In terms of sequence structure there are also two basic models, spin echo and gradient echo.

Figure 12.2 shows the generic pulse sequence family tree, with an indication of acquisition speed and type of contrast. In terms of increasing speed and complexity the spin-echo branch of the family contains turbo or fast spin echo (FSE), turbo **GR**adient **A**nd **S**pin **E**cho (GRASE), single-shot FSE or **HA**lf Fourier **S**ingle-shot

Turbo spin **E**cho (HASTE) and SE-EPI. Other variants include **FL**uid **A**ttenuated **I**nversion **R**ecovery (FLAIR) and **S**hort **TI** **I**nversion **R**ecovery (STIR) and true inver-sion recovery. The family on the gradient-echo side is somewhat more complex: spoiled or incoherent gradi-ent echo, rewound or coherent gradient echo and time-reversed GE and hybrid sequences, most with options for 2D or 3D acquisition. Contrast tends to be T_1- or T_2-weighted and sometimes a mixture of T_1 and T_2. The sequences in this branch will commonly be used for MR angiography (MRA), contrast studies, breath-hold imaging and high-resolution 3D imaging. EPI is the ulti-mate in terms of scanning speed, collecting a whole slice in under 100 ms.

12.3 RARING to go: spin-echo-based techniques

Images with SE-type contrast can be acquired with dra-matic time saving by collecting more than one line of data from a train of echoes formed by multiple refocus-ing RF pulses. This can be achieved over several excita-tions and TR periods (multi-shots) or ultimately from a single shot. The T_2 contrast depends upon the ordering of the PE gradient steps or the filling pattern for k-space.

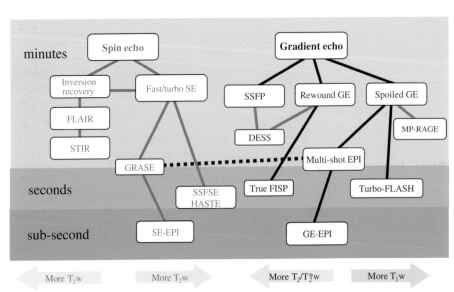

Figure 12.2 The generic family tree. Imaging speed is indicated vertically. The dominant contrast mechanism is indicated horizontally. T_1w and T_2w refer to T_1 and T_2 weighting, respectively; see table 12.1 for further information.

T_1 weighting can be achieved by using a short or intermediate TR as for conventional SE, or by using magnetization preparation usually in the form of an inversion pulse. With TSE some resolution loss, in the form of blurring, may occur. Additionally fat can appear very bright and some slice-to-slice variations in contrast may occur.

12.3.1 Spin echo and multiple spin echo

Spin-echo (SE) formation was considered in section 8.4 and further details are given in the box 'Getting focused on spin echo'. The basic spin-echo imaging sequence is reviewed in figure 12.1. The imaging part resembles the sequence examined in chapter 7 in every respect, except that a 180° refocusing pulse has been added. Phase encoding is applied immediately after the selective 90° pulse. The dephasing lobe of the frequency-encode (FE) gradient between the two RF pulses is now positive. This is because in SE the RF does the rephasing by advancing or retarding the angle of the transverse magnetization components, which continue their phase evolution in the same rotational sense as before. Phase encoding (PE) is applied after the initial 90° pulse.

In multiple spin echo, or 'multi-echo', multiple RF refocusing pulses can be applied to form a train of spin echoes. This process can be repeated for as long as sufficient transverse magnetization remains to form an echo, i.e. as long as T_2 relaxation permits. Each echo has the same phase encoding and thus a series of images each with different T_2 weighting is acquired, with the additional echo time (TE) images acquired for 'free' in terms of overall scan time. The use of a double echo

---

The names game 1: spin echo
Generic name: RARE = **R**apid **A**cquisition with **R**elaxation **E**nhancement
       aka   *Fast Spin Echo* (FSE)
       Turbo Spin Echo (TSE)
       We call it 'fast spin echo' = FSE
Generic name: GRASE = **GR**adient **A**nd **S**pin Echo
       aka   *Turbo Gradient Spin Echo* (TGSE)
       We call it 'GRASE'

---

acquisition with a short and a long TE enables one scan to produce a good anatomical (proton-density-weighted) image and a pathology (T_2-weighted) image.

12.3.2 Fast spin echo

Fast spin echo (FSE), also known as turbo spin echo (TSE) is a commercial version of RARE (**R**apid **A**cquisition with **R**elaxation **E**nhancement) with evenly spaced multiple refocusing pulses (commonly, but not

---

Getting focused on spin echo
In section 8.4 we saw that multiple spin echoes were susceptible to accumulated RF flip angle errors and diffusion effects. For longer echo trains the Carr–Purcell–Meiboom–Gill sequence (CPMG) reduces these errors by changing the phase of the refocusing pulses with respect to the 90° pulse.

CPMG corrects every even echo for B_1 errors and produces echo amplitudes of the same algebraic sign. CPMG also reduces diffusion effects. An alternative scheme is a modified or phase-alternated Carr–Purcell (CP) scheme, where the RF phase angle is kept the same for both the 90° and the 180° pulses, but the algebraic sign of consecutive 180° pulses is alternated. This flips the transverse magnetization forwards (clockwise) and back (anti-clockwise) about the same axis and also assures that every second echo will lie properly in the xy plane in spite of B_1 errors. The sign of the echoes will alternate.

It is not entirely obvious that both CP and CPMG can also produce multiple unevenly spaced spin echoes. An example of a dual echo sequence is shown in figure 12.3. In this case the 'excitation' for the second echo is considered to occur at the time the first echo is formed. In this case

$$TE_1 = 2 \times T_A$$

$$TE_2 = 2 \times T_B \text{ provided } T_B \geq T_A$$

Note that phase encoding is only applied once after the 90° pulse and that the first frequency-encode gradient readout lobe acts as a dephase lobe for the second echo.

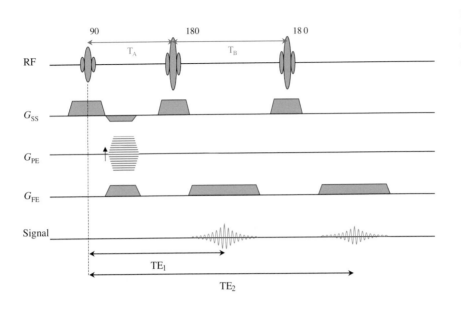

Figure 12.3 Dual spin-echo sequence. The same phase encoding applies for both echoes.

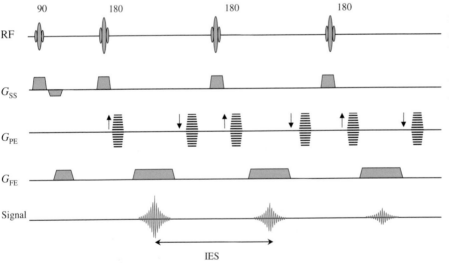

Figure 12.4 Fast (turbo) spin-echo sequence with an echo train length (turbo factor) of 3. IES denotes inter echo spacing, i.e. the time between successive echoes.

always, 180°) forming an echo train. These extra echoes are not used to acquire free images with different TE but are used to acquire multiple lines of data, i.e. to have *different* phase encoding for *each* echo (figure 12.4). The **Inter Echo Spacing** (IES or ESP, echo spacing) is the time between successive echoes. This is always a fixed value as the RF pulses are all evenly spaced apart in time to avoid problems with *coherence pathways*. The echo train length (ETL) or turbo factor (TF) is the number of echoes in the spin echo train.

The total scan time is

$$\text{Scan time} = \frac{\text{TR} \times N_{\text{PE}} \times \text{NSA}}{\text{ETL}}$$

Getting wound up: the details of FSE

In the sequence illustrated in figure 12.4 the formation of the first spin echo is entirely conventional. In FSE the CPMG form of spin echo is used to avoid the accumulation of flip angle errors over the echo train (see section 8.4 or 'Getting focused on spin echo'). However, before we can acquire the second echo, we have to 'rewind' the phase-encoding to undo the dephasing of the spins. To do this a phase encoding step of equal strength but opposite in sign is applied after the completion of the data acquisition. In addition to rewinding, a form of phase correction of the data is required (see also section 16.2). The whole sequence repeats after TR with different phase-encoding steps.

The manner in which k-space may be filled is illustrated in figure 12.5. Each echo is responsible for a portion or segment of k-space. So different lines of k-space will have different T_2 weighting. The echo that contributes the central segment determines the *effective echo time*. By mixing the functions of contrast generation and localization, we have blurred the distinction between contrast and detail. Sequences with high values of ETL/turbo factor may display reduced spatial resolution.

Also we can see from figure 12.5 that we could assign any of the echoes to acquire the centre of k-space, thus changing the effective TE. The order in which phase encoding is applied therefore affects the contrast.

When a refocusing pulse of less than 180° is used, the signal will include contributions from stimulated echoes (see box 'Echoes and coherences: Hahn and stimulated echoes'). These will coincide with the spin echoes but may affect the contrast and cause artefacts. For this reason, the rewinding scheme for phase encoding is applied in preference to 'blipping' (the accumulation of phase encoding from smaller, non-rewound phase-encoding steps) as used in EPI and GRASE (see section 12.3.8 and 16.2.2).

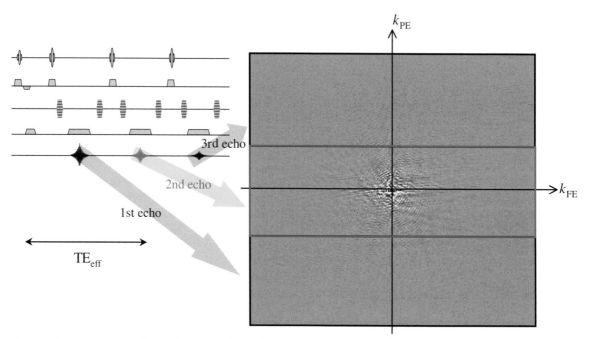

Figure 12.5 Data acquisition (k-space) filling for three echo FSE. The effective TE (TE_{eff}) is given by the time from the initial excitation to the second echo. Each point k_{PE} and k_{FE} represents a spatial frequency in the image.

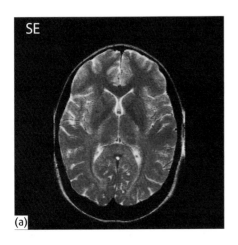

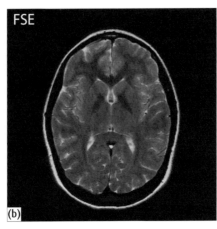

Figure 12.6 Representative images for spin echo (SE) and fast spin echo (FSE) with similar TE. (a) SE: TR = 1500 ms, TE = 120 ms, scan time 4 min. (b) FSE: TR = 2735 ms, TE = 102 ms, ETL = 5, scan time 1 min 46 s. Note the appearance of fat, and the scan times.

Thus an FSE sequence with, for example, 16 echoes, i.e. a turbo factor of 16, will run 16 times faster than the equivalent spin echo. With a TR of 3 s, this means an acquisition requiring 12 min as a conventional spin echo will run in just 40 s. Sometimes FSE has an odd number of phase-encode steps, as the latter has to be a multiple of the turbo factor (ETL). For example, if there are five echoes, the matrix could be 256×255 and a total of $(255 \div 5)$ TR periods or excitations would be required. Details of the k-space segmentation can be found in the box 'Getting wound up: the details of FSE'.

In FSE lines of k-space are acquired from different echoes. So with echoes having a range of TE being used for image formation, what contrast will the images display? In FSE the *effective echo time* (TE_{eff}) is the echo time that dominates the image contrast. We saw in chapter 7 that the overall image brightness is primarily determined by the low spatial frequencies, those acquired with low step values of phase-encode gradient. Thus, the centre of k-space dominates the image contrast. This is exploited in FSE, where TE_{eff} is arranged to coincide with the central parts of k-space. The order in which the phase encoding is applied affects the contrast, and various options are contained in the box 'Getting wound up: the details of FSE'.

Fast spin echo can be PD, T_1 or T_2 weighted in the same way as conventional spin echo. For T_1 weighting, where TR has to be relatively short, a smaller ETL may be required in order to achieve sufficient slice coverage. Dual- and triple-echo FSE sequences are possible where

the echoes of the echo train are divided between the different images with different TE_{eff}. This can be done by assigning the earlier echoes in the train to one image with a shorter TE and the later echoes to form a longer TE image. A more efficient way of achieving dual-echo FSE is by echo sharing, whereby some of the high spatial frequency data are shared between both images and only the low k-space data are encoded for more than one echo. Figure 12.6 shows spin-echo and FSE images.

12.3.3 A compromising situation

So is FSE 'the best thing since sliced bread'? Not quite; there are compromises involved, including reduced slice numbers, higher RF exposure, complicated contrast behaviour and possibly reduced resolution.

The slice number restrictions will be apparent to anyone who has sat at the MR console planning an FSE scan. We saw in section 7.4.3 how slice interleaving within the TR is used to deliver multiple slices within the same overall acquisition time. As the time occupied by the longer echo train in FSE is greater, it reduces the possibility of acquiring a large number of interleaved slices within the TR. The number of slices achievable will be approximately

$$N_{slices} = \frac{TR}{ETL \times IES}$$

To compensate for this, a longer TR can be used with an increased scan time for T_2- or PD-weighted images, but not for T_1-weighted images.

However, even if the required number of slices can be reconciled with the turbo factor and TR required, you often find your plans thwarted by the scanner on account of SAR limits. The SAR introduced in section 10.2.1 is a measure of the RF dose and is subject to national and international standards. FSE techniques with their many large RF pulses can very easily exceed the SAR limit, which is usually implemented by the manufacturer. To reduce the SAR to an acceptable level you need to reduce the number of slices, increase the

---

Turning down the heat: Reducing SAR

The FSE pulse sequence has a high SAR per unit time, particularly on high field scanners since the SAR is proportional to $B_0{}^2$. One way of reducing this effect is to use smaller flip angles during the refocusing echo train. You would think that the expected signal amplitude would be reduced with this scheme. However, a number of extra coherence pathways (see 'Coherence pathways') are formed including stimulated echoes, and these can combine to produce spin echoes with larger signals. Of course, the contribution from stimulated echoes means that the contrast is a function of both T_2 and T_1.

It can be shown that the signal forms a 'pseudo-steady-state' and (ignoring relaxation effects) the signal is proportional to $\sin(\theta/2)$. Furthermore the signal can be 'catalysed' into the steady state by choosing the first few refocusing pulses to have specific flip angles. For example if the *first* refocusing pulse is a $(90 + \theta/2)°$ pulse, and θ is the flip angle of the rest of the refocusing train, the echo amplitude is close to the maximum theoretical amplitude.

The reduced SNR can be further recovered by using 'hyperechoes'. A hyperecho is produced by using a 180° refocusing pulse in a train of reduced θ refocusing pulses. By arranging the timing so that the hyperecho occurs when the centre of k-space is acquired, the overall image SNR will be increased. Figure 12.7 shows a train of seven refocusing pulses, with the 4th pulse a full 180° and the others reduced. The hyperecho occurs after the 7th refocusing pulse, and has an amplitude almost equal to that achieved by a conventional train of 180° pulses.

TR, reduce the ETL or reduce the flip angle of the refocusing pulses (see 'Turning down the heat: Reducing SAR'). This latter is possible on some scanners and usually solves the SAR limitation problem, but at the cost of some reduction in SNR. In a properly constructed sequence it does not lead to artefact.

We have already discussed the complicated contrast behaviour. The low values of phase encoding which fill up the centre of k-space are used to determine the overall contrast of the image. So what of the higher k-space data? They determine the high-frequency or detailed content of the image and their relative strength may be emphasized or reduced, depending on the k-space ordering scheme employed. If the high frequencies are acquired for longer actual TE then they will be attenuated by T_2 relaxation and some spatial resolution will be lost. If they are acquired at a shorter TE than the effective TE they will be emphasized, which may lead to excessive ringing or Gibbs' artefact. For this reason additional filtering may be applied for FSE sequences.

The other major consequence is that the spatial resolution will depend on the T_2 of the tissues contributing to the signal. In practice then an arbitrarily large echo train length cannot be used without impairing the spatial resolution. This is most apparent in single-shot techniques (see section 12.3.7). However, whilst it is true that sequences with large turbo factors may lead to blurring or resolution loss compared with a nonsegmented sequence such as spin echo, FSE offers the opportunity to acquire large matrices (512×512 or even 1024×1024) and therefore produce very high resolution images with a reasonable scan time.

A final issue of compromise relates to the appearance of fat in the images. In FSE fat is extremely bright, as shown in figure 12.6. Bright fat may be useful, particularly in he abdomen where it outlines all of the organs and bowel. However it may also reduce the dynamic range available in the image and therefore obscure subtle contrast changes (e.g. in the knee), or sometimes it may result in a high level of motion artefact (e.g. from the highly motional suborbital fat) or conceal pathology. This can be addressed by applying further prepulses in the form of fat suppression by a number of techniques (addressed in section 6.5). A more detailed explanation is given in the box 'Is FSE the same as SE?'.

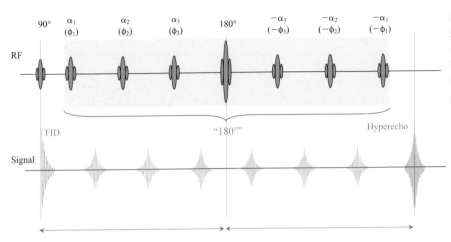

Figure 12.7 TSE echo train showing reduced refocusing angles and the hyperecho formed by making the 4th refocusing pulse a full 180° pulse.

Is FSE the same as SE?

The image contrast in FSE is not the same as for SE. The multiple RF pulses result in the generation of stimulated echoes in FSE which add to the spin-echo component of the signal.

In particular fat appears very bright in FSE. Actually, it is in conventional spin echo that fat is less bright than expected for a tissue with its combination of short T_1 and relatively long T_2. The reason lies with J-coupling, which is an interaction between different nuclei within the fat molecule and results in a shortening of T_2. In FSE the rapid train of refocusing pulses breaks this coupling and thus fat signals have effectively a longer T_2 and appear brighter in the image.

An FSE sequence designed to conserve the J-coupling effect and look more like spin echo is the DIET (**Delayed Interval Echo Train**) sequence, which has a longer IES for the first pair of refocusing pulses. At the time of writing this is only commercially available on Toshiba systems.

The application of various fat-suppression techniques is common for FSE imaging. Additionally there may be slice-to-slice variations in image contrast. This may be due to unwanted magnetization transfer interactions caused by off-resonance RF from adjacent slices.

In GRASE imaging (section 12.3.8) the use of intermediate gradient echoes between each spin echo means that a longer IES (for the 180° pulses) can be employed. This may conserve the J-coupling and produce images that are more spin-echo-like.

12.3.4 Inversion recovery FSE

The use of fast spin echo to obtain T_1 weighting with shorter TR is limited by compromises between the number of slices achievable and the echo train length (ETL). It is possible however to achieve T_1 weighting by the addition of a preparation prepulse in the form of an inversion combined with a high ETL, i.e. as inversion recovery FSE (IR-FSE) or turbo-IR. One of the downsides of conventional inversion recovery is the long scan time involved because of the need for a TR of at

least three (and preferably five) times the T_1 of tissue. The ability to combine an inversion pulse with FSE for spatial encoding makes inversion recovery a clinically applicable technique. The T_1 contrast is conventional and is primarily determined by the inversion time (TI). Clinical applications of this include **S**hort **TI** **I**nversion **R**ecovery (STIR), in which a short TI is used to null the fat signal and something akin to T_2-weighted appearance is achieved in the image (section 3.9), and FLAIR imaging (section 3.10) where a long TI (e.g. 2000 ms) combined with a long TR (up to 10 s) is used to null the cerebrospinal fluid (CSF) signal in neuroimaging. The use of IR-FSE makes the scan time for FLAIR clinically acceptable. Another application is real-reconstruction (or true) inversion recovery, useful for examining the degree of myelination in the immature brain, where the inversion pulse is used to optimize contrast.

Interleaved IR-FSE

The potential for slice interleaving in FSE/TSE sequences is reduced because the data-acquisition time is longer to encompass the whole echo train. This presents special problems for inversion recovery where each slice has to undergo inversion at a time TI before the FSE signal readout/spatial encoding part of the sequence. We have three options for arranging the slices shown in figure 12.8:

(a) Interleave within the TR, i.e. invert and readout one slice before inverting the next one. In this case the maximum number of slices is

$$N_{slices} = \frac{TR}{TI + (IES \times ETL)}$$

For very long TI such as those used in FLAIR this restricts the number of slices obtainable for a given TR and the number is dependent upon the TI you chose. It works best for short TI, e.g. as in STIR. This scheme is sometimes referred to as 'sequential'.

(b) Interleave within TI, i.e. we invert all the slices first within the time TI and then read them all out. The number of slices is now independent of TR but depends upon TI:

$$N_{slices} = \frac{TI}{(IES \times ETL)}$$

Obviously for very high turbo factors, the number of slices is going to be restricted. A compromise between number of slices and speed of acquisition is usually required. This arrangement works best for long TI, e.g. for FLAIR, and is sometimes called 'interleaved'.

(c) In theory, a combination of both methods is possible, but most scanners do not offer this.

The combination of IR with TSE involves certain complications over how slice interleaving is achieved. There are compromises regarding turbo factors (ETLs), TI and TR, which are examined in the box 'Interleaved IR-FSE'. The scan time is given by the same expression as for FSE; however, there may be limitations on the number of slices achievable. With IR-based techniques there are also limitations in the spatial quality of the inversion pulses. It is common in IR-FSE to have a significant gap between slices and to use an interleaved slice order to avoid crosstalk.

12.3.5 Real reconstruction (true) inversion recovery

Inversion recovery offers the possibility of the MR signal being positive or negative. Usually MR images are presented in magnitude form, i.e. with no negative values, the sign of the signal being ignored in the final image (this was to overcome artefact problems arising from phase changes due to susceptibility variations and magnet inhomogeneity). With real-valued ('true') inversion recovery, the image is reconstructed in real rather than magnitude mode, i.e. with positive and negative voxel values. This means that the background is mid- grey and the image values range from black to white. Exceptionally good contrast, particularly in brain tissues, is achievable with true inversion recovery. Figure 12.9 gives an example for a neonatal brain.

12.3.6 Drive time: driven equilibrium

Driven equilibrium is a technique that has been known for a long time in laboratory NMR. The idea is simply to drive the magnetization back to the positive z axis (towards equilibrium) by further RF excitation rather than through longitudinal relaxation, which is a much slower process. Transverse magnetization can be driven back towards equilibrium by a 90° pulse on the -x' axis. This enables a shorter TR to be used in FSE sequences. Examples of this include the DRIVE sequence from Philips and Fast Recovery FSE from General Electric.

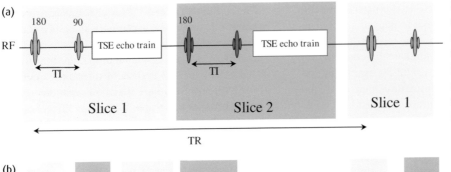

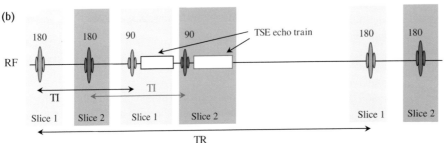

Figure 12.8 Interleaving schemes for inversion recovery FSE: (a) sequential where each TI is completed before incrementing the slice; (b) interleaved where more than one slice is inverted within each TI.

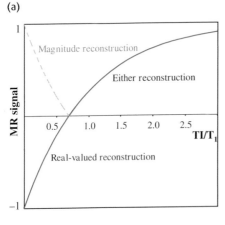

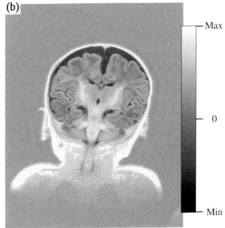

Figure 12.9 (a) Signal dependence of real-valued IR. (b) Example of true inversion recovery sequence of infant brain. The image background is mid-grey, allowing the display of both positive and negative MR signals.

12.3.7 Single-shot FSE and HASTE

The ultimate turbo sequence is single-shot FSE, where there is only one initial RF excitation (90°) pulse followed by a very long echo train over which all the phase-encode steps are acquired. This type of sequence is applied sequentially for multiple slice acquisitions, i.e. a whole slice is acquired at a time before moving on to the next slice. Usually an inter-slice delay (time delay or

TD) is required between successive slices. The scan time will therefore be

$$\text{Scan time} = N_{\text{slices}} \times (\text{scan time for slice} + \text{TD})$$

With this type of sequence there will necessarily be a lot of T_2 signal decay over the course of the acquisition and hence its clinical use is limited to the study of predominantly fluid structures, such as the biliary system, as a

3D FSE

Normally 3D acquisitions use gradient-echo sequences with short TR, required because of the additional multiplication of phase-encode gradient steps. One exception to this is 3D FSE, where a high turbo factor (ETL) can be used to keep the scan time to a reasonable time given by

$$\text{Scan time} = \frac{\text{NSA} \times N_{\text{PE1}} \times N_{\text{PE2}} \times \text{TR}}{\text{ETL}}$$

The sequence gives the geometric and SNR advantages inherent in a 3D acquisition, whilst retaining the FSE features of long TE (T weighting) and long TR.

technique for MR cholangiopancreatography (MRCP). Example images are shown in figure 12.10.

HASTE (Half Fourier single shot TSE) is a form of single-shot FSE available on Siemens scanners, which uses a phase-alternated CP echo train combined with half Fourier acquisition (section 7.7.1). HASTE produces a moderate spatial resolution (256×128 or 240) with a moderate to long TE (60–120 ms) giving T_2-weighted images. It can also be combined with an inversion recovery prepulse to give a single-shot variant of STIR or FLAIR. Often nonselective inversion pulses will be used (see box 'More on RF pulses'). In this case a sufficient interslice delay is required to ensure full

recovery to equilibrium of the inverted magnetization. So why don't we use single-shot sequences all the time? The answer lies in the compromises involved with all segmented spin-echo techniques, of which single-shot-FSE and HASTE are the most extreme examples, and therefore the most extremely compromised. Figure 12.11 shows phantom measurements using FSE and HASTE with the phase-encoding axis vertical. The single-shot method (HASTE) clearly results in massively impaired spatial resolution. However, this limitation must be weighed up against the benefit of taking only 1 s to acquire which effectively eliminates bowel and respiratory motion.

12.3.8 GRASE and SE-EPI

GRadient **A**nd **S**pin **E**cho (GRASE) or Turbo **G**radient **S**pin **E**cho (TGSE) is a fast segmented sequence that combines a multiple spin-echo train and intermediate gradient echoes, each with distinct values of phase encoding (figure 12.12). Although it is a hybrid sequence, we class it in the spin echo section as its behaviour and use are along the lines of spin echo. The scan time for GRASE is

$$\text{Scan time} = \frac{\text{TR} \times N_{\text{PE}}}{N_{\text{spin echoes}} \times N_{\text{gradient echoes}}}$$

Some systems call the number of spin echoes the 'turbo factor' and the number of gradient echoes the 'EPI

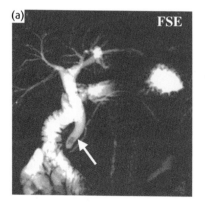
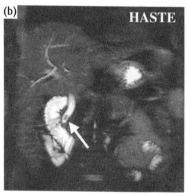
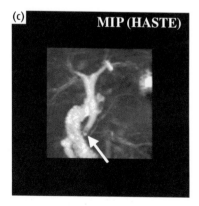

Figure 12.10 Half Fourier single-shot TSE (HASTE) and single-shot FSE (SS-FSE) images (MRCP) showing a dilated common bile duct with a gallstone (arrowed). The pancreatic duct is also visible. (a) "Thick slab" FSE: TE = 1100 ms, ETL = 240, slice thickness 60 mm. (b) HASTE: TE = 87 ms, ETL = 128, slice thickness 5 mm. (c) Maximum intensity projection (MIP) image from the HASTE images.

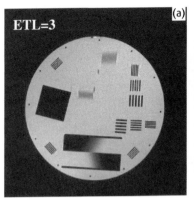
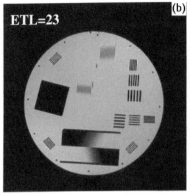
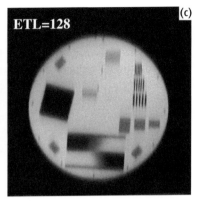

Figure 12.11 Resolution in segmented sequences showing resolution loss in the phase-encode (PE) direction. (a) FSE with 3 echoes (ETL = 3), TR = 600 ms, TE = 12 ms, scan time 52 s. (b) FSE with 23 echoes, TR = 600 ms, TE = 128 ms, scan time = 6 s. (c) HASTE (ETL = 128), single shot ("TR" = ∞), TE = 87 ms, scan time = 1 s. Phase encode is vertical. Note the subtle resolution loss for ETL = 23, and the major resolution loss for HASTE. The phantom fluid had a T_2 of 200 ms.

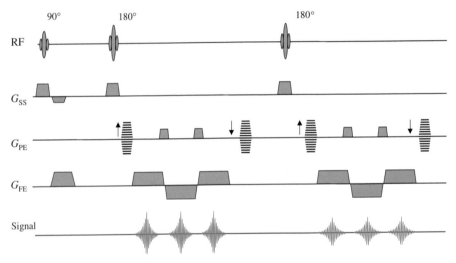

Figure 12.12 GRASE sequence diagram with three gradient and two spin echoes giving six lines of k-space per TR period.

factor'. Typically three gradient echoes will be used for each spin echo. The advantages of this are that much less RF power is used and that higher 'turbo factors' can be achieved. It is sometimes claimed that GRASE contrast is more like T_2-weighted spin echo than FSE (see 'Is FSE the same as SE?'), although its current clinical use is not yet widespread. The complicated k-space scheme (see box 'Grace notes: k-space schemes for GRASE') can lead to substantial ringing artefacts in the phase-encode direction.

Spin-echo-based **E**cho **P**lanar **I**maging (SE-EPI) can be regarded as an extreme case of GRASE, where a single excitation is given and the whole of k-space sampled with gradient echoes under a single spin echo (figure 12.13). It produces sequential slices in less than 100 ms with low spatial resolution, but is prone to artefacts. It is primarily used in dynamic or diffusion-weighted imaging. EPI and its k-space schemes will be considered in more detail in chapter 16. Figure 12.16 shows an FSE, GRASE and SE–EPI image.

More on RF pulses

Selective pulses, as seen in section 7.4, utilize a shaped RF pulse in conjunction with a gradient. If the pulse generates transverse magnetization, i.e. if it is anything but a 180° pulse, it is usually necessary to have a rephase gradient to ensure that the transverse magnetization points in the same direction, i.e. has the same phase to start with. The rephase portion has half the gradient moment of the selective part and the opposite sign. For a 180° pulse, rephasing is not required. In the case of a refocusing pulse (i.e. in spin echo), the gradient is self-rephasing. For an inversion pulse, there is no transverse magnetization (ideally) and the selective gradient ideally produces no phase changes.

Selective slices are not uniform in the selection direction, but have a variation in flip angle perpendicular to the image plane they define, known as the slice profile. A consequence is that for a 180° pulse there will be regions where magnetization is tipped through 90° and unwanted transverse magnetization is created.

For a refocusing pulse a pair of 'crusher' gradients, as shown in figure 12.1, can overcome this problem. These are equal gradients applied either side of the refocusing pulse. Refocused magnetization that goes on to form an echo will have seen both gradients and, because of refocusing, will be unaffected. However, fresh free induction decay (FID) created by the refocusing pulse only experiences one gradient lobe and will be dephased.

In practice it is quite difficult to achieve good inversion, e.g. in inversion recovery sequences. Particularly at higher field strength, 'adiabatic' pulses provide more uniform inversion (see box 'Adiabatic pulses') since they are less sensitive to B_1 inhomogeneities. For single-shot sequences with an inversion pre-pulse, the inversion pulse may be nonselective. A nonselective pulse is applied without a gradient, so it has no spatial localization. Subject to the RF coil's homogeneity and tissue RF absorption, it will have the same effect at all points of space. A nonselective pulse can have any temporal waveform, and it is advantageous to keep the pulse short, a rectangular waveform being common. Such pulses are often called hard pulses.

Composite RF pulses, or 'binomial' pulses (see box 'Binomial pulses'), are often used for spectral excitation, i.e. to obtain a signal from either water or fat. These pulses are made up of a series of either selective or hard pulses and are always followed by spoiler gradients to 'mop up' any residual fat signal.

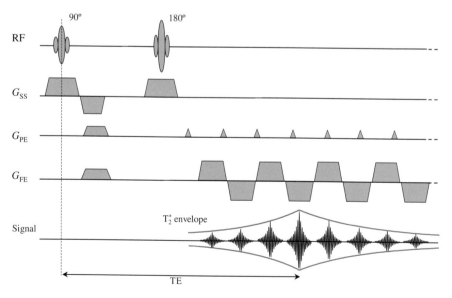

Figure 12.13 SE-EPI sequence diagram. The whole image is acquired from a single spin echo. In practice 64–128 gradient echoes would be acquired.

Adiabatic RF pulses

Adiabatic pulses behave quite differently to the normal RF pulses. They use both amplitude and frequency modulation to pull the magnetization away from the z axis. If this sounds weird, it's because adiabatic pulses are weird! To explain them, we have to go back to the rotating frame and consider how the protons precess around an RF magnetic field.

Previously we have assumed that B_1 is applied at the Larmor frequency along x' or y' in the rotating frame. However if the frequency of the RF is slightly off resonance there is also a component of B_1 in the z' direction. In this situation, the transverse and longitudinal components of B_1 combine to give an effective field B_{eff} at an angle ψ to the z' axis. When the amplitude of B_1 is small or the RF frequency is a long way off resonance, B_{eff} is very close to the z' axis; as the amplitude is increased and the frequency is exactly on resonance, B_{eff} is exactly in the transverse plane.

The protons obey the Larmor equation and precess (in the rotating frame) about B_{eff} (figure 12.14(a)). If we create an RF pulse such that B_{eff} is initially in the z' direction, then gradually change the amplitude and frequency so that B_{eff} slowly rotates towards the transverse plane, the protons will continue to precess about B_{eff} until they are also precessing in the transverse plane. If the pulse is now switched off, lo and behold, the protons are in the transverse plane and can give us an MR signal. The only constraint is that the changing angle of B_{eff} is much less than the precessional frequency about B_{eff}, described mathematically by

$$\frac{\delta\psi}{\delta t} \ll \gamma B_{eff}$$

This can be achieved by choosing a strong effective field (high B_1) or a slow frequency modulation. The term 'adiabatic' comes from Greek meaning 'impassable to heat' and is used in thermodynamics to describe processes where no external energy is used. Returning to the idea that protons absorb energy from a normal RF pulse during excitation, we can think of adiabatic pulses as forcing the protons to use their own internal energy to change their orientation. No energy is absorbed from the RF pulse, so the spin temperature does not change. I warned you these are weird pulses!

Different types of amplitude and frequency modulation can be used to create adiabatic pulses for excitation, inversion or refocusing. For example the hyperbolic secant pulse is popular for inversion: figure 12.14(b,c) shows the amplitude and frequency modulation of the pulse. All adiabatic pulses have the major advantage of being insensitive to B_1 inhomogeneities making them particularly useful at higher field strengths.

Binomial pulses

Binomial pulses are also called composite pulses, because they consist of a short series of RF pulses with short delays between them. The simplest example is a 1:1 pulse used for fat suppression (see figure 12.15). First a 45° pulse is applied along the $+x'$ axis, then the fat and water protons are allowed to dephase. When they are exactly out of phase, a second 45° pulse is applied, taking the water protons into the transverse plane and leaving the fat protons in the longitudinal direction. Other binomial pulses use a 1:2:1 or 1:3:3:1 sequence, i.e. 22.5°–45°–22.5° or 11.25°–33.75°–33.75°–11.25°. Each inter-pulse delay allows fat to dephase by 180° with respect to water. Better fat suppression is achieved with more complex pulses, but there is a time penalty since the pulse takes longer to apply.

The advantages of binomial pulses are that they can be used at low fields, since the suppression does not depend on the frequency separation of the fat and water, and at high fields because they are relatively insensitive to B_1 inhomogeneities. If the component RF pulses are made to be slice-selective instead of hard pulses, the binomial pulse itself becomes slice-selective. This is the basis of the Philips 'Proset' technique.

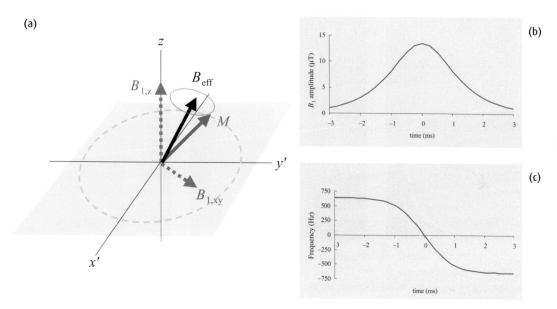

Figure 12.14 (a) When the RF is slightly off resonance, B_{eff} is at an angle between z' and the transverse plane and protons precess about B_{eff}. (b) Amplitude and (c) frequency modulation for a hyperbolic secant (*sech*) adiabatic inversion pulse. Note that the amplitude starts low, increases to a maximum and then returns to zero, and that the frequency is swept from several hundred Hz below ω_0 to several hundred Hz above.

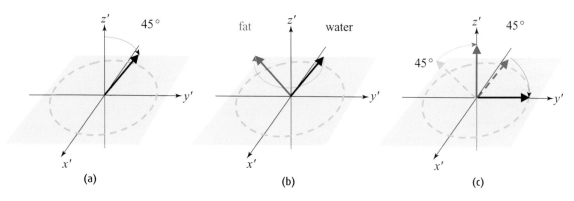

Figure 12.15 A 1:1 binomial pulse suppresses fat by (a) exciting both water and fat, (b) allowing time for the fat to dephase by 180° then (c) applying a second 45° pulse to leave the water protons in the transverse plane and the fat protons returned to the z axis.

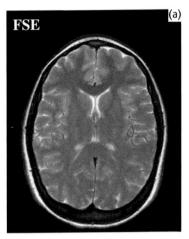
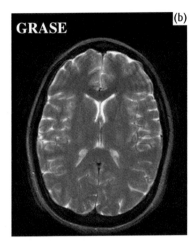
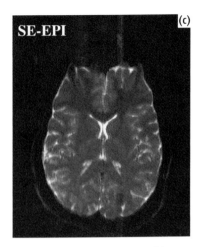

Figure 12.16 FSE, GRASE and SE-EPI images. (a) FSE, ETL = 5, TR = 2735 ms, TE = 102 ms, NSA = 2, scan time 3 min 32 s. (b) GRASE, turbo factor = 7, EPI factor = 3, TR = 3735 ms, TE = 132 ms, scan time 34 s. (c) SE-EPI, single shot, TE = 109 ms, scan time = 0.2 s per slice. Note the different appearance of the scalp fat between the sequences. The EPI uses fat suppression and exhibits significant distortion. Ringing artefacts are evident for GRASE.

Grace notes: k-space schemes for GRASE

Figure 12.17 shows the k-space scheme for the GRASE sequence shown in figure 12.12 with a turbo factor of 3 and an EPI factor of 3. The 180° pulse is followed by a conventional phase-encode gradient, determined by a phase-encode table. However, fixed phase-encode gradients are used for the gradient-echo portion of the acquisition. These cause big fixed-length jumps in k-space, with phase changes being additive from the previous echoes for the current refocusing cycle. The phase encoding is rewound before the next RF and the phase-encode table will increment for the next spin echo. Thus successive lines of k-space will be subject to a T_2 decay envelope with this pattern repeated periodically over k-space in the phase-encode axis. This results in the ringing or ghosting artefacts seen in the image in figure 12.16. As for FSE the contrast is dominated by the echo time used to acquire the centre of k-space.

12.4 Spoiled for choice: gradient echo

Gradient echo (GE) is the other main branch of the sequence family tree. The principles of signal formation are quite different from those of spin echo. In GE speed is enhanced by using a small flip angle so that TR can be reduced dramatically without saturating or driving the signal to zero. After a few RF pulses the magnetization gets into a steady-state where the recovery in each TR period exactly matches the effect of the excitation as considered briefly in chapter 3. GE sequences can be applied to provide proton density (PD), T_2^* or T_1 contrast, and even in some instances T_2. Because of their short TR GE sequences are ideally suited for threedimensional Fourier transformation (3D FT) scanning. In 2D scanning their speed makes them particularly suitable for breath-hold studies, dynamic contrast examinations and angiography (see chapter 13).

The image-formation principles of the basic GE sequence were considered in chapter 7. The echo is formed by the dephasing and rephasing of an MR signal by an imaging gradient. A key point to remember for GE techniques is that the effects of magnet inhomogeneities and local susceptibility changes are not compensated. The time decay of the MR signal is therefore determined by T_2^* not T_2. This means that shorter values of TE are used (less than 10 ms). Additionally there are interesting cancellation effects relating to water and fat signals which are peculiar to GE.

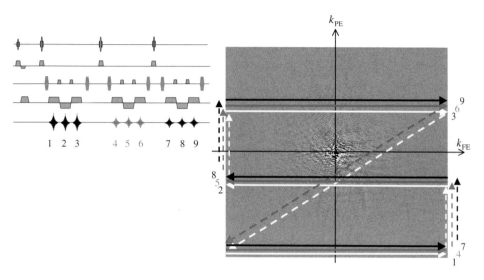

Figure 12.17 k-space acquisition for GRASE with three spin echoes and three gradient echoes. The k-space path corresponding to each echo is numbered.

The names game 2: gradient echo
Generic name: **Gradient Echo** (GE)
      aka   *Field Echo* (FE)
      We call it 'gradient echo' = GE
There are three types:
(a) FID only (T_1 weighted) spoiled or incoherent gradient echo
      aka   *Fast Low Angle SHot* (FLASH)
            SPoiled Gradient Recalled Echo (SPGR)
            T1 Fast Field Echo (T1-FFE)
            RF spoiled Fourier Acquired Steady-state Technique (FAST)
      We call it 'Spoiled GE'
(b) FID and Echo (T_1/T_2) rewound or coherent gradient echo
      aka *Gradient Recalled Acquisition in the Steady State* (GRASS)
            Gradient Recalled Echo (GRE)
            Fast Imaging with Steady-state Precession (FISP)
            Fourier Acquired Steady-state Technique (FAST)
            Fast Field Echo (FFE)
      We call it 'Rewound GE'
(c) Echo only (T_2) Steady state/contrast enhanced approaches
      aka *PSIF* (*FISP* backwards)
            Contrast Enhanced Fourier Acquired Steady-state Technique (CE-FAST)
            T2 Fast Field Echo (T2 FFE)
            Steady-State Free Precession (SSFP)
      We call it 'Time-reversed GE'

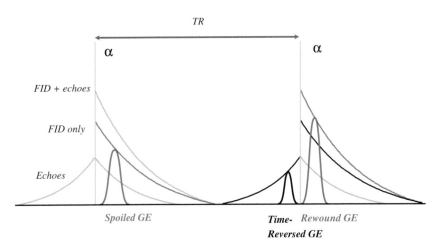

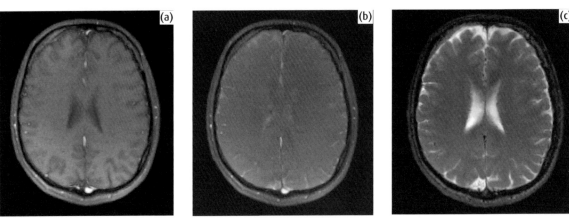

Figure 12.18 Gradient echo: coherent and incoherent signal formation in the steady state resulting from a rapid and regular train of RF excitation pulses. See box 'The names game 2: gradient echo' for an explanation of the terms.

Figure 12.19 Gradient-echo images. (a) Spoiled GE, (b) rewound GE, (c) time-reversed GE. All with TR = 20 ms, TE = 5.8 ms, flip angle $\alpha = 25°$.

12.4.1 Genesis of the GE signal: FIDs, echoes and coherences

If we have a train of RF pulses with TR significantly greater than T_2 as in conventional spin echo, then the transverse component of magnetization will have fully decayed before the onset of the next RF pulse. This means that the RF pulse will always be acting solely on longitudinal magnetization and the strength of the FID signal will depend largely upon T_1. This is normally the case for spin-echo imaging. However, if TR is less than T_2 then a remnant of transverse magnetization will remain as the next RF pulse is applied. This results in 'Hahn' or partial echoes, in addition to the FID. The

origin of these signals is considered in the box 'Echoes and coherences: Hahn and stimulated echoes'.

In a regularly spaced train of RF pulses, the echo signals will coincide with the following RF pulses and therefore add to the FID signal. How these so-called transverse coherences are dealt with determines the contrast behaviour of the GE sequence. 'Spoiling' removes the transverse coherences. 'Rewinding' utilizes them. Conversely they alone, and not the fresh FID signal, may be used in image formation. This gives us three main ways of using gradient echoes, as illustrated in figure 12.18 with example images in figure 12.19.

Echoes and coherences: Hahn and stimulated echoes

We have seen that a 90–180° pulse pair can generate a spin echo. However, any pair of RF pulses, of any flip angle, can form a Hahn or partial echo, and each echo can be further refocused by a subsequent RF pulse. The Hahn echoes are smaller in magnitude than spin echoes and have a T_2 dependence.

The formation of a Hahn echo for a pair of 90° pulses is shown in figure 12.20. We see that it is not a fully refocused echo but that at time TE all the spin vectors are of the same sign and lie in a circle giving an echo magnitude of half of a full spin echo. For angles smaller than 90°, visualizing how the echo is formed is less intuitive. Instead of forming a circle of vectors they lie in an ellipse which refocuses less fully in the $-x'y'$ quadrant.

Stimulated echoes arise when you have three RF pulses. The first pulse generates transverse magnetization which is 'converted' to and stored as longitudinal (T_1) magnetization by the second, and finally refocused by the third. In figure 12.21 we see that three RF pulses will produce five echoes, three Hahn echoes from each pair of pulses, an echo created by refocusing the first echo by the third pulse and the stimulated echo. The stimulated echo has T_1 and T_2 behaviour. Its echo time with respect to the first RF pulse is

$$TE_{STE} = 2 \cdot t_a + t_b$$

In a long RF pulse train, it is not just successive RF pulses that give rise to echoes, but each pair of pulses may do so as well. If the TR is constant, which is normal, these echoes will coincide with the wanted FID signal but, since they arose from earlier excitations, they may have different spatial encoding and contrast – and if left untended may cause artefacts.

GE sequences cope with this by either 'spoiling' the residual transverse magnetization after data acquisition and before the next RF pulse (sometimes called incoherent sequences), or by rewinding the gradients, so that the transverse magnetization at the end of each TR period has no spatial encoding. This results in a rewound (sometimes called coherent) steady-state sequence.

Coherence pathways

The analysis of coherence pathways is of prime importance to the sequence developer, but an understanding of coherence helps to know what the images are about and how the sequences perform. Every time an RF pulse occurs, magnetization will be flipped to both longitudinal and transverse planes resulting in a fresh FID, the possibility of echo formation, and the storing of magnetization for later RF pulses to refocus. Figure 12.22 shows a so-called coherence pathway diagram which can be used to predict the echo-formation properties of trains of RF pulses. In the diagram phase is represented vertically and time horizontally. For simplicity we only consider one component (sometimes called an 'isochromat') of the transverse magnetization rather than multiple vectors fanning out. The rules are simple. Every time there is an RF pulse the magnetization divides into three parts:

(a) A part continues to dephase as if nothing had happened.
(b) A part is converted to longitudinal magnetization which then does not further dephase and runs parallel to the time axis at constant phase.
(c) Another part of transverse magnetization receives the opposite phase, and then continues to dephase (or 'rephase', if it's heading back towards the zero phase axis). Whenever one of the lines crosses the zero-phase axis you get an echo.

Figure 12.22 also shows how a stimulated echo is formed, first by converting the transverse magnetization to longitudinal by α_2, then inverting the phase with α_3 which converts it back to transverse magnetization. You can see that the diagram correctly predicts the existence and timing of the stimulated echo. When the pulse train is regular (i.e. $t_a = t_b$), the stimulated echoes will coincide with the spin echoes. The coherence diagram in figure 12.22 does not show the effect of the imaging gradients, although these can also be included.

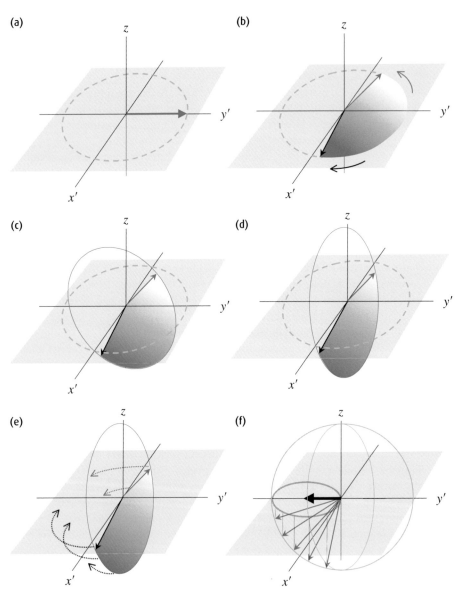

(a)

(b)

(c)

(d)

(e)

(f)

Figure 12.20 Formation of Hahn "partial" echoes. (a) Transverse magnetization after first RF pulse; (b) immediately before 2nd RF pulse; (c) during and (d) immediately after this pulse; (e) continued transverse dephasing before the echo (f). The partially refocused Hahn echo occurs when all the transverse components (shadows) of the magnetization lie in a circular arrangement after a time twice the echo spacing.

Spoiled or incoherent GE utilizes just the FID (i.e. longitudinal magnetization tipped onto the transverse plane) for T_1 or PD contrast. With very low flip angles you get PD weighting and also T_2^* weighting. Rewound or coherent GE sequences contain components from transverse coherences and FID and give mixed contrast depending upon the ratio of T_2 and T_1. They are also subject to T_2^* decay. Time-reversed GE sequences use just the transverse coherence signals to give T_2 weighting. All GE sequences must be constructed to avoid the formation of artefacts from *coherence pathways*.

12.4.2 Spoiled gradient echo

In spoiled gradient echo only the FID signal, generated by the action of the current RF pulse on longitudinal

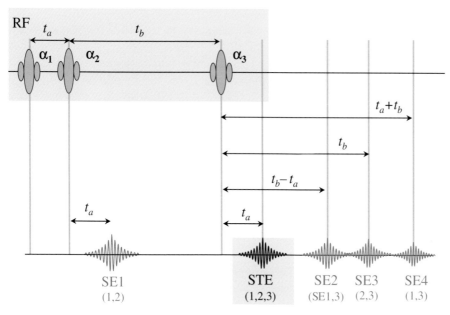

Figure 12.21 Three RF pulses may give rise to four Hahn echoes from each pair of RF pulses SE1, SE3, SE4 and the refocusing of the first echo by the third RF pulse. The stimulated echo STE is generated by all three RF pulses. The times of echo formation are given in terms of t_a and t_b, the time intervals between the RF pulses.

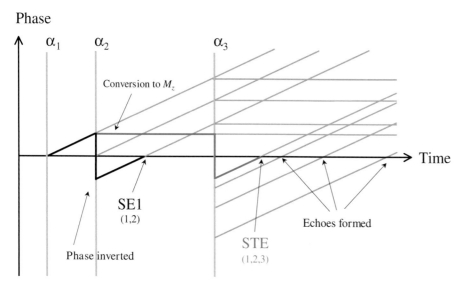

Figure 12.22 Coherence pathway diagram showing the formation of the first spin echo (black line), the stimulated echo (blue) and all the other echoes (grey).

magnetization, is utilized. The residual transverse magnetization remaining after the data-acquisition period (figure 12.23) is removed by gradient spoiling, RF spoiling or both. In all other respects, the image-formation mechanism is conventional, with one line of k-space acquired per TR period. The image contrast is determined by TR and α, as was shown in sections 3.6–3.8. A mathematical expression for the signal is given in the box 'Flash in the pan: signal strength and the Ernst angle'.

Gradient echo does not compensate for magnetic field differences. This includes dephasing from water and fat, which have slightly different resonant

Echo amplitudes

A further way of understanding coherence is to think of an RF pulse of arbitrary flip angle as acting in three separate ways, as follows.

(a) Part of it acts like a 0° pulse. This means it has no effect upon either transverse or longitudinal magnetization. The relative amplitude of magnetization affected by this component is

$$M_{'0°-like'} \propto \cos^2(\alpha/2)$$

(b) Part acts like a 90° pulse, converting longitudinal magnetization into transverse, and transverse into longitudinal magnetization. The amplitude of this component is

$$M_{'90°-like'} \propto \sin \alpha$$

(c) Part of it acts like a 180° pulse, inverting pre-existing longitudinal magnetization and refocusing transverse magnetization by means of a partial or Hahn echo with amplitude

$$M_{'180°-like'} \propto \sin^2(\alpha/2)$$

From this, one can predict that the Hahn echo from two 90° pulses will have half the amplitude of a spin echo. Similarly a true 180° pulse will only invert or refocus, and not cause partial or stimulated echoes, but we can predict that an imperfect 180° pulse will cause unwanted components of magnetization. The nature of the slice profile means that such imperfections will almost always exist for a selective refocusing pulse. This was a source of potential artefact in fast spin echo (FSE) but is avoided by using phase rewinders before each 180° pulse.

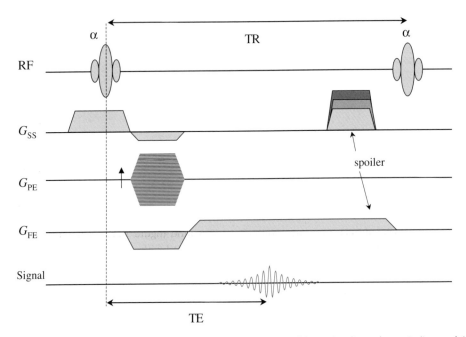

Figure 12.23 Spoiled gradient-echo sequence utilizing gradient spoiling as a table on the slice-select axis (i.e. applying a different gradient for each sequence repetition) and a constant value on the frequency-encoding axis (by extending the read gradient).

Spoil sport: spoiling techniques

Failure to spoil the transverse magnetization can result in two problems: the formation of image artefacts and wrong contrast.

Image artefacts from incomplete spoiling, taking the form of banding, are shown in figure 12.24. This arises due to interference between differently phase-encoded signals from different excitations. A constant spoiling gradient will dephase only non-echo-forming parts of the signal. More thorough spoiling can be achieved by using a pseudo-randomly varying (i.e. the value isn't actually random, but the effect is) spoiler gradient table. Spoiler gradients can be applied on any axis, but the slice-select axis is commonly chosen as this represents the largest dimension of the voxel.

In RF spoiling we apply each α excitation pulse with a random or pseudo-random phase angle (direction in the rotating frame), as in figure 12.25. The effect of this is to accentuate the natural dephasing of the spins, thus giving an apparent reduction in T_2 for the remnant of transverse magnetization from previous excitations.

Figure 12.26 gives an explanation of spoiling in terms of coherent pathways. Gradient spoiling must be sufficient to cause dephasing within a voxel, illustrated by the three lines. This effectively dephases any transverse magnetization that does not lead to a Hahn echo. However, it does not prevent echo formation. To avoid this, RF spoiling must be used. Each RF pulse causes a vertical (phase) offset and if properly randomized the isochromats never add up constructively. The current FID signal is not affected. When RF spoiling is utilized the phase-encode gradients are usually rewound, otherwise unwanted spatial inhomogeneities in the signal can occur.

Flash in the pan: signal strength and the Ernst angle

The signal obtained from a spoiled GE sequence is

$$\text{Signal} = \rho \frac{\sin \alpha \cdot [1 - \exp(-TR/T_1)] \cdot \exp(-TE/T_2^*)}{1 - \cos \alpha \, \exp(-TR/T_1)}$$

and you can see that flip angle α is an important parameter in determining the image contrast.

For each value of T_1 there is an optimum flip angle that will give the most signal from a sequence where repeated RF excitations are made. This angle, known as the Ernst angle, is given by

$$\alpha_{\text{Ernst}} = \cos^{-1}[\exp(-TR/T_1)]$$

At flip angles greater than the Ernst angle you tend to get T_1 weighting. At less than the Ernst angle the contrast is flatter, more PD like. See also figure 5.2(c).

frequencies. Following excitation water and fat signals are in phase but will resonate at different rates, seen as a dephasing over time in the rotating frame of reference. Once the two components get 180° out of phase with each other the signals will subtract from one another. This does not affect the image, unless a voxel contains a *mixture of water and fat*, in which case a partial cancellation will occur. See section 6.5.2 for a full discussion of this artefact and how to avoid it.

12.4.3 Rewound gradient echo

In coherent steady-state sequences, the transverse magnetization left after the data-acquisition period is rewound, i.e. reset to zero by reversing the sign of the gradient pulses. In **F**ast **I**maging with **S**teady **P**recession (FISP) and **G**radient **R**ecalled **A**cquisition in the **S**teady **S**tate (GRASS) only the phase-encode gradient is rewound (figure 12.27). Thus the signal contains FID enhanced with echo and coherent transverse components. This gives more signal than spoiled gradient echo but more complicated weighting. At longer TR values (>100 ms) and small flip angles there is little difference between spoiled and rewound gradient sequences. Also if T_2 is short then there is little opportunity for enhanced contrast due to the coherent component. The ideal contrast behaviour depends only upon the flip angle and the ratio of T_2 to T_1, shown in the box 'On the rewound'.

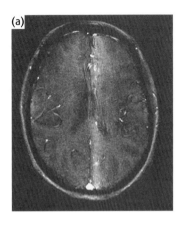
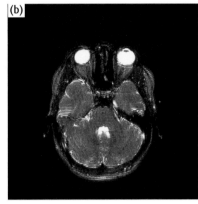

Figure 12.24 Artefacts in GE arising from insufficient spoiling. (a) 'Flash bands' in 'spoiled' gradient echo, (b) resonant offset artefacts in balanced SSFP.

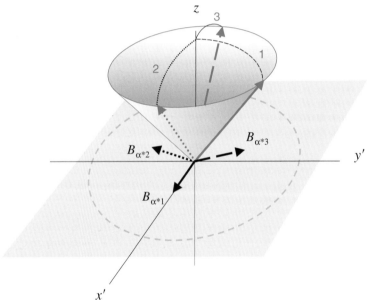

Figure 12.25 Principle of RF spoiling. Changing the RF phase changes the direction of the B_1 field in the rotating frame of reference. RF spoiling is denoted by the asterisks.

As for spoiled sequences, the image-formation principles are completely conventional and the extension to 3D FT is standard, with the same equations for scan time applying. Rewound GE sequences produce good myelographic effect images. Figure 12.19 shows an example of a rewound GE sequence in the brain with very bright CSF and little grey/white matter contrast. Since the signal is relatively independent of TR, rewound sequences are excellent for high contrast between fluid and solid structures in rapid imaging. However, because of the combination of refocused and fresh transverse magnetization, rewound GE sequences are sensitive to motion and flow which can destroy the steady-state transverse coherence.

True FISP or balanced fast field echo (FFE) is a sequence which has balanced, rewinding gradients in all three directions as shown in figure 12.28. An extension to 3D FT can be made by adding phase encoding and rewinding on the slice-select axis in place of the rephasing lobes. True FISP requires high-performance gradient technology to obtain a very short TE and good shimming. If this is not achieved the images become degraded with banding artefacts, which have spacing inversely proportional to the field inhomogeneity. Phase alternation of

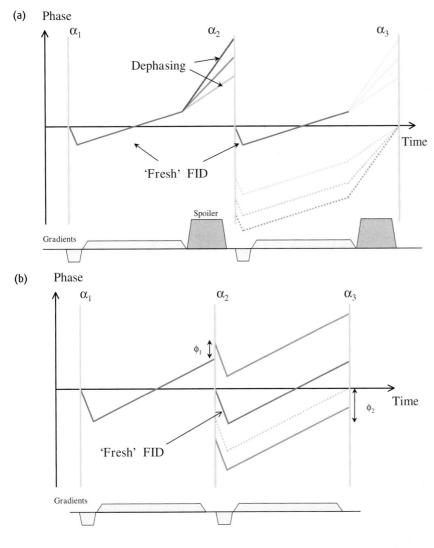

(a) Phase

(b) Phase

Figure 12.26 (a) Coherence diagram showing that gradient spoiling with a constant gradient amplitude dephases the non-echo-forming part of the FID, but that the echo-forming parts (dotted lines) are rephased. (b) Coherence diagram for RF spoiling showing that echo-forming and non-echo-forming parts of transverse magnetization do not form coherences. The dotted line shows the coherence pathway without RF spoiling. Fresh FID is considered to be 'in-phase'.

the RF pulse also helps to achieve a rapid steady-state magnetization and reduces these artefacts. True FISP has found clinical applications in cardiac imaging, where it provides excellent SNR and contrast between blood and the myocardium. An example is shown in chapter 14.

12.4.4 Echoes only: time-reversed gradient echo

Sequences that only utilize the echo component are known as time-reversed gradient echo. An example is the oddly named PSIF sequence (try saying it after a few

gins), an acronym that stands for nothing – but is FISP backwards both in spelling and in function. It is shown in figure 12.30. Strictly speaking it is not a gradient-echo sequence, its signal is of Hahn echo origin. This is how it works: you start with the data acquisition, then you do the phase encoding and finally excite the signal! See 'Getting in a state: how time-reversed GE works' for details. The images (figure 12.19) give a T_2-weighted appearance but with the advantage of a faster acquisition than spin echo. Time-reversed GE has the slightly odd property that the effective TE is approximately

On the rewound

A general solution for gradient echo signal strength is

$$\text{Signal} = \rho \frac{\sin \alpha \cdot [1 - \exp(- TR/T_1)] \cdot \exp(- TE/T_2^*)}{1 - \cos \alpha \exp(- TR/T_1) - \exp(- TR/T_2) \cdot [\exp(- TR/T_1) - \cos \alpha]}$$

Rewound gradient-echo sequences (FISP, GRASS, FFE, FAST) are used with very short TR, much less than T_1 and T_2. In this case the exponential terms can be approximated by Taylor expansions [e.g. $\exp(-TR/T_2) \approx 1 - TR/T_2$], and the above equation simplifies to

$$\text{Signal} = \rho \frac{\sin \alpha \cdot \exp(- TE/T_2^*)}{1 + T_1/T_2 - \cos \alpha \, (T_1/T_2 - 1)}$$

so the signal is ideally independent of TR, dependent only on flip angle and the ratio T_1/T_2. If $\alpha = 90°$ we get

$$\text{Signal} = \frac{\rho}{1 + T_1/T_2}$$

$$\approx \frac{\rho T_2}{T_1}$$

if T_1 is much greater than T_2. As with spoiled gradient echo, there is a flip angle which gives an optimum signal

$$\text{Signal}_{opt} \propto \sqrt{\frac{T_2}{T_1}}$$

sometimes quoted as the 'signal from true FISP'. Unlike spoiled GE sequences, however, the flip angle dependence is only moderate for most practical applications, e.g. imaging of fluids.

A right ROASTing: resonant offsets

The main technical difficulty in true FISP arises from 'resonant offsets' (figure 12.29). The number of RF excitations required to achieve a steady-state magnetization is dependent upon the amount of dephasing during TR. For spins that are not exactly on resonance, e.g. due to main field inhomogeneities, the MR signal will oscillate from excitation to excitation, resulting in banding in the image related to the field inhomogeneity. A simple way of visualizing this is that progressive systematic errors are introduced to the flip angle. Phase-alternating the RF pulse can help to alleviate the problem, as does reducing TR. This problem only arises when all the gradients are balanced, e.g. in true FISP. In rewound sequences that are not fully balanced the degree of residual dephasing is chosen to ensure that each voxel contains a full range of resonant offset angles and the problem is averaged out, i.e. each RF pulse will have the same effect. The term ROAST (**R**esonant **O**ffset **A**veraging **ST**eady State) is sometimes used to describe this technique.

twice TR and that the degree of T_2 weighting is controlled mainly by adjusting TR. Its disadvantages are sensitivity to motion and relatively low signal-to-noise ratio (we are not using the majority of the signal at all). Time-reversed GE images are acquired in sequential mode (slice by slice) or 3D mode. Clinical applications of time-reversed GE are few, but one is as an alternative to echo planar imaging for diffusion-weighted imaging.

12.4.5 3D GE sequences

The extension of spoiled and rewound GE sequences to 3D is relatively straight forward. The scan time is

$$\text{Scan time} = NSA \times N_{PE1} \times N_{PE2} \times TR$$

where, as before, NSA is the number of signal acquisitions and N_{PE} the size of the phase-encode matrix. In practice multi-slab or multi-chunk sequences can be applied,

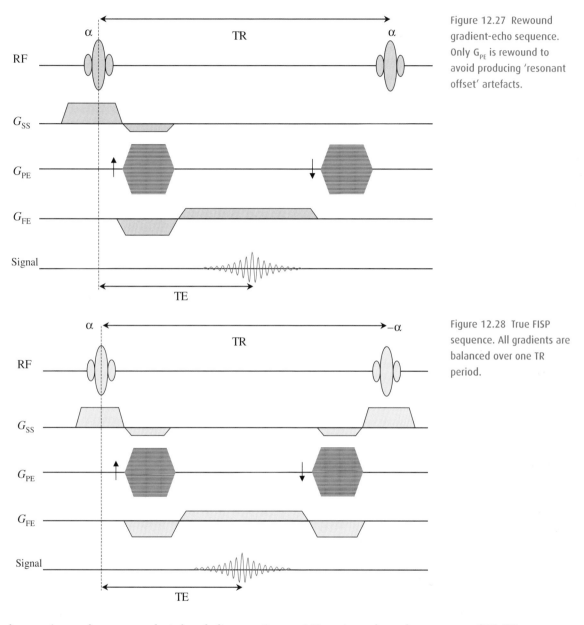

Figure 12.27 Rewound gradient-echo sequence. Only G_{PE} is rewound to avoid producing 'resonant offset' artefacts.

Figure 12.28 True FISP sequence. All gradients are balanced over one TR period.

where various volumes are selected and slices partitioned within them in the manner outlined in section 7.8.

The advantages of 3D sequences are an improvement in SNR over 2D acquisitions of a similar slice thickness and the ability to have well-defined, contiguous slices. Where isotropic resolution is achieved, multi-planar reformatting can be used to advantage.

MR angiography makes great use of 3D GE sequences. Because a second phase encoding is used you have to be careful of two potential problems: phase wraparound in the slice direction (e.g. neck overlying top of brain) and Gibbs slice-to-slice ringing. The solution to the former problem is to increase the field of view, use oversampling or suppress phase wrapped signal with a

If I could turn back time: how time-reversed GE works

Figure 12.31 shows a coherence diagram for time-reversed GE. If we plot out the phase evolution for time-reversed GE we see that the first RF pulse causes the initial excitation of transverse magnetization, and this is dephased by the readout gradient and then partially rephased.

The second RF pulse flips the phase of part of this and the next readout gradient rephases this midway between the TR period to give the echo. Because two RF pulses are involved the behaviour is of a Hahn echo, and hence T_2 weighted in nature. As in other coherent sequences the phase encode requires rewinding. Slice selection is also rewound. As this is a time-reversed sequence, we often consider a 'reverse TE' (figure 12.30) in which case the signal strength approximates to the following:

$$\text{Signal} \propto \exp\left(\frac{-(2 \cdot \text{TR} - \text{TE}_{\text{reverse}})}{T_2}\right)$$

So the T_2 weighting is related to twice TR. For a short reverse TE we can say that the effective TE is approximately twice TR.

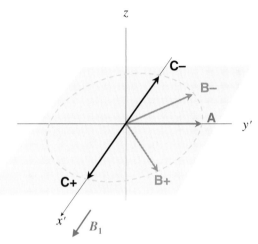

Figure 12.29 Resonance offsets. B_1 has maximum effect upon spins in orientation A, and no effect upon C. Only A is on resonance. In a fully balanced sequence, the spin orientations A, B and C would occur at different positions within the field of view. In an unbalanced sequence the residual spread of phase angles from the gradients will mask differences arising from spatial inhomogeneity.

fat suppression technique since water protons generally have minimal signal. The solution to the Gibbs' ringing problem is to increase the number of partitions or slice direction phase-encode steps.

12.5 Ultra-fast GE imaging

The GE sequences we have examined so far have utilized conventional spatial localization methods. In this section we look at sequences that use segmentation of k-space and non-steady-state methods in their

Double trouble: DESS, FADE and CISS

DESS (**D**ouble **E**cho **S**teady **S**tate) is a Siemens sequence in which two echoes are acquired, one a FISP gradient echo, the other a time-reversed (or PSIF Hahn) echo. The heart of the DESS sequence is shown in figure 12.32. As this is primarily a 3D technique, phase encoding is applied on two axes after prior slab selection. The dephase and rephase portions are arranged such that the FISP echo occurs ahead of the PSIF echo. In the resultant image these two components are combined to give high-resolution images (the FISP part), with strong T_2 weighting (the PSIF part) giving strong fluid signals. DESS is quite sensitive to motion artefacts but is well suited to high-resolution 3D orthopaedic scanning with spatial resolution to significantly sub-millimetre dimensions, as shown in figure 12.33. FADE (**F**ast **A**cquisition **D**ual **E**cho) is a similar sequence available on Marconi (Picker) scanners.

CISS (**C**onstructive **I**nterference in **S**teady **S**tate), another Siemens sequence, is a combination of two true FISP images, one acquired with and one without alternating the sign of the RF pulses. The purpose of the sequence is to avoid banding artefacts that arise in true FISP when the TR is too long. It allows for very high resolution GE images. State-of-the art gradient technology renders this sequence obsolete since we can now use 3D FSE instead.

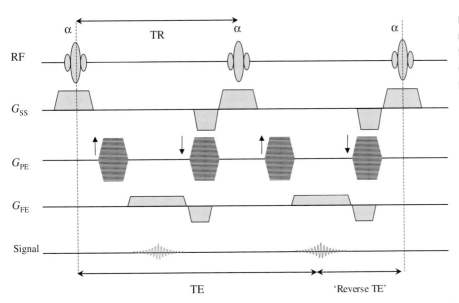

Figure 12.30 Time-reversed GE sequence. The first echo (shown in grey) occurs from an earlier TR period.

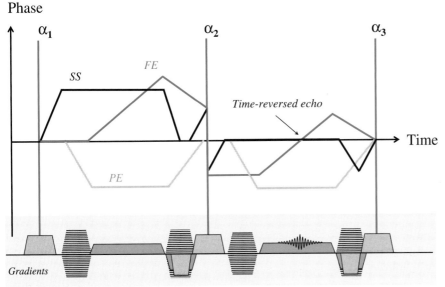

Figure 12.31 Coherence pathway diagram showing echo formation for time-reversed GE. The dephasing effect of each gradient is shown separately. SS denotes slice select, and FE and PE have their normal meanings.

image formation. This, combined with low flip angle techniques, enables them to run 'ultra-fast'. What is ultrafast? Generally scan times of a few seconds or less per whole slice. In addition to these GE sequences, SS-FSE, HASTE and SE-EPI would be considered as ultra-fast.

12.5.1 Turbo-FLASH

Turbo-FLASH is a spoiled technique applied ultra quickly with extremely short TR and very low flip angle.

One of the consequences of a very short TR and low flip angle is that the T_1 contrast is very poor. To get round this problem, turbo-FLASH uses an inversion

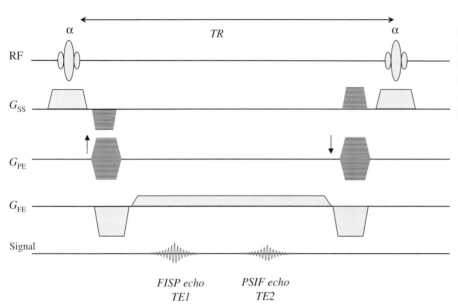

RF

G_{SS}

G_{PE}

G_{FE}

Signal

α TR α

FISP echo   *PSIF echo*
TE1   *TE2*

Figure 12.32 DESS sequence. The "FISP" echo is the rewound gradient echo arising from the most recent RF pulse. The "**PSIF**" echo is refocused from the previous excitation.

pre-pulse followed by a delay to generate T_1 weighting as shown in figure 12.34. As for fast SE, the order of phase encoding affects the contrast, with an effective inversion time TI from the centre of the inversion RF pre-pulse to the centre of k-space shown in figure 12.35. For a linear-ordered phase encoding this is

$$TI_{eff} = TI + \frac{N_{PE}}{2} \cdot TR$$

Therefore with this sequence, changing the matrix size (in the phase-encode direction) changes the contrast.

On some scanners (e.g. the Siemens Syngo platform) the definition of TI has been changed to be the time

from the initial inversion to the middle of k-space: this makes much more sense as now you don't change the contrast if you change the matrix size, you just change the delay between the inversion pulse and the start of the RAGE loop.

Turbo-FLASH can run very fast acquiring a whole slice in 1 or 2 s. When used in a multiple slice mode, it is applied sequentially. That is, the whole of one slice is acquired before the next. A delay, TD, between slice acquisitions must be applied if a nonselective inversion pulse is used. The scan time is therefore proportional to the number of slices:

$$\text{Scan time} = N_{\text{slices}} \times (TI + N_{PE} \cdot TR + TD)$$

Turbo-FLASH can be applied in both single-shot and segmented mode. In single-shot mode the whole of k-space is acquired by the train of RF pulses. This imposes practical limits on the spatial resolution achievable but makes for very rapid (1 s per slice) acquisitions. In segmented turbo-FLASH k-space is divided into segments and the whole sequence repeated a number of times. Typically up to 32 lines of k-space may be acquired per shot. In order to avoid jumps in signal intensity from one segment to the next, interleaving schemes may be employed. Furthermore, the ordering

---

The names game 3: ultra-fast/transient state techniques

Generic name: **Turbo FLASH** (TFL)

aka   *Turbo Field Echo* (TFE)

       Magnetization Prepared Rapid Acquired Gradient Echo (MP-RAGE)

       Fast SPGR (FSPGR)

       IR-prepped FSPGR

       DE-prepped FSPGR (driven equilibrium)

We call it 'turbo-FLASH'.

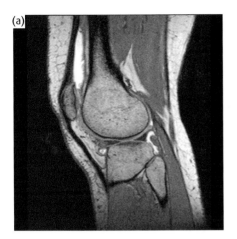
(a)

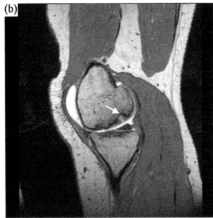
(b)

Figure 12.33 (a) DESS image of the sagittal knee showing bright fluid. (b) Cartilage defect and bone erosion (arrowed) shown by DESS. TR = 26.8 ms, TE = 9 ms, $\alpha = 40°$.

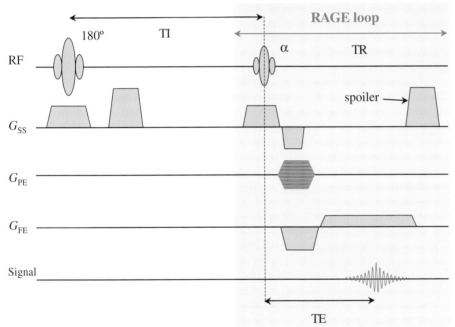

Figure 12.34 Turbo-FLASH sequence. An inverting prepulse and spoiler gradient precede the rapid acquired gradient echo (RAGE) loop for image formation.

of phase-encode steps affects the contrast as shown in the box 'k-space ordering schemes'. Figure 12.36 shows a breath-hold turbo-FLASH abdominal image.

The turbo-FLASH sequence involves RF spoiling to avoid contamination of T_1-weighted contrast by T_2 effects. It is, however, different from spoiled gradient echo in that a steady state is not achieved during data acquisition. The magnetization exists in a transient state, undergoing repetitive very small flip angles while the longitudinal relaxation is recovering from its initial inversion. By appropriately varying the flip angle during the readout portion of the sequence, oscillations of magnetization and, subsequently, inconsistencies of k-space data can be avoided.

Turbo-FLASH is also known as IR-FSPGR (on General Electric scanners) or sometimes T1-TurboFLASH. It is

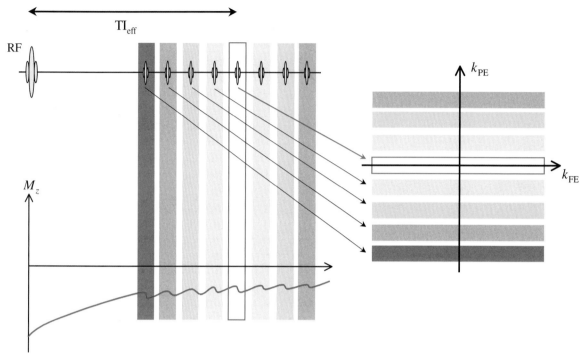

Figure 12.35 k-space acquisition for turbo-FLASH showing how the effective TI (TI_{eff}) occurs.

also possible to have T2-TurboFLASH (DE-FSPGR on General Electric systems), which as the name suggests gives T_2-weighted images. This is achieved by replacing the inversion pulse with a 90°–180°–90° set of preparation pulses. The 90°–180° pair produces a T_2-weighted spin echo, which is returned to the z axis by the second 90°. The turbo-FLASH loop immediately follows to produce the image, so 'TI' now defines the amount of T_2 weighting.

12.5.2 MP-RAGE

MP-RAGE or **M**agnetization **P**repared **R**apid **A**cquisition by **G**radient **E**cho is the same in principle as turbo-FLASH. However, the name has tended to apply to a particular 3D implementation of turbo-FLASH shown in figure 12.38. As a 3D technique there are too many combinations of the two phase-encode gradients to acquire the whole of 3D k-space from a single preparation. The solution is to acquire all the 'slice' or

k-space ordering schemes

In standard spin-echo imaging the order in which the lines of k-space are acquired is generally from maximum negative to maximum positive (or vice versa). This is called linear or sequential ordering. In spin echo the actual order does not matter, as the underlying signal does not change from line to line. The order does matter for segmented k-space and single-shot sequences.

Another commonly used order is centric, where the lowest k_{PE} values are measured first with positive and negative values alternating, i.e. 0, −1, 1, −2, 2, ..., $−N_{PE}/2$, $N_{PE}/2$. This will result in contrast dominated by the beginning of the acquisition period.

Reverse or outer centric is similar but starts from the large values and works backwards. Image contrast will be dominated by the end of the acquisition. These are illustrated in figure 12.37.

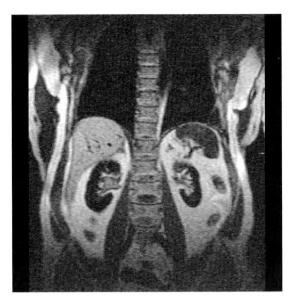

Figure 12.36 Turbo-FLASH image of the abdomen: TR = 8.5 ms, TE = 4 ms, TI = 400 ms, 5 mm slice, acquisition time 1.5 s.

in-depth lines of data from each prep, then introduce a recovery delay (as in segmented turbo-FLASH) before moving on to the next in-plane line of k-space. As a result the in-plane resolution is not compromised, the data being all acquired with the same degree of relaxation. MP-RAGE can produce very high resolution, T_1-weighted images showing very good anatomical detail, particularly of the brain (figure 12.39). The introduction of this delay means that MP-RAGE is not ultra-fast in its scan time (although it uses ultra-fast methods). The scan time is

$$\text{Scan time} = \text{NSA} \times N_{\text{PE}} \times (N_{\text{slices}} \cdot \text{TR} + \text{TI} + \text{TD})$$

12.5.3 GE echo planar imaging

At the time of writing echo planar imaging (EPI) is the fastest pulse sequence, capable of producing a whole slice in under 100 ms. In single-shot GE-EPI the whole train of gradient echoes are acquired following a single

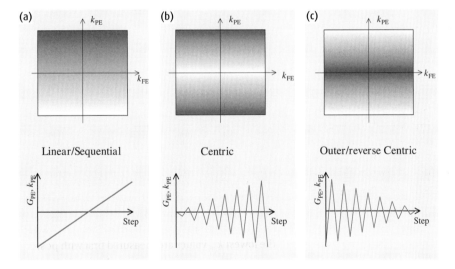

Figure 12.37 k-space ordering schemes: (a) linear or sequential, (b) centric, (c) reverse centric. In centric, the image contrast is determined by the beginning of the acquisition, in reverse centric by the end.

Through the key-hole

A further way of speeding up dynamic imaging is the key-hole technique, which uses data reduction techniques similar to those used in CT fluoroscopy. To acquire a rapid series of images of the same slice position, the whole data matrix is only acquired for the first image. For subsequent images only the centre of k-space is acquired, the edges being copied from the initial data. This technique is only applicable to time series of dynamic images. Figure 12.41 illustrates the principle.

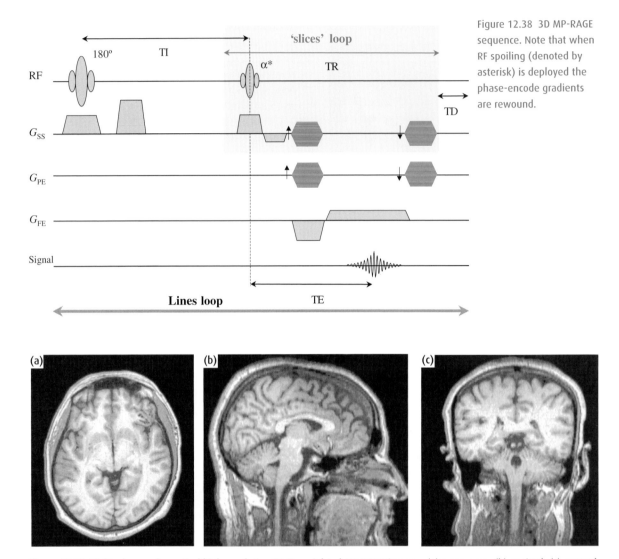

Figure 12.38 3D MP-RAGE sequence. Note that when RF spoiling (denoted by asterisk) is deployed the phase-encode gradients are rewound.

Figure 12.39 Multi-planar reformatted high-resolution 3D T_1-weighted MP-RAGE images: (a) transverse, (b) sagittal, (c) coronal.

RF excitation pulse (figure 12.40). In this instance the phase encoding of each line is acquired by adding a constant-amplitude gradient lobe, or 'blip', after each frequency-encode gradient reversal. To run successfully EPI requires high-performance gradients. EPI suffers from a number of inherent limitations in image quality. Its speed however makes it useful for real-time cardiac imaging and functional MRI of the brain. EPI is considered in greater detail in chapter 16.

12.6 Pulse sequence conversion chart

Needing to choose a pulse sequence? At this point we refer you back to figure 12.2 but this time view it more as a route map than a family tree. First decide your destination – T_1, T_2 or PD weighting, etc. Then decide how you want to get there and how fast you want to go. Finally think about potential pitfalls; for example, what

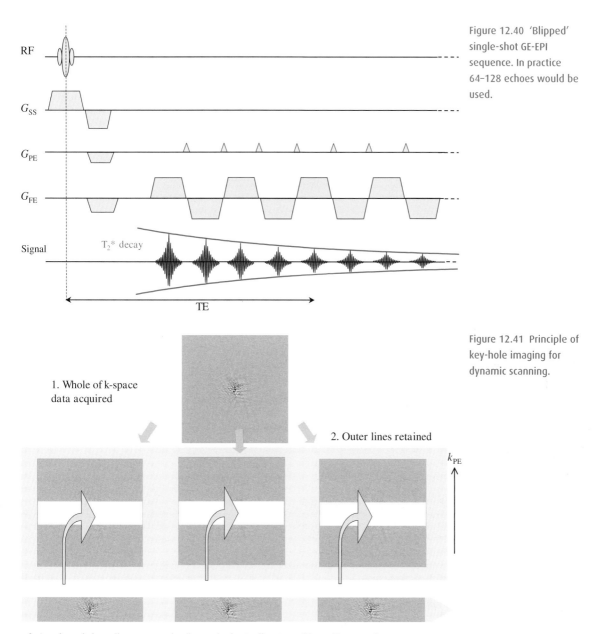

Figure 12.40 'Blipped' single-shot GE-EPI sequence. In practice 64–128 echoes would be used.

Figure 12.41 Principle of key-hole imaging for dynamic scanning.

1. Whole of k-space data acquired

2. Outer lines retained

3. Acquire only inner lines, use previously acquired outer lines to enable rapid scan series

artefacts you might encounter, or what limitations there are on resolution or slice number.

If you get lost you can always ask directions. However, you may be unfamiliar with your manufacturer's language. Table 12.1 contains a 'translation' of manufac-

turer-speak terminology. Beware! Most manufacturers like to coin trendy acronyms for specific combinations of parameters for particular clinical applications. Good examples are VIBE (Siemens), THRIVE (Philips) and LAVA (General Electric). All of these are essentially fast,

Table 12.1 Pulse sequence comparison for major manufacturers

Family	Generic name	General Electric	Marconi (formerly Picker)	Philips	Siemens	Toshiba
Spin echo	RARE (rapid acquisition with relaxation enhancement)	FSE	FSE	TSE	TSE	FSE
	IR-RARE	FSE-IR	Fast IR	IR-TSE	Turbo-IR	Fast IR
	Single-shot RARE	SS-FSE, SSFSE-IR	Express	UFSE	SS-TSE, HASTE	FASE, DIET SuperFASE
	GRASE (gradient and spin echo)	–	–	GRASE	TGSE	–
Gradient echo	Spoiled GE	SPGR, MPSPGR	RF-FAST	T1-FFE	FLASH	RF-spoiled FE
	Rewound GE	MPGR, GRE	FAST	FFE	FISP	FE
	Fully rewound GE	FIESTA (cardiac systems only)	–	Balanced FFE	True-FISP	–
	SSFP (steady-state free precession) GE	SSFP	CE-FAST	T2 FFE	PSIF	–
	Dual echo GE	–	FADE	–	DESS	–
	Constructive interference GE	–	–	–	CISS	–
Ultra-fast gradient echo	RAGE (rapid acquisition with gradient echo)	FGRE, FSPGR, FMPSPGR	RAM-FAST	TFE	Turbo-FLASH	TFE
	MP-RAGE (magnetization prepared)	IR-FSPGR, DE-FSPGR	–	IR-TFE, Sat-TFE	T1-Turbo-FLASH, T2-Turbo-FLASH	Fast-FE

Notes:
Angiography and EPI-based sequences are excluded from this table as they are generally self-explanatory.
General Electric: VEMP (**V**ariable-**E**cho **M**ulti-**P**lanar) and MEMP (**M**ulti-**E**cho **M**ulti-**P**lanar) are both spin-echo sequences found on older scanners. GRASS (**G**radient **R**ecalled **A**cquisition in the **S**teady **S**tate) is an old name for GRE, i.e. GRASS is a rewound GE sequence.
Siemens: MEDIC (**M**ulti-**E**cho **D**ata **I**mage **C**ombination) is a multi-echo FLASH sequence in which the signals are all combined to form the final image; contrast is mixed T_1/T_2^*: VIBE (**V**olume-**I**nterpolated **B**ody **E**xamination) is a another FLASH sequence with zero-filling in the slice-select direction, designed for breath-hold abdomen examinations.

Table 12.1 Notes (*cont.*)

Acronyms anonymous:

CE-FAST contrast-enhanced FAST
CISS constructive interference in steady state
DE driven equilibrium
DESS dual echo steady state
DIET dual interval echo train
FADE fast acquisition with dual echo
FASE fast advanced SE
FAST Fourier-acquired steady state
FGRE fast GRE
FISP fast imaging with steady-state precession
FLASH fast low-angle single shot
FMPSPGR fast MPSPGR
FSPGR fast SPGR

GRE gradient recalled echo
HASTE half-Fourier acquisition with single-shot TSE
MPGR multi-planar gradient recalled
MPSPGR multi-planar SPGR
PSIF reversed FISP
RAM-FAST rapid acquisition matrix FAST
RF-FAST RF-spoiled FAST
SPGR spoiled GE
SS-FSE single-shot FSE
SS-TSE single-shot TSE
TFE turbo field echo
TGSE turbo gradient and spin echo
UFSE ultra-fast spin echo

T_1-weighted, 3D scans for abdomen and breast applications. For a good dictionary of MRI terms, see Liney's 'MRI from A to Z' (full details in Further Reading).

See also:

- How frequencyand phase-encoding gradients work: chapter 7
- Basic image contrast: chapter 3
- Pulse sequences for specialist imaging: chapter 16

FURTHER READING

Bernstein MA, King KF and Zhou XJ (2004) *Handbook of MRI Pulse Sequences* Elsevier Academic Press (ISBN: 0120928612).

Brown MA and Semelka RC (1999) MR imaging abbreviations, definitions and descriptions: a review. *Radiology* **213**: 647–62.

Elster AD and Burdette JH (2001) *Questions and Answers in Magnetic Resonance Imaging*, 2nd edn. London: Mosby-Yearbook (ISBN: 0323011845), Chapters 5 & 12.

Haacke EM and Tkach JA (1990) Fast MR imaging: techniques and clinical applications. *Am J Roentgen* **155**: 951–64.

Haacke EM, Brown RW, Thompson MR and Venkaten R (1999) *Magnetic Resonance Imaging: Physical Principles and Sequence Design.* New York: John Wiley (ISBN: 0471351288), Chapters 18 & 26.

Liney G (2005) *MRI from A to Z* Cambridge: Cambridge University Press (ISBN: 0521606381).

Mansfield P and Maudsley AA (1977) Medical imaging by NMR. *Br J Radiol* **50**: 188–94.

Twieg DB (1983) The k-trajectory formulation of the NMR imaging process with applications in analysis and synthesis of imaging methods. *Med Phys* **10**: 610–23.

13

Go with the flow: MR angiography

13.1 Introduction

Magnetic resonance angiography (MRA) uses the inherent motion sensitivity of MRI to visualize blood flow within vessels. There are two major classes of flow imaging methods that rely on the endogenous contrast of moving spins to produce angiographic images. The time-of-flight (TOF) technique relies on flow-dependent changes in longitudinal magnetization, whilst the phase-contrast (PC) technique relies on flow-dependent changes in transverse magnetization. In addition there are contrast-enhanced MRA techniques that employ exogenous contrast agents, such as gadolinium chelates, to provide vascular contrast. In this situation the intravascular signal is more dependent upon the T_1 shortening properties of gadolinium than the TOF effect. Each method has particular advantages and disadvantages for angiographic imaging which are reflected in their applications.

Before we describe how MRA sequences work, we will look at the appearances of flowing blood in conventional spin-echo and gradient-echo scans. You should read (or review) section 6.4, as a foundation for the material in this chapter. This chapter will explain:

- that flowing blood creates an in-flow or TOF effect in standard imaging, as well as velocity-induced phase artefacts, and how these can be avoided when angio imaging is not required;
- how TOF MRA techniques take advantage of the in-flow effect in blood vessels, and show how it is used in 2D and 3D techniques for carotids, Circle of Willis, and peripheral vessels;

- that 3D TOF needs better background signal suppression and causes spin saturation through the volume. Magnetization transfer and ramped RF pulses are used to avoid these effects;
- how phase-contrast MRA takes advantage of the velocity-induced phase effects in blood flow, and that it offers the possibility of flow quantification;
- how gadolinium-based contrast agents are used as a bolus injection to reduce the T_1 of blood and produce angiograms using rapid 3D gradient-echo sequences;
- how time-resolved MRA can be achieved by repeatedly scanning a volume with a scan time significantly faster than the rate at which a gadolinium bolus passes through the circulation; alternatively long, ultra-high-resolution MRA and detection of internal bleeding is possible using blood pool contrast agents.

13.2 Effect of flow in conventional imaging techniques

Moving spins, such as flowing blood, have a significant influence on the magnetic resonance signal. These effects may be undesirable since they produce degrading artefacts but we can also take advantage of them to produce MR angiograms. As both an artefact and an important source of diagnostic information, it is important to understand the effects of motion.

Unless appropriately controlled, all motion during an MR acquisition will cause artefacts. This is mainly because the Fourier transform (FT) used in reconstructing MR images assumes that the signal within each voxel does not vary from measurement to measurement (i.e.

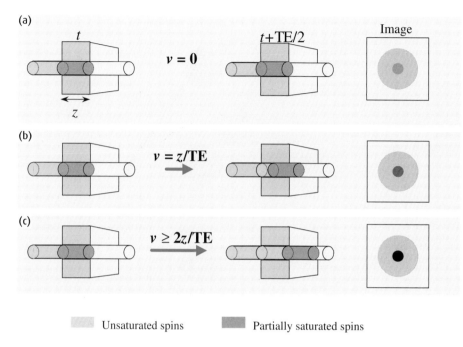

(a)

t $t+\text{TE}/2$ Image

$v = 0$

z

(b)

$v = z/\text{TE}$

(c)

$v \geq 2z/\text{TE}$

☐ Unsaturated spins   ■ Partially saturated spins

Figure 13.1 Time-of-flight effect in spin-echo imaging. If blood is stationary (a) it receives both the 90° and the 180° pulse and produces a spin echo like any other tissue. When $v \geq 2z/\text{TE}$ (c) all the blood that received the 90° pulse has moved out of the slice during TE/2, the time between the 90° and the 180° pulses, so the vessel has a flow void. At intermediate velocities, e.g. $v = z/\text{TE}$ (b), there will be a reduced signal compared to (a) but greater than (c) due to partial wash-out of the blood during TE/2. v is blood velocity and z is slice thickness.

from TR to TR) except in response to the phase-encoding gradient. Any other signal change, e.g. due to flow, is interpreted as arising from the phaseencoding process. This results in signal ghosting and artefact along the phase-encoding direction in the final image, and the exact nature of the signal changes determines the nature of the observed artefact. Methods for reducing motion-induced artefacts therefore usually try to minimize the TR-to-TR variation in signal within a voxel. A simple method of reducing artefacts is to average the data: the signal from static objects will be reinforced whilst the signal from random artefacts will decrease.

Blood flow is one of the most troublesome sources of artefact because of its pulsatility and can cause variations in either longitudinal magnetization (TOF effects) or transverse magnetization (phase shift effects).

13.2.1 TOF effects

The first effect of blood flow is the slice transition, or TOF effect. The TOF effect arises because some or all of the blood within an imaged slice is replaced during the repetition time, TR, or the time between the 90° and 180°

pulses (TE/2). We will consider the latter case, the spin-echo sequence, first. In a spin-echo sequence three types of signal behaviour can be identified depending on the blood velocity (figure 13.1). If blood is 'stationary' the spins experience both the 90° and 180° pulses generating a spin echo, which may be T_1 or T_2 weighted depending on TR and TE. You might think that blood in a living human being is never stationary. However, from figure 13.1 you can see that the signal intensity depends on blood velocity v, the slice thickness z and the sequence TR. If we have a very thick slice, slow flowing blood may appear to be 'stationary' and thus give us a signal.

When the blood velocity is such that the blood within the slice completely leaves the slice between the 90° and 180° pulses (figure 13.1(c)), then a spin echo is not generated and the vessel lumen has no signal; this is known as high-velocity signal loss or wash-out. The third type of signal behaviour occurs at the intermediate stage when the blood is moving at a speed such that only some of the blood leaves the slice between the 90° and 180° pulses. The portion that has left is replaced by blood flowing into the slice. Only blood that remains in the slice for both the 90° and the 180° pulses will

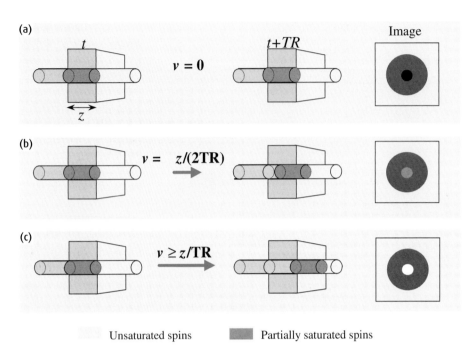

Figure 13.2 Time-of-flight effect in gradient-echo imaging. When blood is stationary (a) it becomes saturated like other tissues with long T_1 and has reduced signal. When $v \geq z/\text{TR}$ (c) maximal inflow of unsaturated blood occurs and therefore maximal signal is observed. At intermediate blood velocities, e.g. $v = z/2\text{TR}$ (b), there will be increased signal compared to (a) but less than (c) due to partial in-flow of unsaturated blood during TR.

produce a signal, so there will be a partial reduction of signal due to the wash-out effect.

Gradient-echo sequences, which have no slice-selective 180° refocusing pulses, only demonstrate flow-related enhancement and never show wash-out signal losses. Instead, depending on the velocity of the blood, differing degrees of flow-related enhancement are observed (figure 13.2). When the velocity v is equal to or greater than z/TR, where z is the slice thickness, then complete replacement of spins within the slice occurs during TR, resulting in maximum signal since these spins will not have experienced any previous RF pulses. When v is less than z/TR there is only partial replacement of spins resulting in a reduced vascular signal intensity. Obviously since flow velocities vary due to pulsatility between TRs then the signal amplitude will also vary resulting in ghosting artefacts.

13.2.2 Phase shift effects

The second mechanism responsible for signal intensity modulation is the spin phase phenomena. You should remember from chapter 7 that stationary spins within a magnetic field gradient acquire a phase shift in proportion to the strength and duration of the gradient. The slice-select and frequency-encoding gradients are balanced so that no net phase shift exists after slice selection and at the echo time. The phase-encoding gradient has to be unbalanced to generate the required phase shifts for spatial encoding. Unfortunately balancing the gradients only works for static protons. Those that move even if the gradient is balanced will acquire a phase shift proportional to the velocity of the spins (figure 13.3). This causes the characteristic flow artefact in the phase-encode direction.

If the spins within a vessel are all moving at the same velocity (a situation known as 'plug flow') then the phase shift across the vessel will be constant. However, there is typically a parabolic distribution of flow velocities across a vessel, with the velocity zero at the walls and maximum in the centre of the vessel. This is called 'laminar flow' since adjacent layers of fluid glide past each other without mixing. In laminar flow there is always some stationary blood at the edges of the vessels, even in vessels with quite fast flow. Since the vessel is typically only a few voxels across, each voxel

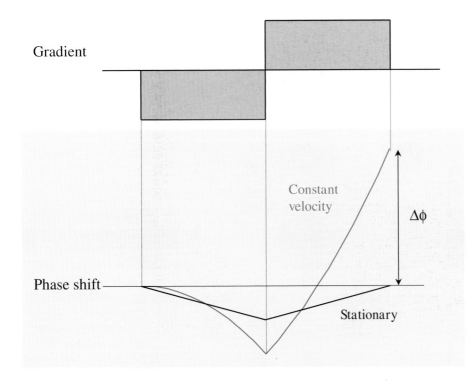

Figure 13.3 Velocity-induced phase shift $\Delta\phi$ due to a balanced, i.e. equal area, bipolar gradient.

will contain a range of flow velocities, particularly those near the vessel wall where the range of velocities can be quite large. Each velocity within the voxel will result in a different phase shift with the net effect being that individual voxels will have different amounts of phase dispersion. Note that the amount of phase dispersion will also depend upon the time for which the spins are allowed to dephase, i.e. the echo time, TE.

If the intravoxel phase dispersion is large enough then complete signal cancellation can occur. This means that the edges of vessels have reduced signal, and so the apparent width of the vessel is less than the true diameter. Furthermore, if flow velocities, whether plug flow or parabolic, vary between TRs (due to pulsatility for example) then the degree of phase shift and hence signal magnitude will vary, again resulting in artefacts in the phase-encoding direction (figure 13.4).

13.2.3 Avoiding flow artefacts

The in-flow effect is most effectively dealt with by eliminating the signal from spins before they enter the imaging slice. This can be achieved using spatial presaturation bands adjacent to the imaging slice. Spins within the presaturation slabs are flipped into the transverse plane and then have their transverse magnetization rapidly dephased by spoiler gradients. When the spins then flow into the imaging slice they are already saturated and give zero signal. A consistent intraluminal signal, zero in this case, from TR to TR means that artefacts are not produced. The disadvantage is that the TR must be increased because of the additional RF and gradient pulses required for the presaturation bands.

Reduction of intravoxel phase dispersion can be achieved by eliminating the phase shifts using a technique called 'gradient moment nulling', also known as 'flow compensation', but perhaps better described as 'velocity compensation', as we will see (see also section 6.4.3). The basic idea is that since spins moving with constant velocity along a bipolar gradient produce a certain phase shift, then this phase shift can be 'unwound' by repeating the bipolar gradient but with opposite polarity. The net phase shifts for both stationary and constant-velocity spins should therefore be zero. This has the

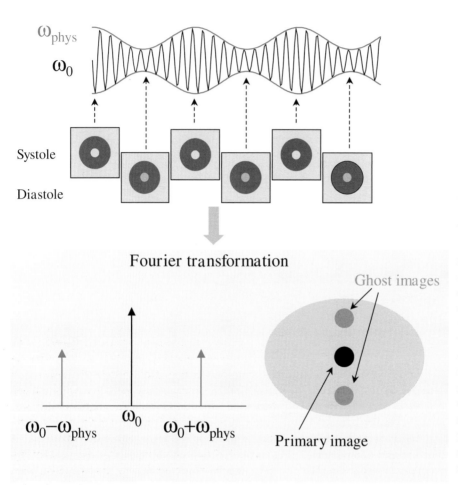

ω_{phys}

ω_0

Systole

Diastole

Fourier transformation

Ghost images

$\omega_0-\omega_{phys}$ $\qquad$ ω_0 $\qquad$ $\omega_0+\omega_{phys}$

Primary image

Figure 13.4 Pulsatile blood flow leads to a modulation of the MR signal during the entire acquisition. This results in sidebands and hence ghosts after Fourier transformation. In this simple example an MR signal at ω_0 is modulated by a sinusoidal physiological process at angular frequency ω_{phys}. Following Fourier transformation sidebands, i.e. ghosts, appear either side of the primary image at $\omega_0 + \omega_{phys}$ and at $\omega_0 - \omega_{phys}$. Note that these ghosts appear in the phase-encoding direction which is anterior-posterior (up-down) in this diagram. In vivo the physiological modulation is often more complicated than a simple sinusoid and the sideband pattern is consequently more complex resulting in multiple ghosts.

effect of reducing the variation in intraluminal signal intensity and therefore decreasing artefacts.

Flow or velocity compensation thus involves inserting extra bipolar gradients into the normal imaging sequence, usually only in the slice-select and frequencyencoding directions (figure 13.5). Why not along the phase-encode direction too? Well, the high-order phase-encode gradients do not contribute to the signal in the image; the low-order phase-encode gradients, which are responsible for the contrast in the image, have an inherently low sensitivity to flow and so do not really need flow compensation. This assumption tends to fail for vessels with fast flowing blood, which may appear misplaced with respect to their true position.

With improved gradient performance 3D TOF sequences are increasingly becoming flow compensated in all three directions.

Velocity compensation has the slight disadvantage of increasing TE because of the increased gradient complexity. Higher order motions, i.e. acceleration and jerk, require three and five lobed gradient waveforms respectively to eliminate the phase shifts from these motions. These additional gradient pulses will significantly increase the minimum TE and so usually only velocity compensation is performed.

Reducing TE is an important factor in minimizing artefacts from intravoxel phase dispersion arising from complex flow phenomena. In particular the flow distal

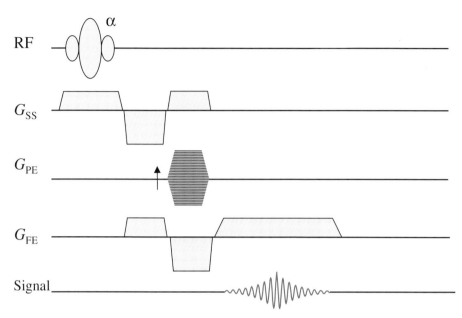

to vascular stenoses may become turbulent, resulting in individual voxels containing a range of velocities and therefore phase shifts. The large range of phase shifts typically causes cancellation and signal dropout within the vessel. Short TEs help to reduce the phase dispersion by reducing the time over which it can occur. TE can be minimized by using partial or fractional echo data acquisition. In this technique the readout prephasing gradient areas are reduced so that the echo is formed earlier in time, i.e. asymmetrically within the data-acquisition window. The missing data from the front of the echo can then be reconstructed using mathematical techniques similar to those used for reconstructing images acquired with half Fourier imaging techniques (see section 7.7.1).

13.3 Time-of-flight MR angiography

Time-of-flight MRA uses gradient-echo sequences with short TRs and TEs to saturate the signal from stationary spins, whilst spins flowing into the imaging slice with full magnetization yield a high signal. Post-processing methods such as the maximum intensity projection (MIP) algorithm accentuate these differences and allow

the MRA data to be displayed so that it resembles conventional X-ray arteriograms. TOF MRA can be performed as either multiple 2D single-slice acquisitions or as a 3D volumetric acquisition. To maximize the inflow effect the slices are acquired perpendicular to the major flow direction. For most applications the flow direction is along the body, so axial slices are used.

Since TOF techniques exploit differences in longitudinal magnetization for contrast care should be taken when imaging vessels that may contain blood breakdown products such as met-haemoglobin, which has a very short T_1. The rapid signal recovery within haemorrhages or thrombus containing met-haemoglobin will result in bright signal on TOF MRA, mimicking flow where there is none.

13.3.1 2D TOF

2D TOF MRA involves the sequential acquisition of many thin (approximately 1–2 mm) 2D slices, followed by MIP of the stacked slices. The advantage of this technique is that the saturation of background tissue is quite effective since high flip angles can be used (typically 60°). The sequence is also sensitive to slow flow since the velocity threshold for complete replacement

(a)

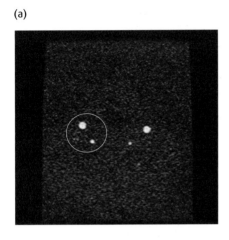

(b)

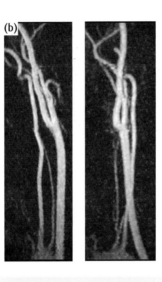

Figure 13.6 2D TOF. (a) Single 1.5- mm-thick slice from a 2D TOF study of the carotid and vertebral arteries. (b) Sagittal and coronal maximum intensity projections (MIP) of the outlined region.

MIP disxplay of MR angiograms

All MRA techniques aim to create images with the maximum possible signal from blood vessels and a near-zero background intensity. Although the modes of data collection may be different, the processing methods for display are the same. The standard method is to use the maximum intensity projection (MIP) algorithm. The MIP produces a projection image by casting 'rays' through the stack of 2D or 3D slices and detecting the maximum pixel value, which is then displayed on the projection. You can think of this as being similar to producing an X-ray angiogram: the X-rays are attenuated by the iodine-enhanced blood vessels and produce a shadow on the image intensifier. You may find the analogy easier to understand if you use 'inverse video' to view an MR angiogram: the bright pixels within the vessels now appear dark on a white background. Some people prefer to see MIPs in inverse video because they look similar to the standard X-ray angiograms.

By rotating the dataset a small amount and performing the MIP again we can obtain another projection from the new viewpoint. Repeating this process at say 5° intervals for a total rotation of 180° and then displaying the images in a movie loop provides the necessary visual cues for a strong 3D impression of the vasculature.

The MIP does however have certain fundamental limitations. First small low-contrast vessels may be masked by higher intensity background pixels along the ray. Second there is no depth encoding, making the separation of different vessels very difficult on static images (e.g. when they are viewed on film hard copy). This problem can be overcome by displaying a series of MIPs rotating the vessels around so the observer develops a 3-dimensional feel for the arteries. Various other algorithms have been proposed and implemented (e.g. volume rendering); however, the MIP is currently the favoured commercial implementation because it is computationally very simple.

of spins ($v = z/\mathrm{TR}$) is low with these thin slices. Selectivity to a particular flow direction (i.e. arterial or venous) can be obtained by closely applying presaturation bands either above or below the imaging slice, depending on the direction of flow to be suppressed. The disadvantages of 2D TOF include relatively long TEs associated with selecting thin slices, which can result in signal loss from metal clips as well as turbulent or complex flow; poor through-plane resolution compared with the in-plane resolution; in-plane saturation with tortuous arteries; slice misregistration artefact from minor motions; pulsatility artefact in arteries with high resistance flow; and poor quality with slower flow which is common in elderly patients and with aneurysmal disease. Figure 13.6 shows a 2D TOF MRA study of the carotid arteries.

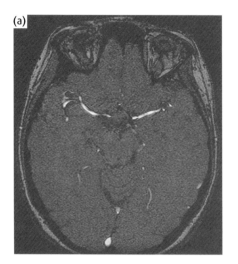

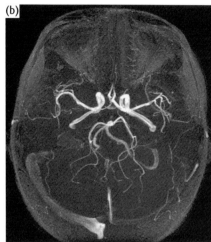

Figure 13.7 3D TOF. (a) Single 0.7- mm-thick slice from a 3D TOF MRA study of the intracerebral circulation. (b) Axial maximum intensity projection (MIP). Note the excellent signal-to-noise ratio obtained with a 3D acquisition.

Using ECG or peripheral pulse gating in combination with short-TR gradient echoes can reduce the problem of pulsatility artefacts in 2D TOF; for example, in the major arteries and at the carotid bifurcation. By acquiring data only during peak systole, the vascular contrast is increased and ghosting artefacts are reduced albeit with the requirement of even longer scan times. 2D TOF methods are best used as rapid vascular localizersand for imaging steady flow, e.g. MR venography, carotid arteries and pedal arteries when there is occlusive disease that obliterates arterial pulsation.

13.3.2 3D TOF

3D TOF methods acquire a volume of data. A relatively thick slab of tissue is excited and then sub-divided into thin slices or partitions by a second phase-encoding process in the slice-selection direction. Image reconstruction is done with a 3D FT instead of the usual 2D FT. The advantage of slice encoding using this method is that much thinner slices can be reconstructed (typically as little as 0.7 mm), which improves the resolution and hence vessel conspicuity by reducing the partial volume effects. The SNR in individual images is also significantly improved compared to 2D methods. However, this improvement in SNR also applies to the background tissue which limits the contrast and visibility of some small vessels in the final MIP. Magnetization

transfer techniques are commonly used to reduce background tissue signal. A further problem with 3D TOF studies is the saturation of slow flow within the slab and various approaches have been adopted to try and reduce this effect. Figure 13.7 shows a 3D TOF MRA study of the intracerebral circulation.

The choice of echo time (TE) is an important factor in optimizing TOF MRA. Whilst short TEs minimize intravoxel dephasing due to turbulent flow, the preferred choice of TE is one at which fat and water are out of phase to provide some reduction in the intense fat signal. At 1.5 T the shortest TE at which fat and water are out of phase is 2.3 ms. However, many imaging systems cannot achieve such a short TE since there are quite a lot of gradient pulses to be played out between excitation and readout. The next shortest time at which fat and water will be out of phase is 6.9 ms. With highperformance gradient systems, this TE allows time for velocity compensation on the phase-encoding axis as well as slice-select and frequency-encoding axes, resulting in a fully flow compensated sequence.

13.4 Phase-contrast angiography

Phase-contrast MRA relies on detecting changes in the phase of blood's transverse magnetization as it moves along a magnetic field gradient. We already know that a

Improving background suppression: magnetization transfer

In order to reduce the unwanted background from stationary tissue, magnetization transfer (MT) is used. MT refers to the process whereby protons associated with unbound, or free, water molecules can exchange their spin energy with other protons bound to macromolecules. Protons that are bound to macromolecules have very short T_2 relaxation times and hence very broad resonances. These protons are therefore essentially 'invisible' to conventional MR imaging. To apply MT background suppression, a high-power, off-resonance (typically 1–2 kHz) RF pulse is used to saturate the magnetization of protons in the bound pool (see figure 13.8). When these protons exchange their magnetization with the free protons, there is a significant reduction in the signal from tissues. In the brain, the signal from grey and white matter can be reduced whilst the signal from moving blood, which does not exhibit a significant MT effect, is relatively unaffected. The result is an overall improvement in vessel contrast. Section 8.7.4 contains more information about magnetization transfer.

The use of MT also has a few disadvantages. First there is increase in RF power deposition because of the high-power MT pulse. Second it is necessary to increase TR and thus the total scan time in order to play out the pulse, although this actually improves in-flow effects. Finally fat tends to be more conspicuous since lipids do not exhibit significant MT effects either. For this reason MT is used primarily in the brain where there is minimal fat. At 3.0 T, MT is less important for background suppression; blood has a longer T_1 and the in-flow effect is more marked at this field strength, so the contrast between the vessels and background is stronger. In addition MT has a very high SAR at 3.0 T, which tends to force a longer TR to keep within the $4\,W\,kg^{-1}$ limit, so most users do not add MT to TOF sequences.

bipolar imaging gradient will give a zero phase shift for stationary spins, but a nonzero phase shift for moving spins. In a phase-contrast pulse sequence additional bipolar gradients are used to create a known linear relationship between blood velocity and the phase of the MR signal. This relationship between velocity and phase angle is adjusted by setting the *velocity encoding* value or 'venc'. The venc is the maximum velocity that will be properly encoded by the sequence.

The scanner computer takes the user-supplied venc and calculates the appropriate gradient amplitudes and durations to yield a phase shift of 180° for that velocity. However, if velocities occur that are higher than the venc then the phase will become 'wrapped' and will appear to flow in the opposite direction! For example, if we set a venc of $100\,cm\,s^{-1}$ then a velocity of $125\,cm\,s^{-1}$ yields a phase shift of 225°. This is indistinguishable from a phase shift of $-135°$, produced by a velocity of 75 $cm\,s^{-1}$ in the opposite direction (figure 13.11). Because phase angles keep repeating themselves every 360°, it's even possible to get velocities aliasing two or three times across a velocity profile. Although this phenomenon of aliasing causes problems in quantifying flow speed and direction, it is less of a problem in routine phase-contrast angiography because of the way images are processed for display. As long as the scanner saves both magnitude and phase data, some aliasing can be unwrapped by post processing. Further details on the use of phase-contrast techniques to quantify blood velocity can be found in section 14.5.

Phase-contrast MRI is most commonly used with gradient-echo acquisitions. This creates a problem because minor variations in static magnetic field homogeneity produce nonuniform phase shifts even for stationary spins. To overcome this problem, two acquisitions are performed with the bipolar velocity-encoding gradients reversed in polarity for the second acquisition. The phase images for each acquisition are then calculated and subtracted. Since the background phase variation due to the inhomogeneous magnetic field is constant, after subtraction the background is zero with positive and negative values (phase shifts) only where the spins are moving. Finally to suppress background pixels, e.g. air, where the phase is essentially random, the phase subtraction image is multiplied, pixel-by-pixel, with the conventional magnitude image.

Phase-contrast MRA is also directionally sensitive, which means only blood moving in the same direction

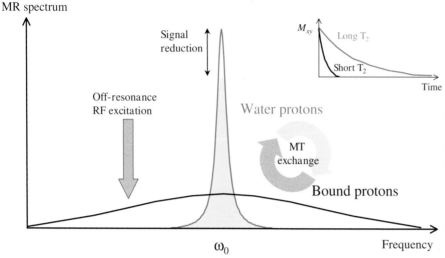

MR spectrum

Signal reduction

Off-resonance RF excitation

Water protons

MT exchange

Bound protons

M_{xy}

Long T_2

Short T_2

Time

ω_0

Frequency

Figure 13.8 The principles of magnetization transfer (MT) for background suppression in 3D TOF MRA. An off-resonance (1–2 kHz) RF pulse saturates bound protons that have a very short T_2. The signal from water protons, which have much longer T_2s, is then reduced as they exchange with the saturated bound protons. Tissues such as brain parenchyma have a strong MT effect, which results in a decrease in the background tissue signal and improved vessel visibility.

Reducing spin saturation 1: ramped RF pulses

A further major disadvantage of 3D TOF techniques is known as progressive saturation (see figure 13.9). Repeatedly exciting a thick slab of tissue means that the signal from flowing spins gradually saturates as the spins penetrate more distally into the volume, i.e. spins progressively experience more RF pulses the longer they remain within the volume. Although the signal loss can be reduced through the use of small imaging flip angles (e.g., 25°), this is at the expense of an overall reduction in vascular contrast. There are two sequence improvements that help to reduce this effect. The first is the use of ramped RF excitation pulses (TONE, **T**ilted **O**ptimized **N**onsaturating **E**xcitation), which are specially designed pulses that increase the flip angle across the 3D acquisition volume. Instead of exciting a flattopped rectangular slab profile, the profile is a trapezoid with a linear variation of flip angle with position through the slab. The ramp direction is set so that the higher flip angles further into the scan are downstream of the blood flow to help compensate for the saturation, whilst the lower flip angles are at the start of the scan to ensure that the spins are not saturated too early.

Reducing spin saturation 2: MOTSA

The second improvement is the use of a 2D/3D hybrid technique, often termed MOTSA (**M**ultiple **O**verlapping **T**hin **S**lab **A**cquisition). This method aims to reduce the saturation effect by reducing the thickness of the 3D slabs, but maintains the volume coverage by using multiple slabs. Continuity is maintained by slightly overlapping the slabs, and discarding the overlapping slices when doing the final MIP. This can sometimes cause an artefact commonly known as the 'venetian blind' effect, especially when ramped RF is used within each thin slab (figure 13.10). The background tends to get brighter at the top of the slab due to increased flip angles, producing a distinct boundary with the lower signal background at the bottom of the next slab. The combination of MT, ramped RF (TONE) and MOTSA allows us to acquire high-resolution TOF angiograms of the intra- and extra-cerebral circulation.

(a)

(b)

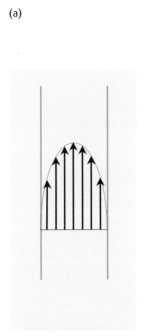

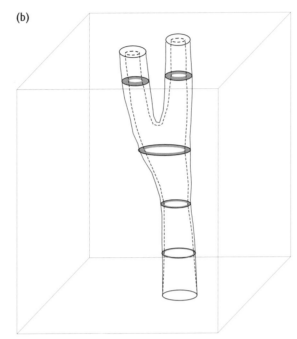

Figure 13.9 Progressive saturation of laminar flow in a 3D volume. (a) Typical parabolic flow profile with slow flow at the vessel wall. (b) When acquiring a 3D TOF study of the carotid arteries, repeatedly exciting a thick slab of tissue means that the signal from flowing spins gradually saturates as the spins penetrate deeper into the volume. This effect is more noticeable in the slower moving streamlines near the vessel wall.

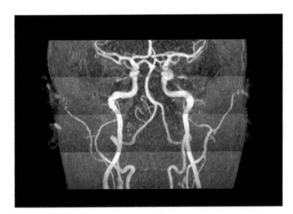

Figure 13.10 Multiple Overlapping Thin Slab Acquisition (MOTSA) to reduce progressive saturation in 3D TOF. Note the venetian blind artefact at the slab boundaries.

as a bipolar flow-encoding gradient will result in a phase shift. Therefore, it is necessary to match the flow-encoding axes to the direction of blood flow. When blood vessels follow a fairly tortuous path throughout the body and we have to flow-sensitize along all three gradient directions. This means that each pair of alternate polarity velocity-sensitizing gradients must be applied along each gradient axis in turn, i.e. slice select, phase encoding and frequency encoding (figure 13.12(a)). Although this means that in principle six acquisitions are required, it is usual to reduce this to four, e.g. one in each direction and one with no velocity sensitizing, although in practice there are more efficient schemes, known as Hadamard encoding, that can improve the signal-to-noise ratio (SNR). Even so, this means that a phase-contrast MRA study with velocity sensitization in all three directions will take at least four times as long as an equivalent TOF study. Even if velocity sensitization is only required in a single direction, e.g. for through-plane flow quantification, we still need two acquisitions.

In order to produce a single angiogram from 3D phase contrast data, the individual phase images for each flow direction are combined (figure 13.12(b)). This involves calculating for each pixel the resultant flow magnitude $|v|$ from the three vector directions x, y and z using the expression

$$|v| = \sqrt{v_x^2 + v_y^2 + v_z^2}$$

The resultant magnitude image has no directional information and is best termed a 'speed' image (figure 13.12(c)). Also since each velocity value is squared in the calculation all the positive and negative velocity information is eliminated and thus any aliasing that might have occurred disappears from the speed image. The result is an image with a background value of zero (black) and positive values only for pixels with flow. Since this processing avoids the problems of flow aliasing, the venc can be set to the average velocity within a vessel, which for laminar flow is about half the peak velocity. This has the effect of increasing the signal from spins near the vessel wall which are travelling more slowly, giving a more realistic visualization of the true diameter of the vessels. Finally, since only moving spins give signals on phase-contrast MRA images, they do not have the same problems with short-T_1 blood-breakdown products as TOF MRA images.

13.4.1 2D phase contrast

Like 2D TOF, 2D phase contrast (2D PC) is a single-slice method, usually used to provide a projection angiogram through a thick slice, i.e. visualization of all vessels within the slab – very similar to an X-ray angiogram. Signal cancellation can occur in regions where vessels with flow in opposite directions overlap along the projection direction. The use of thick slices, however, requires two slight modifications to the technique. First, because blood vessels will only occupy a small proportion of the slice volume, an additional dephasing gradient is applied in the slice-select direction. This has the effect of reducing the large signal from stationary tissue. Second, instead of phase subtraction, a 'complex' subtraction is performed. This doesn't mean the maths becomes complicated! It means that instead of just subtracting the phase angles from each other, vector subtraction is used, as shown in figure 13.13. Complex subtraction produces a better quality image in this situation, compared with phase subtraction. Figure 13.14 shows a set of axial 2D PC thick-slice projection MR angiograms obtained at different velocity encoding (venc) values. Note the improved visualization of the arterial circulation as the venc is increased.

Velocity encoding

Nuclei precess at the Larmor frequency

$$\omega = \gamma B_0$$

Phase (ϕ) is the time integral of frequency (ω), i.e.

$$\phi = \int \omega \, dt$$

In a magnetic field gradient G_x, this phase shift becomes

$$\phi = \gamma \int (B_0 + G_x x) \, dt$$

For spins moving at a constant velocity v in the x direction, the phase shift is

$$\phi = \gamma \int (B_0 + G_x(x + vt)) \, dt$$

If we consider a single gradient pulse of amplitude G and duration T then the phase shift due to velocity will be

$$\phi = \gamma \int_0^T Gvt \cdot dt = \left[\frac{1}{2}\gamma v G t^2\right]_0^T = \frac{1}{2}\gamma v G T^2$$

The product GT^2 is usually called the 'first moment' of the gradient, M_1, and we can write

$$\phi = \frac{1}{2}\gamma v M_1$$

If a second gradient of the same duration (T) but opposite amplitude ($-G$) immediately follows the first then we have a bipolar gradient pulse with a total phase shift of

$$\phi = -\gamma v M_1$$

If we repeat the acquisition with the polarity of the bipolar pulse reversed and subtract the phases, then we have the phase difference $\Delta\phi$, which can be expressed as the difference in the two moments ΔM_1 of the two bipolar pulses.

$$\Delta\phi = \gamma v \cdot \Delta M_1$$

The velocity encoding or 'venc' parameter is defined as the velocity that produces a phase shift of π radians or 180°

$$\pi = \gamma \cdot \text{venc} \cdot \Delta M_1$$

therefore,

$$\therefore \text{venc} = \frac{\pi}{\gamma \Delta M_1}$$

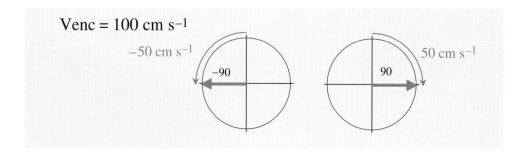

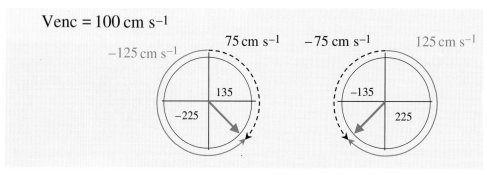

Figure 13.11 Velocity aliasing in phase-contrast acquisitions using a venc of 100 cm s^{-1}. In (a) a velocity of either + or −50 cm s^{-1} will result in a phase shift of + or −90°. In (b) the velocity increases to 125 cm s^{-1} resulting in a phase shift of 225°. However, this is indistinguishable from a phase shift of −135°, produced by a velocity of 75 cm s^{-1} in the opposite direction. A similar effect occurs for a velocity of −125 cm s^{-1}. Since phase shifts from 0 to 180° are assigned to velocities in one direction and 180°−360° to velocities in the other direction the signal will appear aliased in the opposite direction.

Because 2D PC is a single-slice technique, angiograms can be produced quite quickly. Alternatively the sequence can be combined with cardiac triggering to obtain multiphase cardiac images, producing dynamic angiograms. Depending on the choice of venc, images of either slow or fast flow may be acquired. The speed of acquisition also means that they can be used as 'venc localizers' to choose the best venc for a more timeconsuming 3D PC study.

13.4.2 3D phase contrast

3D phase contrast (PC) MRA is a thin-slice volumetric technique with each slice having velocity sensitization in the required directions, usually all three. This means that 3D PC studies are quite time-consuming and usually we have to sacrifice some resolution in the phase-encoding direction for a reduction in scan times. The speed images from each 3D slice are processed by the MIP algorithm as usual in order to produce an angiogram. Figure 13.15 shows a 3D phase-contrast MRA of the intraand extracerebral circulation, obtained with a venc of 60 cm s^{-1}.

In spite of the longer acquisition times, 3D PC produces better quality images than thick-slab projection 2D PC methods since much thinner slices are possible. The use of a low venc means that good 3D images of slow flow can be obtained, which are not possible with 3D TOF techniques due to slow flow saturation. One of the disadvantages of 3D PC is the requirement for all the flow-encoding gradients, which increases the TE resulting in poorer image quality in areas of complex flow or susceptibility. Furthermore, since PC methods are by definition not flow-compensated, there is increased artefact seen around vessels with pulsatile flow.

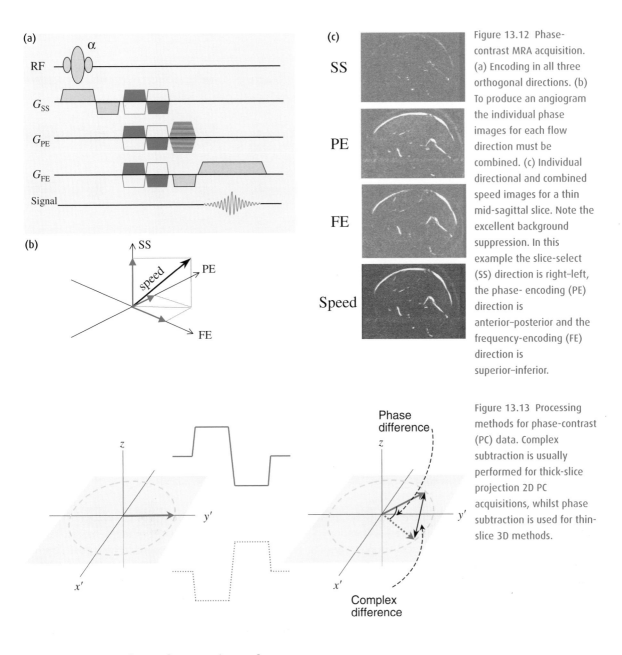

Figure 13.12 Phase-contrast MRA acquisition. (a) Encoding in all three orthogonal directions. (b) To produce an angiogram the individual phase images for each flow direction must be combined. (c) Individual directional and combined speed images for a thin mid-sagittal slice. Note the excellent background suppression. In this example the slice-select (SS) direction is right–left, the phase- encoding (PE) direction is anterior–posterior and the frequency-encoding (FE) direction is superior–inferior.

Figure 13.13 Processing methods for phase-contrast (PC) data. Complex subtraction is usually performed for thick-slice projection 2D PC acquisitions, whilst phase subtraction is used for thin-slice 3D methods.

13.5 Contrast-enhanced MR angiography

Gadolinium-based contrast agents have been used with both TOF and PC MRA in order to improve the SNR and conspicuity of small vessels. The term 'contrast-enhanced MRA' however refers to MR angiograms produced using bolus administration of a contrast agent. This can be considered to be a variant of 3D TOF techniques since we are exploiting differences in the longitudinal magnetization to yield vascular contrast. However, unlike TOF methods, these differences arise

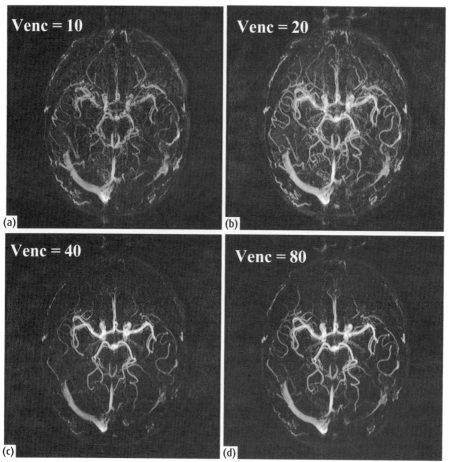

Venc = 10 (a)

Venc = 20 (b)

Venc = 40 (c)

Venc = 80 (d)

Figure 13.14 Axial 2D PC thick-slice projection MRA images through the head, obtained using complex subtraction. These images were obtained with velocity-encoding (venc) values of (a) 10 cm s^{-1}, (b) 20 cm s^{-1}, (c) 40 cm s^{-1} and (d) 80 cm s^{-1}. Note the improved visualization of the arterial circulation as the venc is increased.

because of the shortening of the blood's T$_1$ relaxation time by the contrast agent, rather than the in-flow phenomenon. This means that vascular contrast is relatively independent of flow dynamics and problems associated with saturation effects are considerably reduced. Contrast-enhanced (CE) MRA can therefore be used to acquire large field-of-view 3D angiograms in the plane of the vessels, e.g. coronal or sagittal planes without the problems of spin saturation. A fast 3D gradient-echo sequence, with short TE and TR, is used to capture the first-pass transit of the contrast agent bolus through the area of interest. The TE is usually minimized by not using flow-compensation methods and by employing fractional echo data collection.

Timing is critical in CE MRA studies; the scan acquisition has to be timed to coincide with peak contrast agent concentration in the area of interest. In order to maximize arterial contrast it is important to ensure that the centre of k-space, which primarily contributes to the contrast in an image, is acquired when the arterial contrast agent concentration is at its peak in the area of interest. Since there is a delay between peak arterial and venous enhancement, it is possible, with appropriate sequences and phase-encode ordering, to capture only the arterial phase. Figure 13.17 shows the relationship between circulation time, arterial contrast agent concentration and data acquisition for a centrically phase- encoded (k_{PE}) 3D acquisition. Acquiring data too

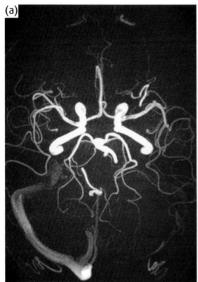

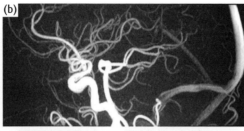

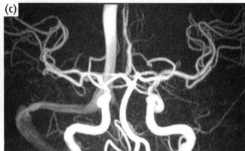

Figure 13.15 A 3D phase-contrast MRA of the intra- and extra-cerebral circulation, obtained with a venc of 60 cm s⁻¹: (a) axial, (b) sagittal and (c) coronal maximum intensity projections. Note the lower intensity of the venous circulation.

Reducing the T_1 of blood

The reduction in T_1 achievable with a paramagnetic contrast agent is given by

$$\frac{1}{T_{1,post}} = \frac{1}{T_{1,pre}} + R_1 \cdot [C_A]$$

where $T_{1,pre}$ is the T_1 of blood prior to administration of the agent (typically 1200 ms), $T_{1,post}$ is the T_1 of blood following administration, R_1 is the longitudinal relaxivity of the contrast agent and $[CA]$ is the concentration of the agent in the blood. Standard Gd-DTPA (see section 8.8.1) has a concentration of 0.5 mol l⁻¹ and an R_1 of approximately 4.5 s⁻¹ mM⁻¹ at 1.5 T.

For first-pass studies the dynamic contrast agent concentration $[CA]$ is given by

$$[C_A] = \frac{\text{injection rate (ml s}^{-1})}{\text{cardiac output (l s}^{-1})}$$

A fast injection rate increases $[CA]$ which in turn increases SNR. A reduced cardiac output also increases $[CA]$ and SNR. So older patients with low cardiac output and slow flow have high SNR on contrast-enhanced MRA. This is the opposite situation to TOF, where older patients with slow flow have low SNR on TOF. Figure 13.16 shows the reduction in the T_1 of blood for standard Gd-DTPA and a cardiac output of 5 l min⁻¹ as a function of injection rate (in ml s⁻¹). Since fat is usually the brightest tissue in T_1-weighted imaging the T_1 of fat at 1.5 T (270 ms) is also shown.

early with respect to the injection can result in poor arterial enhancement and edge artefacts, whilst acquiring data too late not only gives poor arterial enhancement but also unwanted venous enhancement.

Since fat is usually the next brightest structure in CE MRA studies, most techniques also employ fat-suppression methods to reduce the background fat signal. Fat suppression increases TR, so the suppression pulses are usually only played out intermittently during the sequence, i.e. once for every slice-encoding (k_{SS}) loop. The slice loop is therefore performed centrically to maximize the effect of the fat-suppression pulse (figure 13.18).

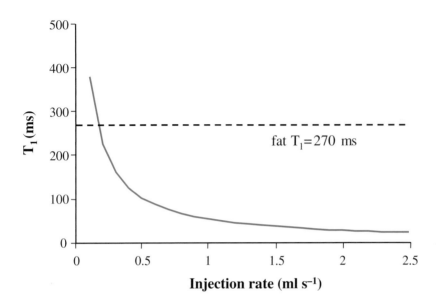

Figure 13.16 Reduction in T_1 as a function of Gd-DTPA injection rate for a cardiac output of 5 l min^{-1} and a Gd-DTPA concentration of 0.5 mol l^{-1}. The figure also shows the T_1 of fat, which will generally be the tissue with the shortest T_1.

Good timing!

Whilst the circulation time can be 'guess-timated' for each patient, the best and most consistent results are obtained by optimizing the timing, either retrospectively or prospectively. The retrospective method involves the injection of a small test bolus, typically 2 ml, of contrast. Rapid repeat (multiphase dynamic) imaging of a slice through the vessel at the level of interest is performed during the injection. Analysis of the multiphase images shows a peak in the signal intensity when the contrast reaches the area of interest (figure 13.19). Thus the circulation time of the contrast through the patient can be calculated.

There are currently two prospective triggering methods. The first uses a rapid one-dimensional (1D) monitoring sequence that detects the increase in signal intensity as the contrast agent arrives in the area of interest (or lower in the arterial path) and starts the 3D MRA sequence automatically. The second method uses rapid 'fluoroscopic' imaging at the level of interest so that the operator can see the contrast arrive and then manually start the MRA sequence. In both cases the system needs to provide a rapid switch over between the monitoring sequence and the MRA sequence. An alternative approach is to acquire multiphase 3D angiograms, i.e. provided the individual 3D acquisitions are very short, they can be rapidly repeated to ensure that the peak arterial concentration occurs at least at one of the acquisitions. Future improvements in gradient technology will probably make this the most convenient method for CE MRA.

Further suppression of background signals is obtained by acquiring a pre-contrast mask that can be subtracted from the arterial phase data. Subtraction is most effective when performed as a complex or vector subtraction on the Fourier data or on both phase and magnitude data so that the final image can incorporate the gadolinium effect on both magnitude and phase data.

The use of very rapid imaging also permits the acquisition of breath-hold MRA studies, especially important for thoracic and abdominal vasculature (figure 13.20). Various imaging strategies have been used to reduce scan time without significantly compromising image quality. The most common methods for reducing scan time in 3D CE MRA are to use the shortest possible TR, to use half Fourier acquisitions and to decrease the resolution, particularly in the phase-encoding and slice-selection directions. The reduction in acquisition resolution can be partly offset through the use of

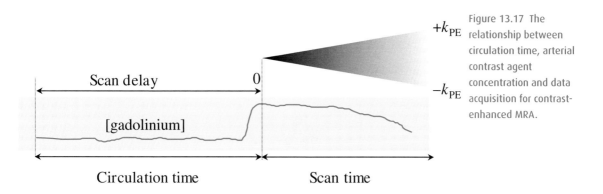

Figure 13.17 The relationship between circulation time, arterial contrast agent concentration and data acquisition for contrast-enhanced MRA.

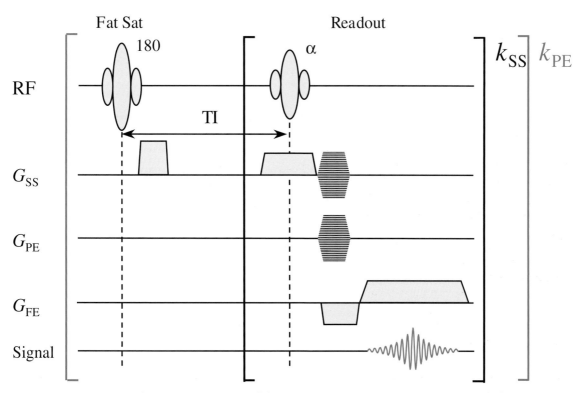

Figure 13.18 A 3D contrast-enhanced MRA sequence with fat suppression. Note that the entire slice encoding (k_{SS}) loop is performed for every one of the in-plane phase-encoding steps (k_{PE}). For fat suppression the k_{SS} loop is centrically ordered, i.e. 0, +1, −1, +2, −2, ..., to maximize the effect of the suppression pulse. The k_{PE} loop is typically also centrically ordered. This diagram shows a SPIR or SPECIAL fat-suppression scheme, with a frequency-selective 180° pulse to invert fat protons with slice-select crushers to spoil any transverse magnetization, followed by a TI such that fat is at the null point when the α° pulse is applied.

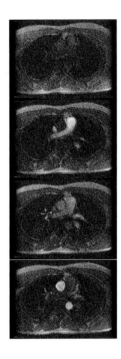

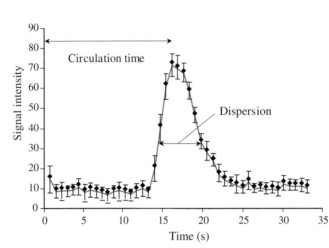

Figure 13.19 Signal intensity within the aorta measured with a rapid multiphase gradient echo sequence approximately every second following a 2-ml bolus of Gd-DTPA at 2 ml s^{-1}. Note the peak at 17 s (i.e. the circulation time) and the dispersion of the 1-s bolus (i.e. the spreading out of the bolus caused by its passage through the right side of the heart, the lungs and the left side of the heart).

Elliptic centric phase encoding

A major factor in the optimization of contrast-enhanced MRA of the arterial circulation is to minimize the signal within the venous circulation. In the abdomen and peripheral circulation this is relatively easy given the difference in circulation time between the arteries and veins. However, in the head and neck the rapid transit of the contrast agent from arteries to veins, typically 6 or 7 s, means that it is very difficult to obtain purely arterial angiograms without some degree of venous enhancement. In order to overcome this problem many techniques use elliptic centric k-space encoding.

We know that the centre of k-space is the most important for controlling the contrast within an image. In a conventional encoded 3D sequence the entire slice-encoding (k_{SS}) loop is acquired before the k_{PE} phase-encoding step is changed. So even if the phase encoding is centrically ordered (i.e. starting at zero and increasing to the maximum, alternating between positive and negative) we would be acquiring an entire k_{SS} line before the next k_{PE} line.

The elliptic centric ordering acquires the k_{SS} and k_{PE} lines in a spiral fashion starting from the centre and moving outwards depending upon the actual spacing in k-space for each k_{PE} and k_{SS} step. In this way all the central k-space lines are acquired together. The k-space trajectories for a conventional and an elliptic centric acquisition are shown in figure 13.21. This ordering means that the centre of k-space is acquired almost a factor of ten times faster. This concentration of the centre of k-space into a very short time helps reduce artefact from the rapidly changing arterial gadolinium concentration during bolus injection The result is high-resolution images of the cranial circulation without venous contamination (figure 13.22).

A further improvement in elliptic centric ordering is to recess the absolute centre of k-space in a few seconds from the beginning of the scan. This prevents excessive ringing artifact in the event that the 3D MRA is initiated prematurely while the arterial gadolinium concentration is still rising. It also enables the scan to take advantage of some of the arterial enhancement occuring before the peak in order to more effectively suppress veins.

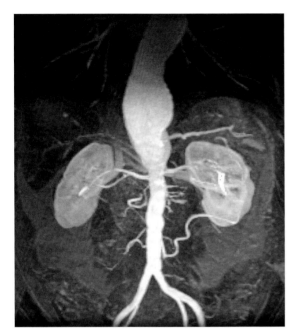

Figure 13.20 Breath-hold, contrast-enhanced MRA study of the abdominal aorta with an aneurysm, displayed as a coronal projection.

zero-filling interpolation methods. Alternatively advanced reconstruction techniques such as SENSE and SMASH (see chapter 17) can also be used to reduce acquisition times.

13.5.1 MRA tricks

In comparison to X-ray angiography CE-MRA is generally a static imaging technique and gives very little information on flow dynamics. A 3D volume could be repeated multiple times but the temporal resolution would be quite poor unless the time for an individual volume is reduced. There are a number of methods by which 4D (three spatial and one time dimension) CE-MRA acquisitions can be performed. As discussed in Chapter 17 parallel imaging techniques such as SENSE or SMASH can be employed to reduce the acquisition time for an individual volume. Alternatively methods that leverage the relationship between the bulk of the image contrast and the acquisition of the centre of k-space can be used to acquire volumes at a greater

temporal resolution. **T**ime **R**esolved **I**maging of **C**ontrast **K**inetic**S** (TRICKS) is a method that segments k-space into a central volume and multiple concentric peripheral volumes. During the TRICKS acquisition the volumes nearer the centre of k-space are repeatedly acquired more rapidly than the outer volumes. Sharing of data then allows multiple volumes to be reconstructed with a high temporal resolution. More advanced versions of this approach utilize spiral or radial data acquisition for oversampling the center of k-space with sliding window reconstruction to obtain temporal resolution which in theory can be as short as the TR.

MRA data acquisition can also be accelerated by repeatedly acquiring 2D images. This allows sub-second data acquisition which has been used for MR fluoroscopy (e.g. BolusTrak) and even for imaging coronary arteries. In order to maximize sensitivity to the contrast agent, pre-contrast mask data is subtracted in the Fourier domain which takes advantage of both phase and magnitude effects of the contrast agent.

13.5.2 Peripheral MRA

Contrast-enhanced MRA is ideally suited to large field of view (FOV) coverage since data can be acquired in the coronal or sagittal planes without spin saturation. However, some regions of the body, e.g. the peripheral vasculature, are much larger than the maximum FOV of most MRI scanners. To overcome this FOV limitation we can use so-called moving table or bolus chase techniques, where the patient is automatically moved through the scanner by a fixed distance and a further MRA acquisition performed. The process is then repeated until the total desired coverage is obtained. The entire peripheral vasculature can be covered in typically three or four slightly overlapping 'stations' (figure 13.23).

CNR is maximized by first performing a mask run without contrast to use for background subtraction. SNR is high on moving table peripheral MRA because a single, large contrast bolus (typically triple dose) is imaged multiple times as it travels down the torso and legs. However, timing can be complicated because it is important for the rate at which the table is moving to roughly match the rate at which contrast flows down the legs. In practice, it is virtually impossible for MRA

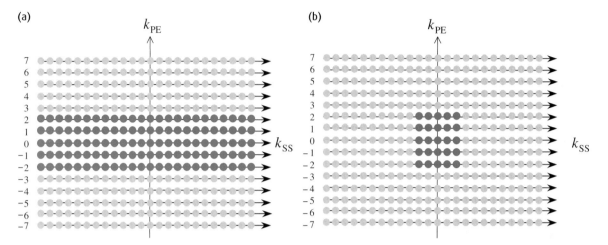

Figure 13.21 Comparison of conventional (a) and elliptical centric (b) 3D k_{SS}-k_{PE} acquisitions for contrast-enhanced MRA. In conventional centrically ordered acquisitions the k_{SS} data and the k_{PE} lines are acquired centrically, i.e. 0, +1, −1, +2, −2, ... However, the data for the whole of each k_{SS} line are acquired for each k_{PE} line. Since only data acquired at the centre of k_{SS}-k_{PE} space contribute to image contrast, these edge data reduce the time-contrast efficiency of the sequence. In (a) the blue points represent the central five k_{PE} lines; note that all k_{SS} data are acquired for these five k_{PE} lines. The elliptical centric ordering, however, acquires each k_{SS}-k_{PE} data point depending upon its distance from the centre. This means that the central part of the k_{SS}-k_{PE} data space is acquired much more rapidly, improving the time-contrast efficiency of the sequence. In (b) the blue points represent the data collection for five k_{PE} lines. Note that now only the central k_{SS} data are also acquired and time is not wasted collecting the edge k_{SS} data points as in (a) which do not contribute to image contrast.

data acquisition and table movement to keep up with the contrast agent flow. The time for table movement between stations should be quite short, typically less than 3 s. In addition, it is useful to place blood pressure cuffs around each upper thigh to compress veins and slow down the flow (figure 13.23a). The blood pressure cuffs are typically inflated to 60 mmHg just before the pre-contrast mask run in order to compress the venous outflow without compressing the arteries. The veins become dilated with blood that has no contrast. If the gadolinium bolus gets ahead of the table motion, gadolinium reaching the veins will dilute and blend into the background. This technique can also be used for imaging the arms.

13.5.3 Direct Contrast MR Venography

Gadolinium taken straight from the bottle is so concentrated that its T_2 shortening effect dominates and it is invisible on MR. When a gadolinium bolus reaches the heart, it is diluted into the cardiac output and become visible. However, if gadolinium is pre-diluted, before injecting into the vein, it is possible to image the vein. This technique is known as direct MR venography. Gadolinium is typically diluted 10 to 20-fold. A simple procedure is to draw 4ml of gadolinium into a 60 ml syringe and fill the rest with normal saline; a second syringe is prepared in the same way. Multiple 3D CE-MRA data sets are acquired before, during and after injecting the two syringes of contrast as fast as possible into an arm vein in order to visualize upper arm and subclavian veins. Both arms can be injected simultaneously to visualize both subclavian veins and the SVC. The large volume of dilute gadolinium and fast injection rate is important to obtain good venous distension and to fill collaterals when there is venous obstruction (see figure 13.24)

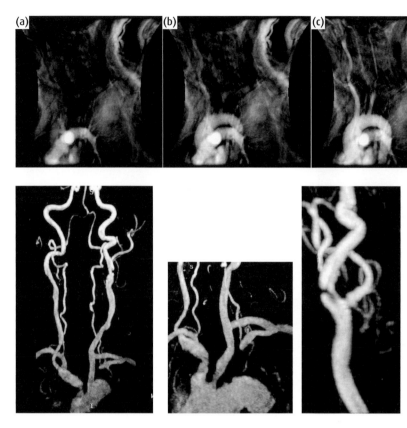

Figure 13.22 A contrast-enhanced MRA study of the carotid and vertebral arteries acquired using elliptic centric encoding. (a) Three frames from the low-resolution fluoroscopy scan showing the bolus passage through the great vessels. (b) MIPs of 3D high-resolution MRA in the coronal plane (and a zoomed view of the carotid origins) and in the sagittal plane. Note the absence of any venous enhancement.

13.6 Novel contrast agents

Current methods of CE MRA rely on reducing the T_1 of blood below that of surrounding tissues during the firstpass of the contrast agent. Rapid volumetric (3D) MR imaging during this period results in 3D images of the vasculature. The primary difficulty with small molecular weight gadolinium chelates, e.g. Gd-DTPA, is that they are quickly cleared from the vascular spaces. Very rapid imaging sequences are required to capture the first-pass of the agent through the arterial circulation. While this approach has been extremely successful, there has also been considerable interest in the development of paramagnetic contrast agents specifically for MRA.

The three main requirements for an MRA contrast agent are: (a) it is safe at relatively high concentrations, (b) it reduces the T_1 of blood to below that of any surrounding tissues and (c) it can be injected as a bolus for first-pass imaging. In addition an MRA-specific agent should also remain exclusively in the blood-pool for a reasonable period of time before excretion. This prolonged vascular residency or steady state can be used to acquire images with a higher signal-to-noise ratio and improved spatial resolution. These features are particularly relevant for imaging structures that require physiological gating, e.g. coronary arteries. Multiple regions could also be investigated following a single administration of agent. A long duration of vascular enhancement has been hypothesized to be useful for MR guided vascular interventions which may take an hour or more to perform. Yet another application of blood pool contrast agents is for detecting internal bleeding. If a blood pool contrast agent is detected in the small bowel an hour after injection, that indicates there is GI bleeding into the small bowel. Similarly, detection of blood pool contrast outside of an aortic stent graft indicates that the stent graft is leaking.

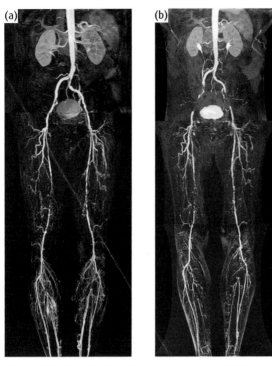

Figure 13.23 A multiple-station contrast-enhanced MRA study of the peripheral vasculature using a moving table technique: (a) with blood-pressure cuffs around the thighs and (b) without BP cuffs.

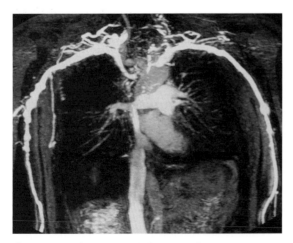

Figure 13.24 Direct contrast MR venography

13.6.1 Increased concentration

The effective gadolinium concentration in the blood may be increased by injecting the contrast at a faster rate and/or by using a higher concentration of the agent. Standard gadolinium chelate agents have a concentration of 0.5 M but a 1.0 M agent was introduced in 1998 (Gadovist™, Schering). This contrast agent was designed for the practical advantages of a smaller injection volume for high-dose applications, e.g. MR perfusion imaging, and it has also been employed in CE-MRA studies and is now licensed for this application in many European countries. The faster injection rate achieved with this higher concentration is particularly useful for time-resolved MRA where the bolus needs to stay compact.

13.6.2 Increased relaxivity

The alternative approach to reducing the T_1 of blood is to increase the effective R_1 of the agent. In simple terms R_1 is primarily affected by the rate at which the paramagnetic compound tumbles in relation to the hydrogen nuclei of water molecules. Standard gadolinium chelates are quite small molecules with molecular weights of only 300–500 Da and have an R_1 around 4 – 5 mmol^{-1} s^{-1}. Therefore, the major thrust for blood-pool agents has been in the development of large molecular weight paramagnetic agents.

One way to increase molecular weight is to bind the gadolinium chelate to a large macromolecule in vivo. Gadobenate dimeglumine (MultiHance™, Bracco) is an example of an agent that weakly and reversibly binds to human serum albumin (HSA), increasing the R_1 value to around 11 mM^{-1} s^{-1}. The agent was originally developed for liver imaging because its protein binding leads to increased hepatobiliary excretion. It is now also being evaluated for MRA applications. MS 325 C (EPIX Medical) is another agent that binds more strongly (80–96%) to HSA. Giving an R_1 between 30 and 50 mM^{-1} s^{-1} in the bound state. This agent is now commercially available as VasoVist™ (Schering).

R_1 may also be increased by rigidly attaching the gadolinium ion to a large molecular weight synthetic polymer. An example is Gadomer-17 (Schering), a

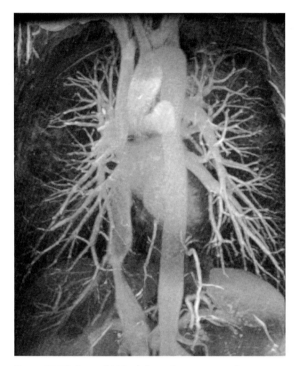

Figure 13.25 Coronal MIP of the pulmonary vasculature obtained 10 min after administration of Clariscan™ (Nycomed Amersham) at a dose of 5 mg Fe kg^{-1}. Both arteries and veins are shown in this steady-state image.

5–200 nm, can also be used as blood-pool agents. These agents were developed as T_2 contrast agents for liver imaging and have a large value of R_2 (the T_2 relaxivity analogous to R_1). Interestingly the ratio R_2/R_1 for a SPIO particle decreases with decreasing particle size, making the ultra-small (USPIO) particles much better T_1 agents. Even so, these agents are primarily T_2 agents and the degree of T_1 shortening achievable may be limited in practice. One example of an USPIO developed originally for MRA is Clariscan™ (GE Healthcare Bioscience), which contains starch-coated single USPIO crystals with a diameter of 5–7 nm, an R_1 of 20 mM^{-1} s^{-1} and an R_2 of 35 mM^{-1} s^{-1}. A similar USPIO agent from Schering (SH U 555 C) has recently completed phase I clinical trials.

While it is possible to obtain a degree of arterial selectivity using a blood-pool agent by imaging during the first-pass, a disadvantage when imaging in the steady state is that all vessels enhance (see figure 13.25). This offsets the benefits of longer imaging times for higher spatial resolution and considerable work is therefore in progress to develop techniques to effectively segment images and separate arteries from veins.

See also:

- Flow artefacts: chapter 6
- Contrast agents: section 8.8

FURTHER READING

Graves MJ (1997) Magnetic resonance angiography. *Br J Radiol* **70**: 6–28.

Prince MR, Grist TM and Debatin JF (1998) *3D Contrast MR Angiography*, 2nd edn. Berlin: Springer Verlag (ISBN: 3540625771).

socalled cascade polymer that has an effective molecular weight of 35 000 Da and an R_1 of 19 Mm^{-1} s^{-1}. Guerbet are also developing a macrocyclic gadolinium agent (G792-12) for MRA, but so far none of these agents is licensed for clinical use.

13.6.3 SPIO particles

Super-paramagnetic iron oxide (SPIO) agents, comprising iron oxide particles with typical diameters of

A heart to heart discussion: cardiac MRI

14.1 Introduction

Since the first MR images of the heart in the late 1970s there has been much commercial and academic development of cardiovascular MRI techniques, but clinical usage has been relatively limited compared with neurological and musculoskeletal MRI. However, in recent years improvements in MR system hardware, most notably vector ECG gating and high-performance gradients, has led to robust and reliable imaging techniques capable of providing high-quality morphological and functional imaging of the heart. MRI now offers the potential to provide, in a single investigation, more accurate and repeatable data than could be obtained using a combination of other tests, with the added advantage of providing some unique methods for the qualitative and quantitative evaluation of cardiac function.

In this chapter we will:
- review the main artefacts from heart, blood and respiratory motion on standard images and the methods available to avoid them;
- show that cardiac-gated spin echo is used for morphological information;
- show that retrospective or prospective gating of gradient-echo techniques can be used to create cine images which show cardiac function, such as wall contraction and valve motion;
- see the use of velocity mapping using phase-contrast MRA can be used to measure ejection fractions and stroke volumes;
- describe new techniques for myocardial perfusion imaging;

- discuss the difficulties in producing high-quality images of the coronary arteries, one of the biggest challenges in cardiac MRI.

14.2 Artefact challenges

The major challenge in cardiac MRI is the motion of the heart, pulsatile blood flow and respiratory motion. Artefacts arise because of changes in signal intensity or phase as a function of time and commonly result in ghosts (see chapter 6 for an introduction to these problems). Blood flow within the cardiovascular system can produce differing signals depending upon the pulse sequences employed, the scan timings and options and the characteristics of the flow. Depending upon the required image contrast, i.e. dark or bright blood, various schemes are available to improve image quality.

14.2.1 ECG gating

Artefacts due to cardiac motion are most effectively controlled by synchronizing imaging to the patient's electrocardiogram (ECG), so that each phase-encoding step is performed at exactly the same point in the cardiac cycle. Successful gating requires a good-quality ECG waveform for the MRI system to detect the QRS complex and trigger the scanning sequence. The standard three-lead ECG (or four with a reference electrode) is based on the three electrode locations forming the points of an equilateral triangle (Einthoven's triangle). The components of the mean QRS vector are detected in each of the three standard limb leads, I, II or III. For

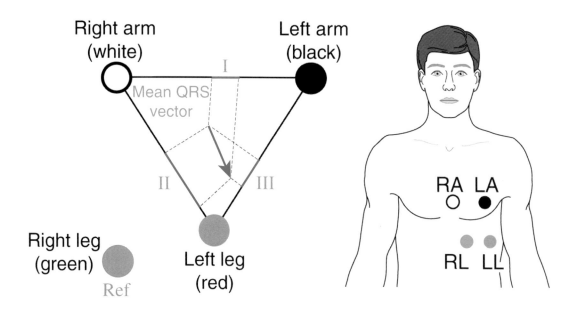

Figure 14.1 Einthoven's triangle and suggested ECG electrode positioning on the patient's chest to reduce the differential voltage being induced in the ECG leads from gradient and RF pulses. LA denotes left arm; LL, left leg; RA, right arm; RL, right leg.

diagnostic ECG monitoring, the electrodes are usually physically spaced as far apart as possible to maximize the ECG signal; however, this is not recommended during MRI since the magnetic field gradients across the body will induce differential voltages in the leads.

Therefore, electrodes are usually placed relatively close together to minimize the gradient-induced voltages (figure 14.1).

A further difficulty in obtaining good-quality signals from within the magnet is the additional voltage that is induced as a result of a conducting fluid (blood) moving within a magnetic field (the magneto-hydrodynamic effect, see section 10.4.1). Since major blood flow in the aorta occurs at the time of ventricular ejection this additional voltage is superimposed on the T-wave of the ECG (figure 14.2), which may exceed the gating amplitude resulting in a false trigger. Proper electrode positioning and skin preparation to maximize the amplitude of the observed R-wave is important to reduce this possibility. The historical problems of gradient and RF interference induced in the ECG leads is reduced through sophisticated filtering of the ECG

waveform; however, this filtering effectively renders the ECG nondiagnostic and it should not be relied upon to monitor the patient's condition.

More recently ECG gating has been made significantly more reliable through the use of vector cardiac gating (VCG). Instead of using the electrode positioning in Figure 14.1 the four electrodes are placed in a cross arrangement so that there is a left-right signal component (x) and an superior-inferior signal component (y). Simultaneously acquiring both the x and y components allows the direction of the QRS vector to be tracked as it moves with the cardiac cycle. It has been shown that the electrical vector of the heart tracks a different path to that of the magneto-hydrodynamic artefact. Appropriate signal processing of both the spatial and temporal changes of these 2D vectors therefore significantly improves the gating reliability compared to using just the 1D or scalar value from a single lead, e.g. I, II or III in the conventional ECG arrangement. The standard lead positioning for VCG also minimises patient set-up times, although skin preparation is still important.

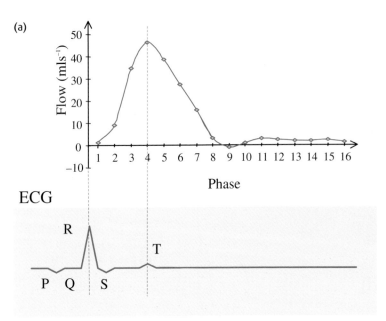

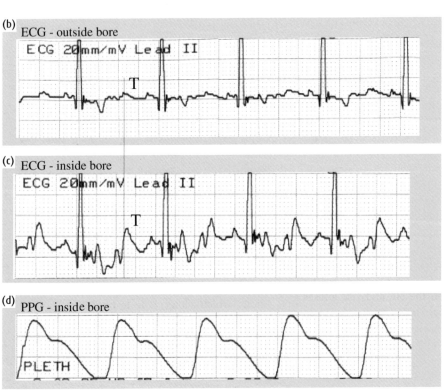

Figure 14.2 (a) The relationship between aortic blood flow and the electrocardiogram (ECG). (b) ECG trace with the patient outside the bore of a 1.5 T magnet. (c) ECG trace with the patient in the centre of the bore. Note the increased amplitude of the T-wave when the patient is placed inside the magnet. (d) Peripheral-pulse-gated (PPG) waveform from inside the bore shown for comparison. Note the delay between the R-wave of the ECG and the peak of the PPG waveform.

14.2.2 Peripheral gating

Peripheral pulse gating (PPG) using a photoplethysmo-graph, often just called the 'pleth' or 'pulse ox', positioned on a finger or toe may be used for triggering, although it should be remembered that there is a significant delay (150–500 ms) between the R-wave of the ECG and the peak of the peripheral pulse (figure 14.2(d)). The shape of the pulse may also be modified by the time it is detected in the finger or toe. ECG gating will in general produce better cardiac images; however, where there is difficulty in obtaining a suitable ECG waveform then PPG will often produce acceptable images. This is because the PPG signal simply reflects the change in blood volume through the vessels in the finger or toe and is therefore insensitive to magnetic field effects. Note that images acquired immediately after the PPG trigger will fall in diastole and that systole may be lost in the arrhythmia rejection (AR) period at the end of the PPG cycle.

14.2.3 Respiratory motion

The problems of respiratory motion are most effectively addressed through the use of fast breath-held or respiratory-triggered acquisitions. Alternatively several cardiovascular imaging sequences, e.g. gated spin echo, employ respiratory compensation schemes to reduce respiratory artefacts. However, this method does require that the patient breathes regularly throughout the acquisition.

14.3 Morphological imaging

Conventional spin-echo imaging produces good dark-blood contrast for relatively fast flowing blood since spins will washout between the 90° and 180° pulses (TE/2) resulting in a signal void (see section 13.2). Lengthening TE will therefore improve the dark-blood appearance at the expense of poorer SNR. However, for slow flowing blood, signal enhancement (sometimes called paradoxical enhancement) may occur, as unsaturated spins move into the imaging slice between TRs and are too slow to wash-out during TE. Spatial satura-

Navigating the pulse sequence

Navigators involve some unusual methods for pulse sequence programming. The first question is how do you excite a column? There are two possibilities: you can use a spin echo sequence with orthogonal slice selective gradients on each RF pulse. The column can be freely positioned and angled, and the excitation creates a well-defined square column. This technique has the disadvantage of creating black bands where the navigator selection intersects with the main image – possibly right through the anatomy of interest.

The alternative is a spiral excitation, shown in figure 14.3. The alternating gradients during the RF pulse excite a circular column, often known as a pencil beam. Since it's a gradient echo, it can be used with a shorter TR and less SAR than the spin echo technique. And since it avoids the cross-banding artefacts, it is easier to set up extra pencil beams to correct for motion in 2 or more directions.

In order to work properly, navigator echoes need to be interleaved with the imaging sequence to minimise the chance of motion between the navigator and the data acquisition. For cardiac imaging the image slices are usually double-obliques, so the navigators are excited by a separate RF pulse. However navigators are also useful for other motion correction e.g. head motion during fMRI or for multi-shot EPI scans. In these cases a linear navigator is insufficient and 2D acquisition is necessary, which can be either a spiral or a second EPI readout. Each navigator shares the slice excitation of the main image acquisition, and the navigator itself can be placed either before or after the main acquisition. In multi-shot EPI, the navigator is used to reject data if too much motion has occurred. In general navigators can be extended to 3D acquisitions, which allows them to be used to track the motion and adjust the main image acquisition accordingly. This is most useful for coronary artery imaging or interventional techniques. Navigators are also been used to monitor bolus arrival in contrast-enhanced angiography, and for B_0-shift correction.

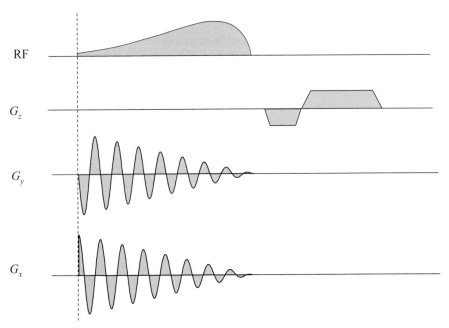

Figure 14.3 Spiral excitation for navigator echoes

RF

G_z

G_y

G_x

tion bands can be used outside the slice range to satu-rate blood before it moves into the imaging region but their effectiveness decreases the further away they are from the actual imaging slice. Since blood flow is pul-satile it is also possible to select the time period over which imaging is performed to coincide with maximum systolic blood velocity, and therefore maximum washout effect.

It is usual to acquire cardiac scans in double-oblique orientations which show the various anatomies of interest. Learning to plan these reliably takes some practice, see figure 14.4 for some basic views. Starting from a standard axial scout, you can plan 2-chamber views on both the left and right side of the heart (showing the atrium and ventricle of each side sepa-rately). From the left 2-chamber view, plan a 4-chamber (almost axial) view. Finally from the 4-chamber view with the left 2-chamber view as a second reference, you can plan a short axis multi-slice stack.

Since the sequence is synchronized to the patient's ECG, in conventional spin-echo imaging one line of raw data is acquired per heart beat, i.e. per repetition. Thus the effective TR is the R–R interval, e.g. 1000 ms if the heart rate is 60 bpm or 750 ms if it is 80 bpm. Interleaved

multi-slice imaging is possible, with the maximum number of slices determined partly by the patient's heart rate. Due to hardware limitations there is always a short delay between detecting the R-wave and actually starting the first slice excitation, often called the trigger delay. At the other end of the R–R interval, the scanner must stop acquiring data and start looking for the next R-wave. This period is sometimes called the arrhythmia rejection window or 'trigger window' and may be expressed as a percentage of the R–R interval. So the available imaging time may be considerably shorter than the R–R interval and may permit only a few slices. It should be remem-bered that in conventional ECG-triggered spin-echo imaging of the heart each image is acquired not only at a different spatial position but also at a different temporal position in the cardiac cycle (figure 14.5).

The scan time using ECG gating is several minutes, resulting in artefacts from respiratory motion, even when respiratory compensation is used. Respiratory artefacts are made worse by the use of dedicated tho-racic surface coils, e.g. torso and cardiac phased array, which accentuate chest wall fat near to the coil.

Fast spin echo (FSE) imaging techniques (see section 12.3.2), which can acquire multiple lines of raw data per

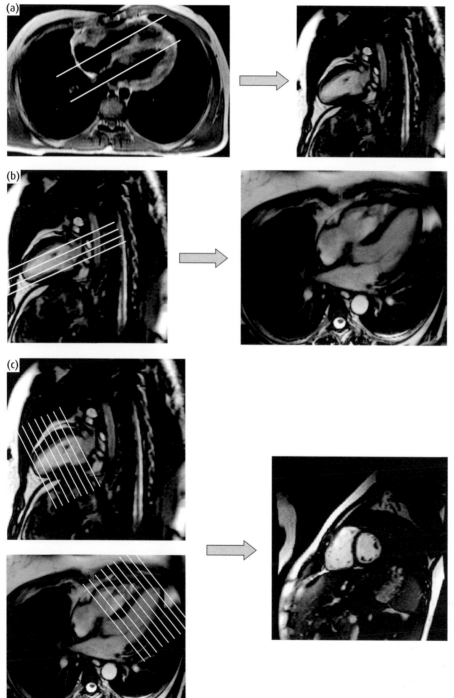

Figure 14.4 Basic cardiac planning. (a) From an axial scout, plan two oblique slices on each side of the heart, producing a 2-chamber view. (b) Plan another oblique scan on the 2-chamber view to create a 4-chamber view. (c) On the 4-chamber view you can plan a multi-slice short axis scan.

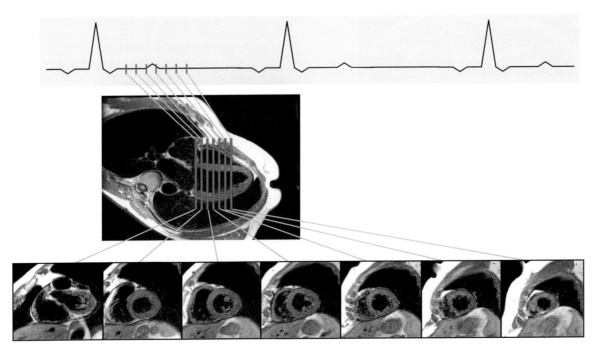

Figure 14.5 ECG-triggered spin-echo imaging of the heart. The figure shows seven short cardiac axis slices prescribed on a four-chamber long axis view. Note that each short cardiac axis image is acquired not only at a different spatial position but also at a different temporal position in the cardiac cycle.

repetition, have revolutionized conventional MRI. The FSE sequence, when combined with ECG gating, has the ability to acquire an entire cardiac image within a single breath-hold. For example, acquiring a matrix of 256×160 with an echo train length (ETL) of 32 requires 5 shots (160/32). With a TR of two R–R intervals, this would take ten heartbeats. The need to acquire a train of echoes during each heart beat limits data acquisition to diastole, when cardiac motion is at a minimum since the readout period will be typically about 200 ms in total. However, diastole is also the period when blood flow is slowest, resulting in a high signal from the blood pool. Employing a blood suppression preparation (BSP), or black-blood technique reduces this signal.

14.4 Functional imaging

Global and regional ventricular contractile function can be imaged using cine (dynamic) gradient-echo (GE)

sequences, synchronized to the patient's ECG. Since rapidly moving blood appears bright on GE images, there is generally excellent contrast between the blood pool and the myocardium. In addition, GE sequences have very short repetition times (TR) permitting data from the same slice location to be acquired at different time points, or phases, throughout the cardiac cycle (figure 14.6). (Rather confusingly, the word 'phase' in the context of cardiac imaging often has nothing to do with angles!)

Cine GE images may be acquired either prospectively or retrospectively. In prospective gating the pulse sequence is triggered by the R-wave of the ECG, and the end of the cardiac cycle, typically 10–15%, is not sampled to allow for variations in R–R interval (figure 14.9(a)). This is known as the arrhythmia rejection (AR) period. Depending on the heart rate, number of cardiac phases required and the TR, one or two slice locations may be acquired.

Looking into the void – black-blood imaging

The BSP (**B**lood **S**uppressed **P**reparation) or 'black-blood' method involves a double inversion preparation scheme applied at an inversion time (TI) prior to the FSE acquisition. A spatially nonselective 180° pulse inverts the entire imaging volume, and is immediately followed by a slice-selective 180° de-inversion (figure 14.7). The overall effect is to invert all spins outside of the imaging slice, whilst the spins within the slice experience both the inversion and the de-inversion, i.e. they are effectively unchanged. The TI period is calculated to be the time for the longitudinal magnetization of blood to reach zero from the initial inversion. Therefore, at the time of the FSE readout, blood that has flowed into the imaging slice will be nulled, resulting in a dark-blood pool (figure 14.8). The delay means that all the slices will be acquired during diastole. Note that blood that is not replaced during the TI period, i.e. very slowly flowing blood, or blood flow that is mainly in-plane, may not be completely suppressed. Note also that the TI time will require adjustment if the study is performed after administration of a contrast agent that shortens the T_1 of blood. The pulse sequence may be combined with a third slice-selective 180° pulse to give a **S**hort **TI** **I**nversion **R**ecovery (STIR) contrast mechanism. This permits fat-suppressed images to be obtained with the benefits of a blood-suppressed, breath-hold, FSE acquisition.

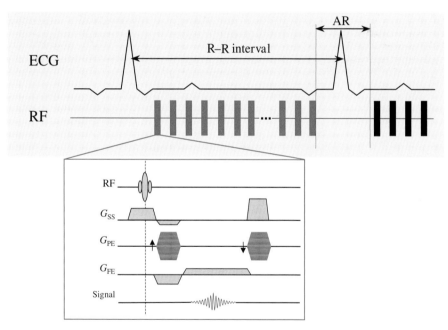

Figure 14.6 ECG-triggered gradient-echo (GE) imaging. Once triggered the GE sequence is repeated continually throughout the cardiac cycle acquiring one line of data for each phase. AR denotes arrhythmia rejection window.

Beware of the flasher!

Since data are not collected during the arrhythmia rejection period in prospective gating, there is T_1 recovery of the magnetization and therefore a very bright first image following the R-wave. This 'flashing' artefact can be reduced by performing a 'dummy' acquisition immediately following the R-wave, i.e. playing out the sequence but disabling data acquisition. This has the slight disadvantage of losing an image close to the R-wave.

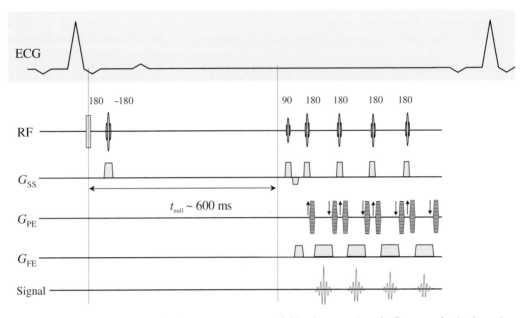

Figure 14.7 ECG-triggered fast spin echo (FSE) imaging sequence with blood suppression. The first nonselective inversion pulse inverts all spins within the coil. The second selective inversion pulse de-inverts the spins within the imaging slice. During the inversion time (TI) period, inverted blood flows into the imaging slice. The FSE readout is performed when the longitudinal magnetization from blood crosses zero, yielding no signal. The TI is optimized to null the signal from blood depending on the patient's R–R interval.

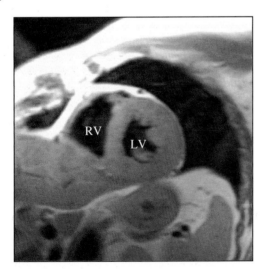

Figure 14.8 Image of a patient with a hypertrophied left ventricle acquired in the short cardiac axis using a breathheld, blood-suppressed FSE imaging sequence. LV denotes the left ventricle; RV, the right ventricle.

14.4.1 Retrospective gating

In retrospective gating, data are acquired continuously throughout the cardiac cycle, with the R-wave causing a real-time update of the phase-encoding gradient. With this method the cardiac waveform is recorded for the whole scan time (figure 14.9(b)) and the data sorted after acquisition (i.e. retrospectively) to account for variations in R–R interval. This requires more processing before Fourier transform (FT) reconstruction than prospective gating, as follows.

First the computer takes the recorded trigger signals and divides each cardiac cycle into the required number of phases, N, chosen by the operator. This is achieved by measuring the duration of each cardiac cycle then the time of each temporal phase is calculated as a percentage of that R–R interval. This provides a linear expansion or contraction of each cardiac cycle to account for variations in the length of individual heartbeats (figure 14.10). The nearest acquired phase-encoding step to each of the N temporal phases is placed in the raw data matrix for the

(a)

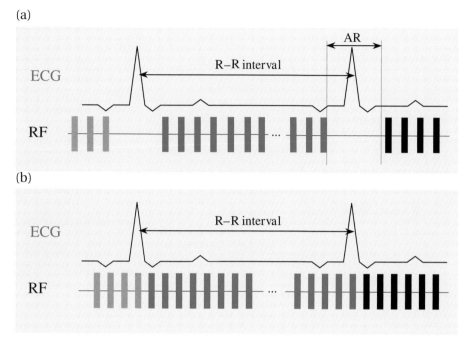

(b)

Figure 14.9 Comparison of prospective and retrospectively gated cine imaging. (a) In prospective triggering a user-defined arrhythmia rejection period (AR) is employed in which the sequence is not played out to allow variations in the subject's heart rate. (b) In retrospective gating the sequence is allowed to run independently of the heart rate, with the ECG merely serving to trigger and update the phase-encoding gradient for the next line of data. The position of the data within the cardiac cycle is determined after data collection, i.e. retrospectively.

image at that phase (figure 14.11). Once all the temporal phases have been filled with their nearest phase-encoding steps the reconstruction can proceed as normal. Note that each acquired phase-encoding step may be used for more than one of the N phases. Retrospective gating results in a cine study with N equally spaced temporal phases throughout the cardiac cycle with no arrhythmia rejection window dead-time (figure 14.12). If a heart beat falls outside the arrhythmia window then the data are simply thrown away and the acquisition is repeated, so sometimes the scanner keeps acquiring data beyond the end of the scan time! Movie loop display of these multi-cardiac-phase or cine images clearly shows the dynamic contraction and relaxation of the ventricles throughout the cardiac cycle without any flashing artefacts.

14.4.2 Flow compensation

Bright-blood sequences can suffer from signal loss due to intravoxel phase dispersion. It is possible to reduce this phenomenon using flow compensation. This technique incorporates additional gradient pulses in the sequence to eliminate the velocity-induced phase shifts, thereby improving blood signal uniformity. As discussed in chapter 13, flow compensation actually only compensates for spins that are moving with a constant velocity, flow with higher orders of motion, e.g. acceleration or turbulent flow, will not be compensated. A more effective method to reduce the signal loss from intravoxel phase dispersion is to reduce the TE. It should be noted that to visualize some pathologies, e.g. turbulent flow arising from valvular insufficiency, it is desirable to lengthen the TE to make the signal loss more obvious.

14.4.3 Fast prospective cardiac imaging

A major problem with cine cardiac imaging is that only one line of raw MRI data for each cardiac phase image can be obtained in each heart beat. This means that for typical image matrices the acquisition of a cine study takes 128–192 heart beats depending upon the total number of phase-encoding steps required. Whilst ECG gating successfully eliminates artefacts from cardiac motion, the patient's breathing during the acquisition

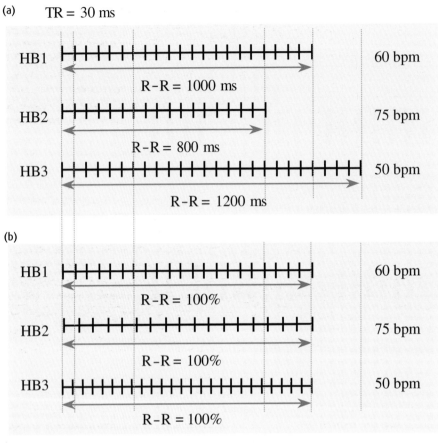

(a)   TR = 30 ms

HB1   R–R = 1000 ms   60 bpm

HB2   R–R = 800 ms   75 bpm

HB3   R–R = 1200 ms   50 bpm

(b)

HB1   R–R = 100%   60 bpm

HB2   R–R = 100%   75 bpm

HB3   R–R = 100%   50 bpm

Figure 14.10 Retrospective processing. (a) Three heart beats (HB1–HB3) are shown of differing lengths. Data are acquired using a gradient-echo (GE) sequence with a TR of 30 ms shown as the vertical tick marks. (b) In retrospective processing each heart beat is made the same nominal length, by either stretching the cardiac cycle as for HB2 or contracting the heartbeat as for HB3. Note how the position of the nominal 30-ms TR has been changed.

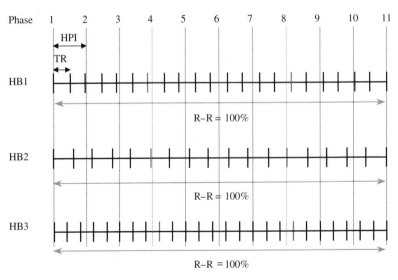

Phase 1 2 3 4 5 6 7 8 9 10 11

HPI

TR

HB1   R–R = 100%   60 bpm

HB2   R–R = 100%   75 bpm

HB3   R–R = 100%   50 bpm

Figure 14.11 Nearest neighbour interpolation. In retrospective processing the user defines the number of equally spaced phases throughout the cardiac cycle. The nearest acquired data line to each of the desired phases is then used for that phase. For example, for phases 4 and 8 the nearest acquired data lines are shown in blue.

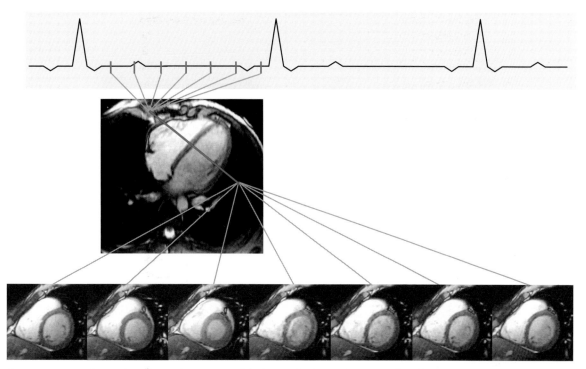

Figure 14.12 ECG-triggered gradient-echo imaging of the heart. The figure shows a single short cardiac axis slice prescribed on a four-chamber long axis view. Note that the short cardiac axis image is acquired at the same spatial position but at different temporal positions (phases) throughout the cardiac cycle.

results in image blurring and ghosting. Techniques to reduce respiratory artefacts by modifying the order in which the raw data lines are acquired have only limited success. It was not until the development of 'segmented' data acquisition that image quality has been significantly improved by allowing data to be acquired within a single breath-hold.

In this technique the raw MRI data lines for each cardiac phase are divided up into a number of groups or segments. GE sequences with very short TRs are then used to acquire all of the raw data lines for each segment in the same heart beat. If, for example, the total number of data lines for each cardiac phase was 128, and this was divided up into 32 segments, then the sequence would acquire four lines of raw data (i.e. four phase-encode gradients) for each cardiac phase in a single heart beat (figure 14.13). This is typically referred to as using four views-per-segment. The total acquisition would then only require 32 heart beats, which

could be accomplished by most subjects in a single breath-hold. Figure 14.14(a) shows a single phase from a conventional cine MRI study requiring 128 heart beats and acquired during normal respiration, and figure 14.14(b) shows a segmented cine acquisition requiring 16 heartbeats (i.e. eight views-per-segment) acquired during a breath hold. Note the improved image quality with the segmented acquisition technique.

The first implementations of segmented data acquisition were prospectively gated, resulting in a 'flashing' artefact in the first image. To avoid this phenomenon, without the use of dummy excitations that would miss the important end-diastolic time point, the technique of uniform TR excitation was developed. In this method the gradient and RF pulses for the segments are played out during the arrhythmia rejection period, to maintain the spin system in steady state. This permits the first phase to be acquired immediately after the R-wave and thus capture end-diastole.

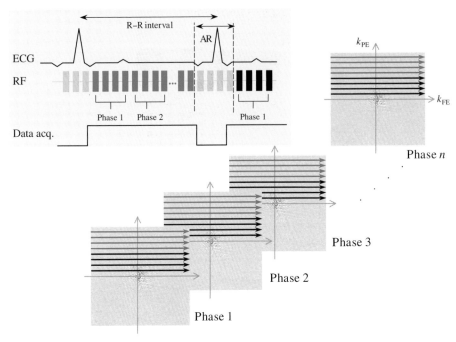

Figure 14.13 Segmented k-space data acquisition. In this example four lines of raw data for each temporal phase are acquired in a single heart beat. This reduces the overall acquisition time by a factor of 4.

View sharing

A further limitation of fast prospective cardiac imaging is the relatively poor temporal resolution compared to conventional cine studies. If an acquisition was made using eight views-per-segment and the TR was 10 ms then this would still result in a temporal resolution of 80 ms, potentially producing only ten cine images during a 1000 ms R–R interval with a 200 ms arrhythmia rejection window. This problem is addressed by 'view sharing' (also known as 'echo sharing'), a technique in which the lines of raw data from adjacent temporal phases are combined to synthesize an intermediate temporal phase image. For example, using four views-per-segment the last two views of phase n could be combined with the first two views of phase $n + 1$ to produce a segment with four views positioned at a time point $1/2(t_n + t_{n+1})$ (figure 14.15). Using this equal sharing, the total number of temporal phases could be increased from N to $2N - 1$. There is of course no reason why views could not be asymmetrically, or variably, shared; for example, the last two views from phase n with the first six views of phase $n + 1$ to generate a new segment positioned at $3/4(t_n + t_{n+1})$.

14.4.4 Fast retrospective cardiac imaging

The development of uniform TR excitation means that the first temporal phase is as close as possible to the R-wave, whilst the view sharing technique improves the temporal resolution so that short features such as end-systole can be depicted more clearly. However, the prospective nature of the sequence still means that there is a blind-spot during the arrhythmia rejection window and the movie display of breath-held data 'jumps' at the end of the movie loop. An alternative rapid dynamic technique is fast retrospective cine cardiac imaging. This sequence acquires data continuously throughout the cardiac cycle, using the R-wave to update the phase-encoding value, in the same way as conventional cine imaging. Following data collection, the images are retrospectively sorted into a user-defined

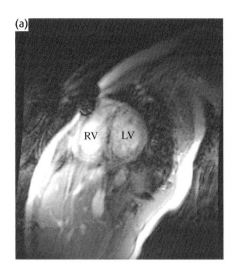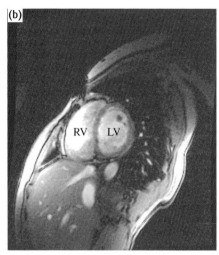

Figure 14.14 Single phase, in the short cardiac axis, from (a) a conventional cine MRI study acquired in 128 heart beats, showing artefacts from respiration, and (b) a segmented fast cine MRI study acquired in a 16-heart-beat breathhold clear of respiratory artefacts. LV denotes left ventricle; RV, right ventricle.

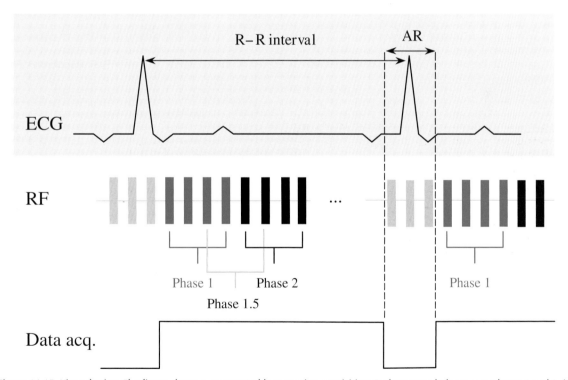

Figure 14.15 View sharing. The figure shows a segmented k-space cine acquisition. Each temporal phase, e.g. phases 1 and 2, is comprised of four views per heart beat. The effective temporal resolution is therefore $4 \times TR$. An intermediate phase, 1.5, is also shown. The phase is produced by sharing two views from phase 1 and two views from phase 2 resulting in an intermediate phase temporally positioned halfway between phases 1 and 2. Sharing views to synthesize phases at intermediate temporal points effectively doubles the temporal resolution.

number of phases taking into account the variation in R–R interval. In this case, the retrospective interpolation is achieved through the use of variable view sharing, as described above. The advantage of this technique over the original retrospective cine sequence is that more cardiac phases are possible with better temporal resolution.

Since systole is usually fixed and it is the diastolic period that either lengthens or shortens, linearly stretching or contracting data depending on the length of the heart beat is not physiologically realistic. This problem can be resolved by using an empirical model relating the duration of systole (t_s) to heart rate (HR). This model can then be used to define the diastolic period over which data are to be stretched or contracted.

14.4.5 Functional analysis

These high-quality breath-hold images can be used to provide both qualitative and quantitative evaluation of myocardial function with a number of advantages over conventional imaging techniques such as contrast ventriculography and echocardiography. Since MRI is a tomographic imaging technique it is possible to acquire multiphase cine images in any plane. Global and regional ventricular function can then be studied by acquiring a stack of multiphase images encompassing the ventricles, for example, in the short cardiac axis. The volume of the ventricular blood pools can be directly measured and summed across all slices at each phase. This allows us to determine the end-diastolic and end-systolic ventricular volumes and to calculate the ejection fraction without resorting to simplistic geometric models such as those used in echocardiography or ventriculography. A number of research groups are working on computer processing techniques to make the detection of the endocardial and epicardial borders semiautomatic (i.e. it needs minimal user interaction), in order to measure global ventricular function, e.g. stroke volume and ejection fraction, and regional function, e.g. systolic wall motion and thickening.

Breath-hold cine imaging can also be used to qualitatively demonstrate pathologies resulting in flow disturbances, e.g. valvular regurgitation or stenosis. Figure 14.16 shows the first 15 phases from a cine study in an oblique plane through the left ventricular outflow of a patient with mixed aortic valve disease. In the early systolic phase a small proximal region of signal loss can be seen. This signal loss is due to turbulence caused by a jet of blood being ejected through the narrowed orifice of the stenotic aortic valve. In the subsequent diastolic phases a region of much greater signal loss is observed distally due to regurgitation of blood back into the left ventricle through the incompetent aortic valve causing turbulence and hence signal loss.

14.4.6 Improving myocardial/blood contrast

Currently fully rewound gradient echo sequences, such as true FISP (see section 12.4.3), are popular for functional cardiac imaging. In this sequence all the gradients are balanced between TR periods and the image contrast is more dependent upon the ratio of T_2/T_1 rather than the inflow effect. This produces images with very good contrast between the blood-pool and the myocardium. Figure 14.17 shows a comparison of two four-chamber long axis views obtained using both a conventional segmented fast GE sequence and a segmented true FISP type sequence.

14.4.7 Myocardial tagging

Myocardial tagging sequences allow us to visualize directly the contractility of the ventricle walls. These methods use a cine GE sequence which is preceded by special selective excitation pulses to spatially modulate the magnetization within the imaging slice. This is sometimes known as SPAMM (**SPA**tial **M**odulation of **M**agnetization). The tagging can be applied in the form of either a 1D (lines) or a 2D (grid) structure. The tagging pattern is produced immediately following the R-wave trigger and then as the tissue moves and deforms throughout the cardiac cycle the tagging pattern will also move. Tagging techniques in combination with breath-hold segmented cine sequences have been shown to accurately measure displacements as small as 0.1 mm. For example, in a patient with hypertrophic cardiomyopathy (HCM), tagging using a grid pattern with 7 mm spacing (figure 14.18) shows that the thickened septum has significantly reduced contraction. Since the tag lines

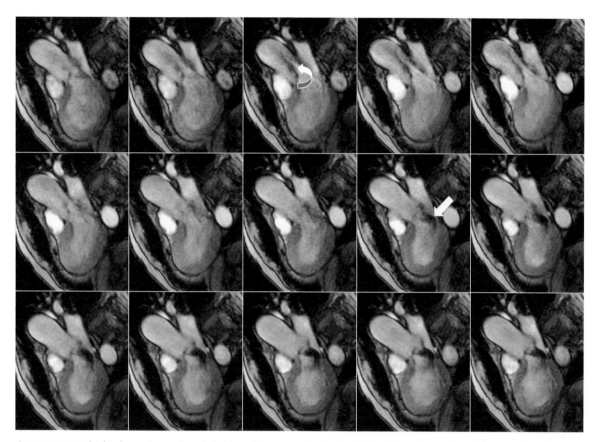

Figure 14.16 Multiple phases from a breath-held gradient-echo cine study obtained along the left ventricular outflow showing signal loss secondary to mild aortic valve stenosis (curved arrow) and more significant aortic regurgitation (straight arrow).

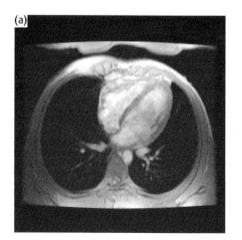

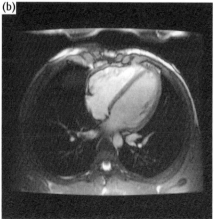

Figure 14.17 Comparison of two four-chamber long axis views obtained using (a) a conventional segmented k-space fast gradient-echo sequence and (b) a segmented k-space true FISP type sequence with improved blood-pool/myocardial contrast.

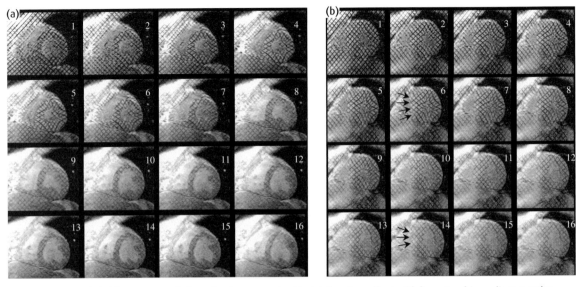

Figure 14.18 Breath-hold cine myocardial tagging in a normal subject (a) and a patient with hypertrophic cardiomyopathy (HCM) (b). Sixteen phases are shown covering the cardiac cycle. Note the relative lack of motion in the hypertrophied septum of the patient (straight arrows) compared with the same region in the normal. Also note how the tag lines fade through the cardiac cycle.

Taking the strain

Whilst the qualitative tagged images are useful, their real power lies in the potential for quantitative analysis of myocardial strain. By sampling the displacements over the entire heart it is possible to calculate the full 3D strain tensor over the myocardium. The quantification of the magnitude and direction of myocardial strain is, for example, a sensitive indicator of ventricular remodelling postinfarction.

are simple modulations of magnetization they will fade, due to T_1 recovery, throughout the cardiac cycle.

14.5 Cine phase-contrast velocity mapping

The principles of phase-contrast imaging for MR angiography are discussed in chapter 13; if you haven't read it yet, you should do so before continuing with this section. As a reminder, the phase shift along a particular axis is proportional to the velocity in that direction.

Simple subtraction of the phase images obtained with the positive and negative velocity encoding will therefore yield a phase image whose pixel value is directly proportional to velocity, and major background phase errors are removed.

Quantitative velocity mapping is usually performed using a cine imaging sequence with the slice angled perpendicular to the vessel of interest. The velocity encoding is then performed in the slice-select direction to quantify the velocity through the slice. The positive and negative velocity encoding is usually interleaved within the same heartbeat to minimize misregistration (figure 14.19). Velocity mapping can also be performed in the other in-plane directions as well by applying the flow-encoding gradients on the appropriate axis. If necessary flow can be encoded on all three axes simultaneously to give full seven-dimensional velocity quantification (three velocity components, three spatial components and one time component).

As in routine phase-contrast angiography the resultant of the three velocity-encoding directions can be generated to produce a speed image. Since the

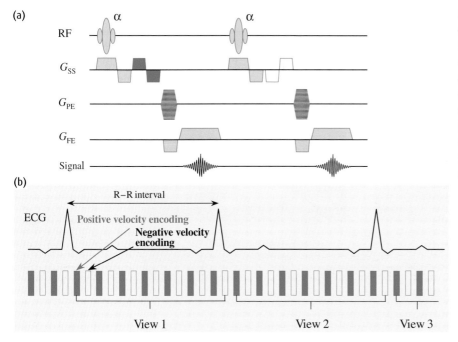

(a)

(b)

Phase imaging

MRI data are acquired in phase quadrature. Following Fourier transformation each voxel value is actually complex valued, i.e. it has a real ($\Re$) and an imaginary ($\Im$) component. Usually the magnitude (M) of the signal is reconstructed where

$$M = \sqrt{\Re^2 + \Im^2}$$

However, the phase (ϕ) of the signal can also be reconstructed from

$$\phi = \tan^{-1}\left(\frac{\Im}{\Re}\right)$$

In a phase-contrast study the measured phase shift ϕ is related to the velocity v through the relationship

$$v = \frac{\phi \cdot \text{venc}}{\pi}$$

venc is discussed in the box 'Velocity encoding', in section 13.4.

calculation of phase is effectively random in areas of very low signal, i.e. air, the images are made more aesthetically pleasing by multiplying the phase image with the conventional magnitude image. This produces a useful qualitative way of evaluating flow during the cardiac cycle, but obviously quantification requires the original phase images.

When phase images are displayed using the conventional greyscale, stationary tissue is depicted as midgrey, flow in one direction is depicted as shades of mid-grey to black and flow in the opposite direction is in shades of mid-grey to white (remember that phase-contrast data are also directionally sensitive). The actual directions depend upon how the flow-encoding gradients are played out. It should also be noted that even though the phase images from positive and negative flow encoding are subtracted to eliminate background phase errors, there may be residual errors due to the different eddy currents produced by the two different flow-encoding polarities. The data may need to have a background phase correction applied.

Figure 14.20 shows a cine phase-contrast velocity mapping study in the ascending aorta. The phase image

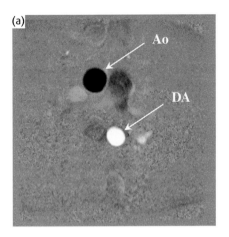

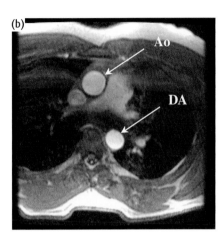

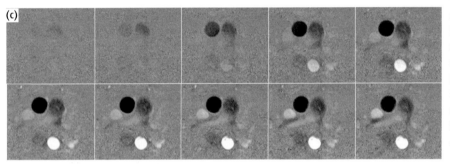

Figure 14.20 Cine phase-contrast velocity mapping through the chest. (a) The phase image shows stationary tissue as mid-grey whilst flow in the ascending aorta (Ao) is depicted as darker shades of grey and flow in the descending aorta (DA), moving in the opposite direction through this slice, is depicted as brighter shades of grey. Note that this image has been multiplied by the modulus image (b) to suppress random phase values in regions of low signal. Image (c) shows the first ten phases from a cine study showing the change in velocity through the cardiac cycle.

(figure 14.20(a)) has been multiplied by the magnitude image (figure 14.20(b)) to remove the background noise. Figure 14.20(c) shows the phase images from the first ten images from the cine study demonstrating the change in signal intensity with blood velocity in the ascending and descending aorta. Remember that the velocity-encoding parameter (venc) is the constant of proportionality linking the measured phase shift and the actual velocity. Therefore, measurement of the phase shift within a voxel can be directly converted to a velocity in m s^{-1}. Usually the boundary of the vessel is outlined and the mean phase shift within the region is measured. This value is then converted to a mean velocity. Multiplication of the mean velocity by the area of the region, in m^2, gives the instantaneous flow within the vessel in m^3 s^{-1}, or l s^{-1}. The flow versus time curves (figure 14.21) are obtained by calculating the instantaneous flow in the ascending and descending aorta in each of the cine images. The area underneath the ascending aorta curve represents the total blood ejected by the left ventricle during a cardiac cycle, i.e. the left ventricular stroke volume.

14.6 Myocardial perfusion imaging

MRI offers a number of advantages over the conventional method of radionuclide scintigraphy for the evaluation of myocardial perfusion, including improved spatial resolution and the absence of overlying tissue attenuation effects. Cardiac perfusion MRI involves imaging the heart during the bolus administration of a contrast agent, usually containing gadolinium, e.g. Gd-DTPA. The most common technique uses 'T$_1$-enhancement', in which the myocardial signal increases as the contrast agent perfuses the heart. Regions of ischaemia with poor perfusion will show a significantly delayed enhancement compared to the normal regions.

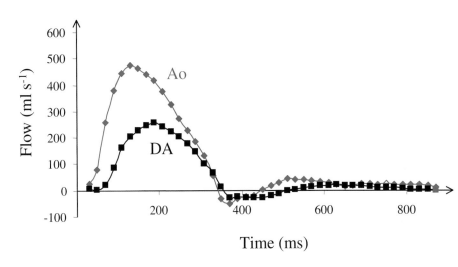

Figure 14.21 Flow versus time curves for the ascending (Ao) and descending aorta (DA) obtained from analysis of the cine phase-contrast velocity mapping study shown in figure 14.20. The area under the ascending aorta curve represents the left ventricular stroke volume of 99 ml.

Since the first pass of the contrast agent through the myocardium is very rapid, typically of the order of 10 s or less, the imaging requirements are extremely demanding. Ideally it would be preferable to achieve whole heart coverage with a temporal resolution of one heartbeat, however currently it is necessary to trade-off temporal resolution with poorer coverage, e.g. only 3–4 slices per heartbeat, or greater coverage, e.g. 6–8 slices every other heartbeat. As in other areas of MRI, the development of parallel imaging techniques will likely approach the idea of whole heart coverage with a temporal resolution of every heartbeat. Figure 14.22 shows four phases from a multi-slice imaging acquisition using an interleaved gradient-echo planar imaging sequence. This sequence first applies a spatial presaturation pulse, e.g. a nonselective 90° pulse to suppress the myocardial signal so that the inflow of the contrast agent can be seen more clearly. The saturation pulse also provides a degree of arrhythmia insensitivity to allow for any differential recovery if the heart rate varies. Note the first-pass enhancement as the contrast agent passes through firstly the right ventricle (from an antecubital intravenous injection), followed by the left ventricle and finally through the myocardium. This study shows a region of sub-endocardial ischaemia as an area of reduced contrast agent uptake. Care must be taken in viewing these perfusion images to try and ensure that apparent perfusion 'defects', particularly those in the subendocardium, are not actually due to susceptibility effects from the high concentration of agents in the left ventricle, or motion artefacts due to the myocardium moving during the readout period.

Getting stressed

Since the symptoms of impaired myocardial blood flow are usually only apparent when the patient is exercising it is also necessary to 'stress' the patient whilst the perfusion study is being performed. Physical stress (exercise!) is difficult to perform in the confines of an MRI magnet so the patient is usually stressed pharmacologically, by infusing an agent such as adenosine or dobutamine, which causes vasodilation, increases cardiac output and increases myocardial blood flow. Perfusion images are also acquired with the patient in the resting state to identify regions of fixed or reversible perfusion. Note, however, that since MR perfusion imaging is not dependent upon transport into the myocytes, as is the case with radionuclide perfusion imaging, infarcted myocardium may not have any residual resting perfusion defect. Interpretation of MR perfusion images is therefore not entirely straightforward and thus is generally performed in combination with viability imaging to identify infarcts.

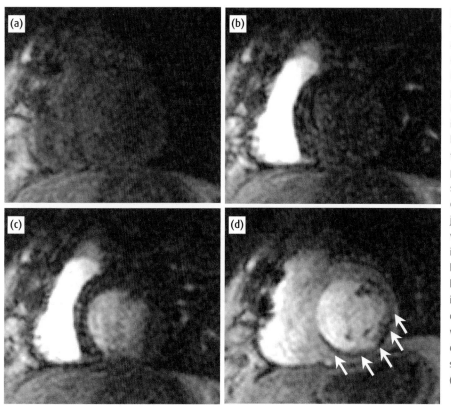

Figure 14.22 Four phases from a multi-slice imaging acquisition, in the short cardiac axis, using an interleaved gradient-echo planar imaging sequence. In the first image (a) the image signal intensity has been suppressed through the use of a saturation preparation pulse. In the second image (b) the contrast agent can be seen just entering the right ventricle. In the third image (c) contrast can just be observed entering the left ventricle. In the fourth image (d) enhancement can be seen in the left ventricular myocardium except in the region of subendocardial ischaemia (arrowed).

Qualitatively MRI myocardial perfusion imaging has shown good sensitivity and specificity compared with conventional radionuclide techniques, although admittedly in limited studies. There have been some investigations into semi-quantitative indices of perfusion that may offer improved sensitivity and specificity above simple qualitative reading of the data. A popular evaluation is to compare the maximum upslopes of the myocardial signal intensity curves at both stress and rest in order to calculate a myocardial perfusion reserve index (MPRI). However since the patients' haemodynamic status is very different between rest and stress, the data is normalised to the upslope of the left ventricular blood pool signal (the input function). More sophisticated analysis involves modelling the myocardial tissue response using a Fermi function and the input function as a gamma-variate.

A problem with all quantitative analyses of myocardial perfusion data is the necessity to ensure that all the temporal phases are properly co-registered. Providing the patient holds their breath for at least the first 20–30 seconds then upslope analysis is fairly straightforward, otherwise each phase needs to be co-registered. Analysis may be further confounded by ectopic beats that may occur in patients undergoing pharmacological stress. Absolute quantification of myocardial perfusion in ml g^{-1} min^{-1} of tissue is more difficult because of the non-linear relationship between signal intensity and the concentration of the contrast agent in the blood and the distribution of the contrast agent during the first pass. At low concentrations the relationship between signal intensity and contrast agent concentration can be considered linear, which is why many groups inject a lower dose, e.g. in the range of 0.05–0.075 mmol kg^{-1}, than would be used for qualitative imaging, e.g. 1.0 mmol kg^{-1} or even higher. In addition, all clinically approved contrast agents distribute in both the vascular and extracellular space, affecting the amount of signal enhancement.

Lack of knowledge about the relative volumes of these tissue spaces makes absolute quantification difficult. However, initial animal studies using purely intravascular contrast agents show very good correlation with the 'gold standard' of radiolabelled microspheres. Alternative approaches are being developed using magnetization-labelling techniques to act as endogenous contrast agents (see also section 16.4.2).

14.7 Myocardial viability

An important clinical question concerns the assessment of myocardial viability, which is technically defined as the presence of living myocytes (specialized cardiac muscle cells), regardless of whether these myocytes are able to contract. A region of the myocardium that contains living myocytes but has impaired function at rest, as a result of reduced myocardial blood flow, is known as hibernating. It is postulated that this reduction of cardiac function to cope with reduced myocardial blood flow is an act of myocardial self-preservation, in which the limited oxygen supply available is used just to maintain cell integrity. The identification of viable or hibernating myocardium is important since restoration of myocardial blood flow, by either coronary bypass surgery or coronary angioplasty, can result in the recovery of myocardial function.

A diagnostic imaging test therefore has to distinguish hibernating myocardium and scar tissue from infarcted myocardium. For tissue to be classified as viable it should demonstrate a reversible wall motion abnormality in the presence of chronic hypoperfusion. Hypoperfusion can be demonstrated using MR perfusion whilst wall motion abnormalities can be demonstrated using conventional resting cine imaging. However, in order to identify hibernating myocardium a dobutamine stress MRI study is required. In this examination multiple slice cine imaging sequences are acquired during increasing doses of dobutamine. Dobutamine increases myocardial contractility so that any myocardial segment that has a wall motion abnormality at rest which subsequently improves with low-dose dobutamine is regarded as viable. Further increases in the dobutamine dose result in the myocardium becoming ischaemic and ceasing to contract.

An alternative and extremely powerful approach is the direct imaging of nonviable myocardial regions using the technique of myocardial delayed-enhancement (MDE) imaging. Recent evidence has shown that delayed hyper-enhancement is exclusively related to irreversible injury, irrespective of contractile function or age of injury. In this technique a simple ECG-gated, inversion-recovery-prepared fast gradient-echo sequence is used to acquire images more than 10 min after contrast administration. If the inversion time is chosen to approximately null the myocardium then regions of hyperenhancement can readily be seen. If the cine studies shows a region of wall motion abnormality that is 'bright' and transmural on MDE imaging then the myocardium will not recover function following revascularisation Conversely, if the wall motion abnormality does not demonstrate hyper-enhancement on MDE then this most probably represents viable tissue that is likely to recover function after revascularisation. The technique is sometimes called 'infarct sizing' since the region of hyperenhancement correlates with the region of infarction. Figure 14.23 shows a myocardial delayed enhancement image with a

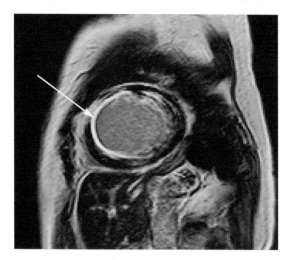

Figure 14.23 A myocardial delayed-enhancement image acquired in the short cardiac axis 10 min after administration of 0.2 mmol kg^{-1} Gd-DTPA. In this sequence the signal from normal myocardium is nulled through the use of an inversion recovery preparation pulse, whilst regions of myocardial infarction (arrowed) appear hyperenhanced.

region of hyperenhancement correlating with an infarct.

As well as chronic infarcts, MDE can be used to detect acute myocardial infarction. In this situation the hyperenhancement represents regions of necrotic myocytes due to compromised myocardial blood flow at the capillary level, despite having a patent coronary artery. This is termed 'microvascular obstruction' or 'no-reflow' and is an important prognostic indicator for future cardiac sequelae. MRI is the only noninvasive imaging technique that that can detect microvascular obstruction associated with an acute infarction. This technique also readily detects mural thrombus which can complicate acute infarction and cause embolic stroke.

14.8 Coronary artery imaging

The visualization of the coronary arteries using MRI presents numerous technical challenges. Coronary vessels have small calibres, follow tortuous paths within the epicardial fat, and move significant distances during the cardiac and respiratory cycles. (Just take a look at coronary X-ray angiography to see how difficult the problem is!) The simplest approach to coronary MRA is to use breath-hold (segmented k-space) gradient-echo imaging with a short acquisition window in diastole.

Multiple 2D slices with fat saturation are prescribed parallel to the coronary vessel. Whilst this method produces quite good results, complete coverage generally requires multiple breath-holds, and the slice thickness limits the spatial resolution achievable.

Better results can be obtained using ECG-gated 3D gradient-echo sequences; however, the extended imaging time generally makes breath-holding impractical and thus respiratory gating is required. This can be done using bellows placed around the thorax, but a more accurate method is to track the motion of the diaphragm directly using a navigator echo positioned at the dome of the right hemi-diaphragm (see section 6.3.1 and 'Navigating the pulse sequence'). The navigator signal may be used to gate the data either prospectively, i.e. before data acquisition, or retrospectively, i.e. after data acquisition but before image reconstruction. Although navigator techniques allow the patient to breath freely during the acquisition they are relatively time-inefficient since useful data are only acquired on average during 50% of the heart beats. Various novel acquisition strategies have also been investigated for coronary imaging, in particular spiral k-space acquisitions which provide an efficient way to sample k-space with good signal-tonoise ratio whilst minimizing artefacts from flow.

To achieve good contrast between the coronary blood-pool signal and the surrounding myocardial

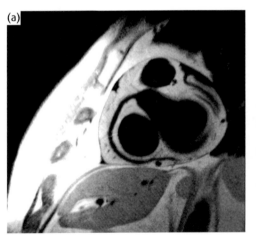 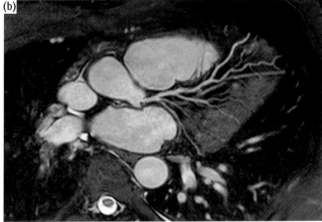

Figure 14.24 (a) Black-blood coronary MRA angled through right coronary artery. (b) Maximum intensity projection of the left coronary artery tree from navigator-gated 3D balanced-FFE.

tissue, a number of techniques have been developed. In gradient-echo sequences the coronary blood-pool signal arises due to the time-of-flight effect, and the background myocardium can be reduced using magnetization transfer or T_2 ('driven equilibrium') preparatory pulses. Steady-state techniques such as true FISP also improve image contrast and look promising for coronary artery imaging. Figure 14.24 shows the right and left coronary arteries obtained with a black-blood and a balanced-FFE sequence respectively.

Blood-suppressed FSE techniques, in which the coronary lumen is suppressed in contrast to the high signal of surrounding tissue, have also been explored. Contrast agents, based on both gadolinium and superparamagnetic iron oxide, have also been employed for coronary MRA. These have the advantage of allowing inversion preparation pulses to be used to effectively suppress the surrounding tissue. Conventional gadolinium chelates such as Gd-DTPA require rapid

imaging within a single breath-hold whereas blood-pool agents allow acquisitions over much longer time periods (see section 13.6).

See also:

• Flow appearances and MR angiography: chapter 13

FURTHER READING

Higgin CB, De Roos A and Sakuma H (1999) *Journal of Magnetic Resonance Imaging* Special Issue: Cardiovascular MRI' *J Magn Reson Imaging* **5**(5)

Lardo AC, Fayed ZA, Chronos NAF, Fuster V (2003). *Cardiovascular Magnetic Resonance: Established and Emerging Applications.* London: Martin Dunitz (ISBN: 1 84184 202 8)

Manning WJ and Pennel DJ (2002) *Cardiovascular Magnetic Resonance.* New York: Churchill Livingstone (ISBN: 0443075190)

Partian CL Ed. (2004) *Journal of Magnetic Resonance Imaging* Special Issue: Cardiac MR & CT. *J Magn Reson Imaging* **19**(6)

It's not just squiggles: in vivo spectroscopy

15.1 Introduction

By now you are familiar with the chemical shift between fat and water in the human body, which can cause artefacts. It occurs because protons in different environments experience shielding of the magnetic field by the electron clouds of neighbouring atoms. Chemists use magnetic resonance to investigate the structure of molecules by measuring very precisely the position of peaks in a spectrum (although they still call it 'nuclear magnetic resonance'). The area of each peak is a measure of the relative number of protons in that particular position. In the chemical soup of the human body, the number of water and fat protons is several thousand times higher than the number of protons on other molecules so we can't usually distinguish the metabolites. In vivo spectroscopy is a combination of imaging and spectroscopy, using gradients to selectively excite a small volume of tissue, then recording the free induction decay (FID) and producing a spectrum from that voxel rather than creating an image of it. For several years this technique was technically difficult and results were unimpressive, but recently it has become much more reliable and is now considered by many to be an essential part of a brain MR examination. Phosphorus spectroscopy is another well-developed application of in vivo spectroscopy, used mainly for looking at muscle metabolism.

In this chapter we will mainly describe proton brain spectroscopy, which is the most common clinical application at the moment. We will include the following:

- the main features of a proton spectrum for normal brain include metabolite peaks for N-acetyl aspartate,

An MRS dictionary

MR spectroscopy has its own language too, which will be unfamiliar to users who have only done MR imaging.

Peaks on the spectrum are also called *resonances*. Some metabolites do not have simple resonances, but may be split into two (called a *doublet*), three (*triplet*) or even more sub-peaks. Efficient *water suppression* is essential to allow the metabolite peaks to be detected.

Shimming refers to the process of adjusting field gradients to optimize the magnetic homogeneity over the voxel, and may be *automated* or *manual*. Voxel homogeneity is usually measured as the *linewidth* (the full-width at half-height) of the water resonance and may be quoted in Hz or ppm. Anything which reduces the homogeneity is described as causing *line broadening*, i.e. increasing the linewidth of the peaks.

The FID is detected in *quadrature* and produces a spectrum with both real and imaginary components. The pure real spectrum is known as the *absorption* spectrum; the imaginary part is called the *dispersion* spectrum and is not used in clinical MR spectroscopy. Processing of the FID usually includes *zero-filling* to improve the spectral resolution and *apodization* to improve the signal-to-noise ratio. *Phase correction* is necessary to remove *baseline roll* from the spectrum, and the residual water peak may be need to be removed.

creatine and choline. Typically *N*-acetyl aspartate is reduced and choline is increased in most of the conditions for which spectroscopy is currently used (tumours, dementia and stroke);

- either PRESS or STEAM sequences can be used for single-voxel spectroscopy, PRESS has the advantage of better SNR but STEAM has better localization;
- combining spectroscopy with phase-encoding gradients in 2 or 3 directions allows us to create chemical shift images, useful for complete metabolite information over the whole brain;
- spectroscopy can also be performed with other nuclei in-vivo, for example carbon fluorine and phosphorus, but these techniques remain in the research domain;
- lung imaging can be achieved by having subjects breathe hyperpolarized gases such as xenon or helium.

15.2 Some basic chemistry

A proton spectrum is shown in figure 15.1(a) from a specialist spectroscopy phantom. The peak from water has been suppressed so that the lower-concentration metabolites can be seen. The reference frequency (zero ppm) is that of the standard tetra-methyl silane Si-$(CH_3)_4$, which has a single proton resonance because it is a completely symmetrical molecule). All other metabolites have a unique pattern of peaks at specific chemical shifts, and the presence and concentration of these chemicals can be found by detecting peaks at the appropriate ppm. Notice that the zero frequency is on the right-hand side of the spectrum, and it is usual to 'read' a spectrum from right to left. Above 4 ppm the spectrum becomes unreliable, since the suppression of the water peak at 4.7 ppm tends to destroy the neighbouring portions of the spectrum too. (Note that the phantom temperature is considerably lower than human body temperature, which causes a shift in the spectrum of about -0.1 ppm, i.e. to the right.) The most important peaks are as follows:

- 1.3 ppm: lactate (Lac) is a doublet and a very specific marker of cell death and tissue necrosis. If both peaks of the doublet can be seen, it is a good indication that the resonance is indeed lactate and not lipid contamination. Lipids have very broad resonances at 0.9 and 1.4 ppm (not seen in the phantom spectrum).
- 2.0 ppm: N-acetyl aspartate (NAA) is regarded as a marker of neuronal integrity and will be reduced if neurons are being destroyed by a disease process.

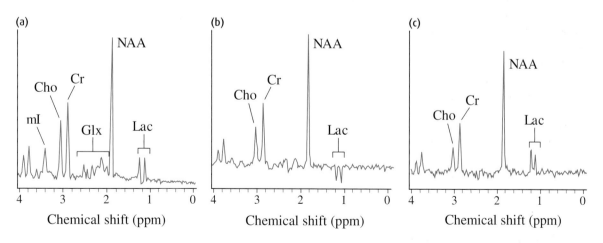

Figure 15.1 (a) A spectrum (TE = 30 ms) from an MR spectroscopy phantom containing the main brain metabolites in normal concentrations, plus lactate. Echo times of (b) 135 ms and (c) 270 ms produce spectra with different appearances. (All spectra are 0.1 ppm lower than in vivo spectra due to the temperature difference.) Cho denotes choline; Cr, creatine; Glx, glutamine and glutamate complex; Lac, lactate; mI, myo-inositol; NAA, N-acetyl aspartate.

• 2.1–2.5 ppm: glutamine and glutamate complex (Glx) is a mixture of peaks that may be elevated or decreased in conditions related to liver function.

• 3.0 ppm: creatine (Cr) is the total peak from phosphocreatine and creatine and is often taken as a reference level, as it is relatively constant throughout the brain and it tends not to change significantly in disease processes. However, there is evidence that it can change particularly in malignant tumours, and we may be missing subtle changes in other diseases.

• 3.2 ppm: choline (Cho) is considered to be an indicator of membrane activity since phosphocholines are released during myelin breakdown, and it is often elevated if malignant processes are present.

• 3.6 ppm: myo-inositol (mI) is a sugar alcohol which is thought to be a product of myelin breakdown and its peak is often higher in conditions such as Alzheimer's disease and malignant tumours.

Just as image contrast is highly dependent on the sequence chosen and the timing parameters, so the height of peaks depends on the MR spectroscopy sequence and on the TE and TR used. Each metabolite has T_1 and T_2 relaxation times which, for brain spectra, are reasonably independent of the tissue in which they are present. In spectroscopy we are only interested in maximizing the signal-to-noise ratio of the spectrum peaks, so we need to avoid signal loss due to T_1 relaxation and T_2 decay. Ideally TR should be at least 2000 ms and certainly no less than 1500 ms. TE should be short, usually 30 ms, but for historical reasons TEs of 135–144 ms and 270–288 ms are also used (see section 15.3.2). Figures 15.1(b) and 15.1(c) show spectra from the same phantom at these TEs; in both spectra the NAA, Cr and Cho peaks are still visible, and you can see that the signal-to-noise ratio is reduced (look at the baseline between 0 and 1 ppm). A spectrum at TE = 144 ms is particularly useful to separate lactate from lipid contamination: not only is the lipid signal lost because it has a short T_2, but the lactate peak is inverted making it easily identifiable.

Currently the main clinical applications for in vivo spectroscopy are stroke, dementia, tumours and multiple sclerosis. Epilepsy shows marked changes in proton spectra, but consistently acquiring high-quality spectra is difficult because the epileptic focus is often in the temporal lobe (see 'Technical challenges of proton spectroscopy'). There are many other possibilities and the interested reader is referred to the end of this chapter for further reading. We will only give a simplistic guide to the main MR spectroscopy findings in these conditions, as follows.

15.2.1 Stroke

In acute stroke the infarct core rapidly shows signs of cell death and a spectrum from this area has the characteristic lactate peak, often with a broad lipid peak too (figure 15.2(a) shows lipids at 0.9 and 1.4 ppm, with the lactate doublet overlying the latter). Lactate may also be present in smaller concentrations in the ischaemic penumbra, the region around the core which, if reperfused sufficiently quickly, may recover its function. Other features are reduced NAA and Cr peaks and elevated Cho (the latter feature is not shown in figure 15.2(a)). Chemical shift imaging (CSI, see below) is probably the best way of getting metabolite information about the penumbra, but this technique is still relatively rare in clinical centres.

15.2.2 Dementia

In Alzheimer's disease (which accounts for around 70% of dementias) proton spectra show decreased NAA and elevated mI and Cho, although Cho also tends to increase with age so this must be interpreted with care. Figure 15.2(b) shows an example from a patient in the early stages of disease, where the main diagnostic feature is the increased mI. Other dementias do not show elevated mI, allowing a differential diagnosis to be made. There are variations between different parts of the brain, and CSI is probably going to be particularly useful in dementia.

15.2.3 Tumours

Spectroscopy may be helpful in the differential diagnosis between various lesions. Broadly speaking, low-grade lesions and meningiomas show reduced NAA and elevated Cho (figure 15.2(c)), features that progress in more malignant tumours (figure 15.2(d)) where Lac

(a)

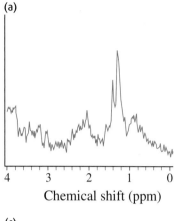

Chemical shift (ppm)

(b)

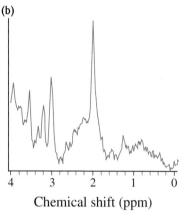

Chemical shift (ppm)

Figure 15.2 Typical spectra from patients with (a) stroke, (b) Alzheimer's disease, (c) low-grade glioma and (d) grade III astrocytoma.

(c)

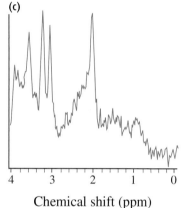

Chemical shift (ppm)

(d)

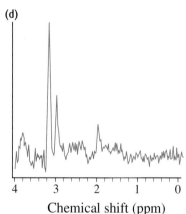

Chemical shift (ppm)

Technical challenges of proton spectroscopy

The frequency separation of peaks in the spectrum depends on the field strength and on the magnetic field homogeneity. At low fields or with a poor shim the peaks tend to overlap and that causes difficulty in interpretation and in measuring peak heights. It is generally thought that a field strength of 1.5 T is the minimum necessary for in vivo spectroscopy, although there is work at 1 T that is surprisingly good. However, it is not obvious that the highest field strengths will give much better results, as at 3 T and above patient susceptibility becomes the dominant inhomogeneity and thus spectral resolution may be degraded unless there is good local shimming, probably involving higher-order shim coils.

Regardless of the pulse sequence used for proton spectroscopy, good water suppression and high magnetic field homogeneity are essential to produce a good spectrum. The water peak is at a much higher concentration than the peaks of all the other metabolites, and without suppression those peaks cannot be seen. Typically a very narrow bandwidth frequency-selective pulse, often called a **CHE**mical **S**hift **S**elective (CHESS) pulse, is applied at exactly the Larmor frequency of water using a low-power Gaussian pulse to give a 90° pulse, followed by gradient pulses to spoil any transverse magnetization. Optimization of the strength and central frequency of the water suppression is essential, as inaccurate CHESS pulses can leave too much water (figure 15.3) and suppress neighbouring metabolite peaks.

Careful shimming is also essential. It helps if the magnet has a very good homogeneity to start with, ideally less than 0.5 ppm over the central 20 cm DSV (diameter of a spherical volume). However, the patient introduces a large inhomogeneity due to magnetic susceptibility variations within the head (air-filled sinuses and nasopharynx, and dense bone in the skull), and the superconducting shim coils cannot be modified for each patient. First-order shimming can be applied using constant currents through the gradient coils, applying a specialized shimming algorithm to optimize the homogeneity over the desired voxel. Some manufacturers offer a set of higher-order room temperature shims that allow a more precise shim.

To be clinically useful the automated shimming done by the scanner must give good reproducible results. Manual shimming (where the operator adjusts the currents while observing the FID or the water linewidth) is a tricky technique to perform well and adds a significant time penalty to the scan time. Research studies, however, may require skilled operators to check the automated shimming and adjust it manually if necessary.

may also be present. Many researchers have found a correlation between the levels of NAA and Cho with the tumour grading, and lipids are also found in necrotic tissue or cysts. Creatine may be reduced but there have been inconsistent findings to date, which may be partly due to the common practice of using Cr as an internal reference peak.

15.2.4 Multiple sclerosis

Spectra from multiple sclerosis plaques show reduced NAA and increased Cho, with Lac appearing occasionally. The time course of plaques from their active phase to the chronic stage has been studied with MR spectroscopy, which shows that the Cho and Lac peaks gradually return to near-normal levels over a period of weeks, while the NAA tends not to recover. Spectroscopy may be particularly useful for monitoring drug therapies in multiple sclerosis.

15.3 Single-voxel spectroscopy

15.3.1 STEAM

STEAM stands for 'STimulated Echo Acquisition Mode' and uses three selective 90° pulses, each with a gradient on one of the three axes (figure 15.4). A total of four echoes is produced from this set of pulses (or five if the first two RF pulses are closer together than the second and third), one of which is a stimulated echo and this is the signal that is acquired for spectroscopy. For many

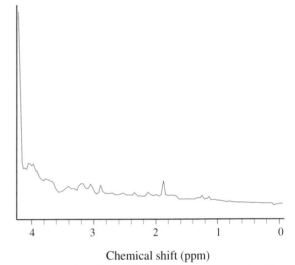

Chemical shift (ppm)

Figure 15.3 The effects of inaccurate water suppression. The large residual water peak at the left of the spectrum dominates the signal and none of the metabolite peaks can be reliably detected.

years STEAM was the only sequence capable of short echo times (down to 30 ms), which show the Glx and mI peaks, and so it has been used for many research studies. Because there is such a large body of literature about a range of conditions it is still popular with many researchers, especially those with long-term studies. However, it has a lower signal-to-noise ratio than PRESS (section 15.3.2) and does not show the useful Lac inversion at TE = 144 ms.

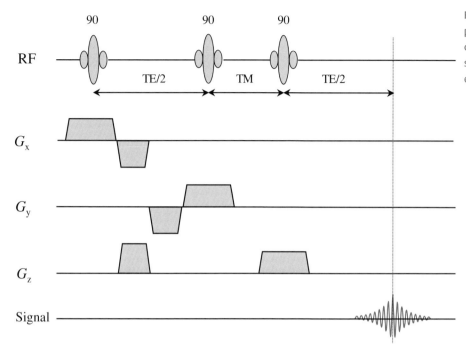

Figure 15.4 The STEAM
pulse sequence. TM
denotes the mixing time –
see box 'Stimulated
echoes'.

Stimulated echoes

Stimulated echoes were first described in 1950 in an important paper by Hahn, which also contributed greatly to the understanding of spin echoes. To understand how they are produced, consider a series of three 90° pulses with unequal spacing (figure 15.5). Some dephasing occurs after the first pulse, and the fan of protons is turned through 90° by the second pulse, leaving some components in the transverse plane which refocus to produce the first spin echo. Other components are put into the longitudinal direction where they relax with T_1 only, until the third RF pulse is applied. These components are turned into the transverse plane again, where they refocus to produce a stimulated echo. The maximum height of the stimulated echo can be calculated from the expression

$$S \propto \frac{M_0}{2} \cdot \sin \alpha_1 \cdot \sin \alpha_2 \cdot \sin \alpha_3 \cdot \exp\left(\frac{-TE}{T_2}\right) \cdot \exp\left(\frac{-TM}{T_1}\right)$$

i.e. it is affected by both T_2 relaxation during the first inter-pulse period and T_1 relaxation between the second and third pulses (known as the mixing time, TM). If we assume that TE and TM are both short compared with the relaxation times and provided each pulse is a perfect 90°, the maximum possible signal is 50% of M_0. To use stimulated echoes for spectroscopy, it is only necessary to add slice-selective gradients to each axis so that only protons within the required voxel experience all three RF pulses.

In order to understand the formation of echoes with multiple RF pulses of an arbitrary flip angle it is helpful to use coherence pathway diagrams, as described in chapter 12. Note that if $TE/2 > TM$ four echoes will be produced in total, whereas if $TE/2 < TM$ there will be five, the extra one being the second refocusing of the spin echo due to RF pulses 1 and 2.

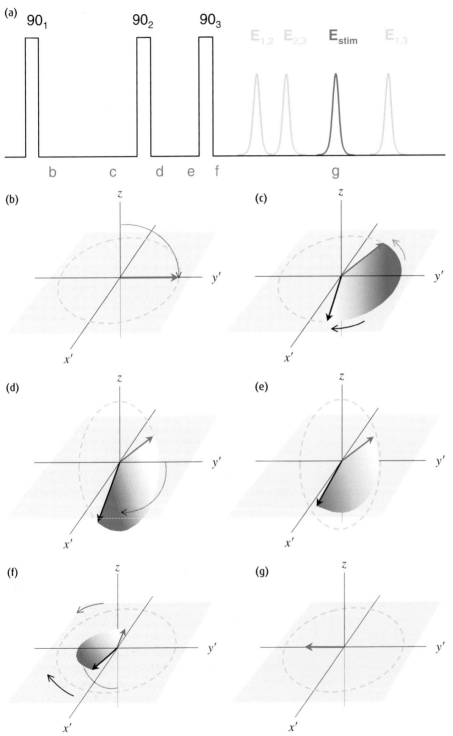

Figure 15.5 (a) Three RF pulses at uneven spacing produce three primary spin echoes and one stimulated echo. (b) The components which form the stimulated echo are flipped first into the transverse plane where they dephase with T_2 relaxation (c), then into the longitudinal plane (d) where dephasing stops and T_1 relaxation occurs (e), then finally flipped back into the transverse plane (f) where they re-phase and form an echo (g).

15.3.2 PRESS

PRESS stands for 'Point-RESolved Spectroscopy' and is based on the spin-echo sequence. A 90° pulse is followed by two 180° pulses so that the primary spin echo is refocused again by the third pulse. Each pulse has a slice-selective gradient on one of the three principle axes (figure 15.6(a)), so that protons within the voxel are the only ones to experience all three RF pulses.

The signal intensity depends on the pulse spacing and relaxation times, and is intrinsically twice as high as STEAM, so spectra can be acquired with good signal-tonoise ratio (SNR) in a relatively short time.

When PRESS was first developed on clinical scanners, its minimum TE was rather long, typically 144 ms, with a resulting loss of SNR so that often only NAA, Cr and Cho could be reliably detected. At an echo time of 144 ms lactate is completely out of phase with the rest of the spectrum and appears as an inverted peak (refer back to figure 15.1(b)). At 288 ms TE it is back in phase again (although SNR is even lower), and the acquisition of two spectra could be used to confirm the presence of Lac (figure 15.1(c)). Modern sequences are able to produce short-echo-time PRESS, however, and a 30-ms TE PRESS spectrum is almost indistinguishable from a 30-ms TE STEAM spectrum (figure 15.6(b)).

15.3.3 Voxel positioning

The choice of voxel position is critical to achieving a good-quality diagnostic spectrum. Obviously it is important to put the voxel in an appropriate place to detect the pathology under investigation. For example, within a single brain lesion there may be necrosis, active tumour and oedema. Appropriate contrast images are needed for planning the voxel. In order to grade a tumour the voxel should be in the active tissue, but it can be difficult to distinguish these regions on standard T_1-weighted or T_2-weighted scans. It has been shown that gadolinium has only a small effect (causing a small amount of line broadening), so postcontrast T_1-weighted scans can be useful. However, this is only true if the concentration of gadolinium within the voxel is relatively low: at higher concentrations the T_1 and T_2 shortening effects must

be considered. The question of whether to perform MR spectroscopy before or after gadolinium administration is a controversial one and there are strong opinions either way.

A good shim over the voxel is absolutely essential to produce a good spectrum, and a linewidth of less than 0.08 ppm (5 Hz at 1.5 T) is ideal. Voxels in inhomogeneous regions of the brain are always difficult to shim, in particular the temporal lobes, the base of the brain and the cortex near the skull. For nonfocal diseases a good choice would be the occipital grey matter or white matter (figure 15.7). Obviously lesions and stroke infarcts do not always place themselves in positions that are easy to shim, and we just have to live with that. If the prescan results in a higher linewidth, a repeat prescan can sometimes bring it down as the automated shimming technique improves on its starting point. Linewidths of 0.15 ppm (9 Hz) or higher are probably not worth acquiring, as the resulting spectrum will be poor quality (figure 15.8) and unlikely to help a diagnosis. In general smaller voxels are easier to shim than larger ones, but the signal also depends on volume so a voxel with 1-cm sides is often considered the practical minimum size to achieve a reasonable SNR. If the volume of the voxel is further reduced in order to help the shim, then the number of signal averages recorded (also known as transients) should be increased.

Whatever criteria are chosen for positioning MR spectroscopy voxels, consistency is the key to obtaining reliable spectra. Don't be tempted to change the timing parameters, as the resulting spectrum will not be comparable with a normal reference spectrum. The only exception to this rule is the number of signal averages, which may be increased to improve SNR in small voxels. Short echo times are preferred because the improved SNR allows more peaks to be seen, and a second spectrum with long echo time (144 ms) may be used to confirm the presence of Lac if necessary. Alternatively a second short-echo spectrum could be acquired from a contralateral site to provide a 'normal' reference, although this really only works if lesions are truly focal (even a stroke may cause changes on the contralateral side if the blood supply is altered).

(a)

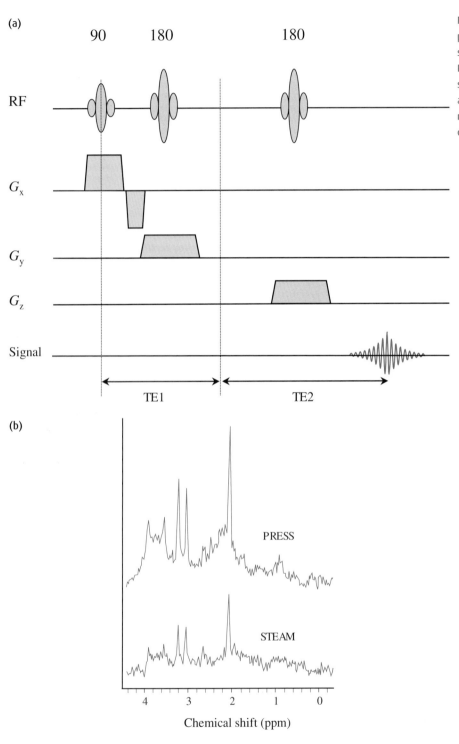

Figure 15.6 (a) The PRESS pulse sequence. (b) In vivo spectra acquired with PRESS and STEAM with the same timing parameters are only subtly different, mainly around the Glx complex.

(b)

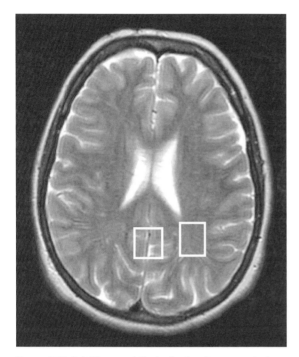

Figure 15.7 Axial image of the brain showing suggested voxel locations for grey matter (occipital midline) and white matter (parietal).

STEAM versus PRESS: the debate continues

Since PRESS is now able to achieve short echo times and produces twice as great SNR as STEAM, you might wonder why anyone is still using STEAM. While it might seem like reluctance to change, there are good reasons to continue with STEAM. Spectroscopy is a difficult technique to do well because there are so many potential errors in the shimming, the water suppression and in quantification. In addition even small changes in the acquisition can produce large differences in the spectra, so it has become accepted practice to use fixed parameters especially for TE. Institutions which started with STEAM have built up local expertise with the acquisition and interpretation of the spectra, with large databases of both normal and abnormal spectra with which to compare new patients' data.

PRESS has slightly different characteristics to STEAM and is sensitive to different technical problems, especially when quantification of metabolite concentrations is important. Thus switching to PRESS would require building up new expertise and a new database of normal spectra, and it can be difficult to find a good time to change when there may be long-term research studies using STEAM. Institutions which are new to spectroscopy should start with short-echo PRESS and stick to it, in the authors' opinion, using a second PRESS acquisition at TE 144 ms to confirm the presence of Lac if necessary.

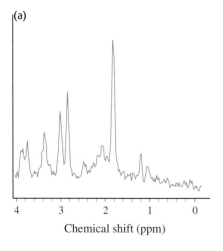
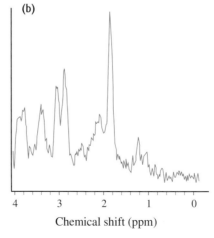

Figure 15.8 The effects of shimming on a phantom spectrum: (a) well shimmed and (b) badly shimmed.

Chemical shift effect in excitation

A significant problem of voxel excitation is sharpness of the voxel edges. Taking water and fat as a simple example, a frequency-selective pulse (figure 15.9(a)) will excite slices of water and fat at slightly different locations due to the chemical shift of 3.6 ppm. In three dimensions, the fat voxel will be offset with respect to the water voxel (figure 15.9(b)). With the added complication of the excitation profile caused by imperfect selective pulses, you can see that the edges of the voxel become rather poorly defined. This is sometimes known as 'voxel bleed', and if the voxel is positioned close to the scalp it can lead to contamination of the spectrum with lipid signals. Similarly a voxel which overlaps the ventricles will have reduced SNR because the cerebrospinal fluid (CSF) contains almost no metabolites but contributes to the water peak.

In order to see the selected voxel directly, it can be imaged instead of acquiring a spectrum from it. This is done by replacing the slice-selective pulse of a standard gradient-echo imaging sequence with the three selective pulses from either STEAM or PRESS. Line profiles can be obtained from the voxel image to examine the sharpness of the edges, and by comparing it with a standard image its position can be confirmed. Adding spatial saturation bands on all six sides (right, left, superior, inferior, anterior and posterior) can improve the voxel profiles.

15.4 Processing of single-voxel spectra

Several specialized processing steps are performed on the acquired FID to produce a high-quality spectrum. Whether they are done in the time domain or the frequency domain (i.e. before or after the Fourier transform) depends on which is computationally easier. All the figures in this section are from a simulated acquisition of a spectrum with two narrow resonances and one broader peak: the raw 'FID' and its spectrum are shown in figure 15.10.

The FID is usually digitized for only a few tens of milliseconds. Extending the digitization time would just increase the noise level in the spectrum, as the FID has decayed away. It is common to zero-fill the data at this stage, i.e. extra data points all set to zero are added to the end of the acquired data (figure 15.11). This corresponds to interpolating between data points in the frequency domain giving a smoother looking spectrum, but is much easier to do before the Fourier transform. Apodization is applied before Fourier transform of the FID. This means multiplying the acquired FID by a smoothly varying function such as an exponential decay or a Gaussian function (figure 15.12). Apodizing has the effect of suppressing the noisier tail-end of the FID, which therefore improves the SNR. However, it also makes the peaks slightly broader in the frequency domain, and so is also called line-broadening. It corresponds to convolving the frequency spectrum with a Lorentzian or Gaussian function, and is computationally easier in the time domain.

After Fourier transformation, the spectrum will be phase-corrected. A zeroth-order phase correction compensates for any mismatch between the quadrature receive channels and the excitation channels (figure 15.13) to produce the pure absorption spectrum. This is usually done using the residual water peak which is still the largest peak in the spectrum. The need for localizing gradients means that there is always a delay between excitation and turning on the receivers. During this delay the nuclei will dephase by an angle that is proportional to their frequency, which then needs to be corrected by a first-order phase correction (i.e. a linear phase shift across the spectrum, figure 15.13). Unfortunately the first-order phase correction introduces

(a)

(b)

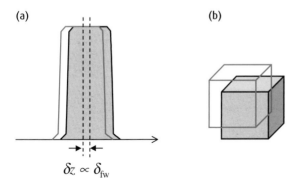

$$\delta z \propto \delta_{\mathrm{fw}}$$

Figure 15.9 (a) The chemical shift effect causes fat and water to have slightly offset slice locations. (b) In three dimensions and with a small voxel size, the offset may be significant.

(a)

Signal

Time (ms)

(b)

Spectrum

Chemical shift (ppm)

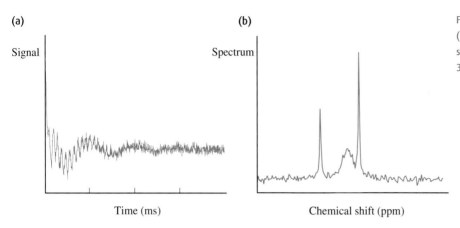

Figure 15.10 The raw FID (a) and spectrum (b) from simulated data (PRESS, 30 ms TE).

(a)

Signal

Time (ms)

(b)

Spectrum

Chemical shift (ppm)

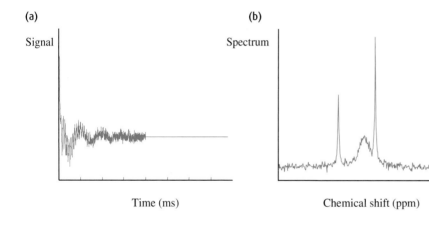

Figure 15.11 (a) Zerofilling the FID is equivalent to interpolating between points in the frequency spectrum (b).

(a)

Signal

Time (ms)

(b)

Spectrum

Chemical shift (ppm)

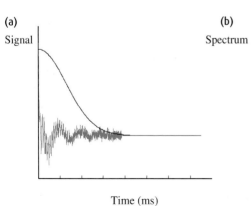
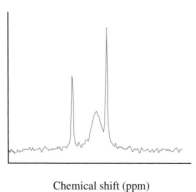

Figure 15.12 (a) Apodization (multiplication of the FID by a special function) improves SNR at the expense of a little line-broadening (b).

(a)

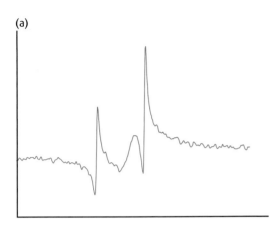

Chemical shift (ppm)

(b)

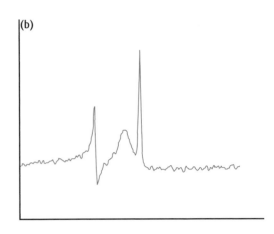

Chemical shift (ppm)

Figure 15.13 (a) A real spectrum may not be correctly phased immediately after Fourier transform (FT). (b) Zeroth-order phase correction has correctly phased the right-most peak, but first-order phase correction is now necessary to correct for hardware delays.

another feature, a slowly varying baseline known as baseline roll. This can be corrected by fitting a spline or polynomial function to the spectrum between the metabolite peaks and then subtracting the resulting function (figure 15.14).

At this stage the spectrum is presented to the user and is ready for qualitative interpretation. Simple ratios are calculated by finding the area under the spectrum between defined ppm limits for the main metabolites, and these are also presented on the screen. Further quantification is usually done by moving the raw data off-line onto an independent workstation. For example, to measure absolute concentrations of the metabolites a model of their known resonances can be fitted to the data using a specialist software package. As with the other processing steps, fitting can be done either in the time domain or the frequency domain.

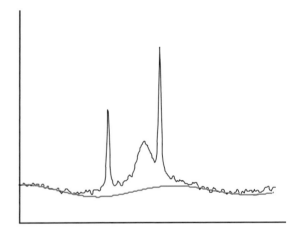

Chemical shift (ppm)

Figure 15.14 Baseline correction is achieved by fitting a spline function (a smoothly varying polynomial function) to the portions of the spectrum known to contain only noise, then subtracting that function.

15.5 Chemical shift imaging

Chemical shift imaging (CSI) uses phase-encoding techniques to acquire spectra from a matrix of voxels. Each slice-selective gradient is replaced with a phase-encoded gradient, which works in the same way as the slice-select gradient in 3D imaging sequences (see section 7.8). In principle this can be done for all three directions, but it is more usual to leave one direction as a straightforward slice select, i.e. to perform 2D single-slice CSI.

CSI can be done either with PRESS or STEAM. Instead of producing an echo from a small voxel, the 'voxel' is now a chunky slab. The phase-encoding rephase lobes then sub-divide the slab into a grid of voxels of the required size. The first phase-encoding gradient must step through all its values for each value of the second phase-encode gradient, so the acquisition time will be $TR \times N_{PE1} \times N_{PE2} \times NSA$. If $15 \times 15 \times 15$ mm^3 voxels are required with a head-sized field of view (FOV) of 24 cm, the matrix required is 16×16. Since TR should be at least 1500 ms to avoid T_1 effects in the spectra, the minimum scan time is thus 6 min 24 s. The good news is that although the voxel size is rather small, the SNR is similar to the equivalent single voxel acquisition thanks to the repeated excitations (in this case $16 \times 16 = 256$). Multi-slice CSI can be done in an interleaved fashion by changing the frequency of the slice-select RF pulse (just as 2D multi-slice images can be produced). Alternatively Hadamard encoding can be used, which offers improved slice profiles and further improves the SNR of the whole acquisition. This is preferable to phase encoding in the third direction, which would push up the scan time to 25 min for just four slices.

Significant time savings in CSI can be made by using a few tricks from normal MR imaging. A simple example is to use a rectangular FOV and reduce the number of phase encodes accordingly. For a typical axial brain CSI, this can reduce the scan time by 20 - 25%. It is also possible to use a RARE-like echo train with different phase encoding for each echo, known as Turbo SI. The acquisition time for a PRESS echo is a lot longer than for imaging, typically 200 ms, so the turbo factor is only 2-4 in order to avoid T_2 blurring. Even a small turbo factor allows significantly higher matrix sizes within a reasonable scan time, for example a 28×28 matrix with a turbo factor of 4 and TR of 2500 ms takes 8 m 10 s, and offers significantly improved voxel resolution.

New parallel imaging techniques (such as SENSE and GRAPPA) offer further time savings with multi-element receive coils, by using coil sensitivities to reduce the number of phase encoding steps required. Both Turbo-SI and parallel imaging have disadvantages of course: they both involve a reduced spectral resolution because the echo has to be acquired more quickly, and parallel imaging reduces SNR in the final images.

Having produced a matrix of spectra, the usual way to display the data is as a series of maps, usually of the main metabolite peaks NAA, Cr and Cho, or other important metabolites (figure 15.15, see colour section). In these maps the intensity of the voxel depends on the area of the relevant peak in that position's spectrum. Software is available which allows the user to define a chemical shift range from which to produce a map; for example, a 'lactate' map could be created from the range 1.2–1.4 ppm. As a 'rainbow' colour scale is often used for these maps they need careful interpretation as even small changes in peak area can produce dramatic colour changes.

15.6 Phosphorus spectroscopy

Like proton spectroscopy, phosphorus spectroscopy is also well developed for acquiring in vivo spectra. Phosphorus (^{31}P) has a lower Larmor frequency than hydrogen, which means that a higher field strength is necessary to achieve good spectral resolution. Some manufacturers offer phosphorus spectroscopy on 1.5 T scanners (at a price – it involves a second RF subsystem), but much of the research has been done at field strengths of 4–7 T. Phosphorus is also much less abundant than protons, with a whole-body concentration 1000 times smaller, and so SNR is relatively poor. Since phosphorus is a major component in adenosine triphosphate (ATP), consumed and renewed during the conversion of sugars to energy, ^{31}P spectra are often used to study muscle metabolism.

In vivo ^{31}P has much shorter T_2 than protons, and echo-based sequences such as STEAM and PRESS, even at short echo times, are unsuitable; instead sequences are used that acquire the FID immediately after excitation. ISIS (**I**mage **S**elective **I**n vivo **S**pectroscopy) is a subtractive technique that uses $\pm 180°$ selective pulses in all possible combinations on the three axes such that the final signal is only from the required voxel. Although it is a good voxel-selective technique, eight TRs are required for each signal acquisition, so it is rather slow. DRESS is also used for ^{31}P MRS, which stands for '**D**epth-**RES**olved **S**pectroscopy'. This relies on the characteristics of a surface coil or phased array of coils to

Technical difficulties in CSI

CSI has all the technical problems of single-voxel spectroscopy and a few more of its own! A major problem is the difficulty of shimming an entire slice to the level necessary for good spectra from every voxel in the matrix. In fact this is so difficult that it is usual to define a sub-region within the brain which is used for shimming (figure 15.16). Outside of this region the shim is allowed to remain poor and spectra in these voxels will be very low quality. When setting up a CSI scan, the edges of the region of interest should lie well within the skull to avoid the susceptibility changes associated with bone.

Since the 'imaging' matrix is so small (usually only 16×16), the Fourier transform produces large ringing (Gibbs') artefacts across the field of view and smoothing is usually applied in an effort to reduce this. However, the smoothing introduces smearing across the voxels, making the voxel bleed much worse than in single-voxel MRS. The resolution of CSI is therefore not just the size of the pixels as in normal MRI, but is always worse. It is now measured using the point-spread function (PSF), which can be calculated if you know the k-space sampling and postprocessing filters. Absolute quantification of metabolite concentration is difficult and relative quantification is more useful, not least because there are so many voxels in a single CS image.

Residual field inhomogeneities across the field of view may cause incorrect water suppression, as the suppression pulses are applied to the wrong part of the spectrum. Phase errors in the selective RF pulses are significant over the larger volume in CSI, and vary from voxel to voxel across the field of view. Baseline correction is often compromised and spectra will rarely be as high a quality as those obtained from single-voxel techniques. This makes it particularly difficult to produce reliable metabolite maps from short echo time CSI, where the baseline is also compromised by short-T_2 macromolecules. Interpretation of CSI maps should include inspection of the underlying spectra to decide whether or not a 'deficit' or 'elevation' is actually present.

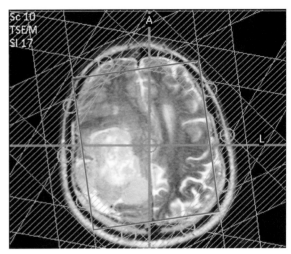

Figure 15.16 When planning CSI, a sub-volume is defined for shimming (blue box). Multiple saturation bands (hatched white bands) are placed over the scalp and skull bone marrow to reduce lipid contamination.

excite a region of tissue at a certain depth within the body. DRESS volumes are large compared with voxel techniques such as ISIS, so signals from small tumours may be hidden by those of normal tissues, and spectra can be contaminated with signals from surface tissues. A normal ^{31}P spectrum from muscle is shown in figure 15.17. Notice that the spectral width is nearly 20 ppm in contrast with that of proton spectra, which is only about 5 ppm. Reading from right to left, ATP has three main resonances at about –15 ppm, –8 ppm and –4 ppm labelled βATP, αATP and γATP respectively, one for each phosphorus atom in the molecule. Phosphocreatine (PCr) is used as the reference chemical shift at 0 ppm. The other main peaks are phosphodiesters (PDE) at 3 ppm and inorganic phosphates (Pi) at 5 ppm.

During and after exercise, ^{31}P spectra show changes reflecting the initial decrease in ATP then its recovery during aerobic exercise. The main changes during aerobic exercise are a reduction in the PCr peak accompanied by an increase in the Pi peak, which returns to normal gradually when exercise ceases. In diseases such as muscular dystrophy ^{31}P spectra show a high Pi/PCr ratio at rest, and during exercise abnormal patterns are seen. [31]P spectroscopy is similarly useful to investigate the energetics of the heart; for this the

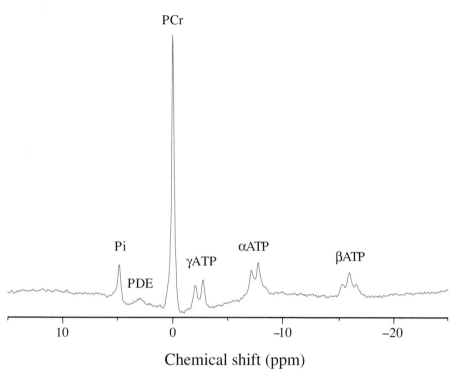

Chemical shift (ppm)

Figure 15.17 Phosphorus spectrum from normal muscle showing the main metabolite peaks. PDE denotes phosphodiesters; Pi inorganic phosphate and PCr phosphocreatine. Courtesy of Dr F. Howe, St George's Hospital Medical School, London.

patient is placed prone on a specially designed phased array coil, so that the heart rests on the anterior chest wall and is close enough to produce a good signal.

[31]P spectroscopy is also used to investigate the liver, where the main difference in the appearance of the spectrum is that PCr is not present in the liver; a PCr peak in such a spectrum indicates contamination with overlying muscle. Repeated ^{31}P spectra can be acquired to study the metabolism of the liver, in the normal state and in hepatitis and cirrhosis, and to monitor the response of malignant lesions to therapies.

15.7 Other nuclei

Other nuclei, primarily from carbon, fluorine and sodium, are often used by research groups for CSI rather than single-voxel spectroscopy.

Only the isotope ^{13}C of carbon is MR-visible, which only comprises 1.1% of naturally occurring carbon. By labelling glucose with ^{13}C, it is possible to examine glucose metabolism in the brain, where studies of stroke patients have shown that lactate turnover is higher in the ischaemic penumbra compared with the infarct core. Spectra from the liver can be produced without using the labelled glucose, with an SNR of about 15:1.

[23]Na is MR visible, although it is present at very low concentrations in vivo. There have been several CSI studies of the brain, in which it can be used to measure intraand extracellular levels of sodium ions.

Fluorine is present in high concentrations in the bones and teeth, but is not detectable because in this form it has an extremely short T_2. However, if pharmaceuticals can be labelled with [19]F (an MR-active isotope), any detected signals are known to arise from these substances, which is a considerable advantage. Such studies can be used to investigate the pharmacokinetics of drugs; for example, the breakdown products of a chemotherapy drug have been measured in the liver. ^{19}F-CSI of the brain is possible using ^{19}F-tagged deoxyglucose ([^{19}F]DG), which is taken up by tissues from the blood supply in the same way as glucose. This technique has the potential to become very important over the next few years, since many perfusion MRI studies rely on [^{18}F]DG positron emission tomography (PET) studies as the 'gold standard' for brain perfusion; [^{19}F]DG CSI may provide the same information without the radiation dose associated with PET.

15.8 Hyperpolarized gases

With hyperpolarized xenon and helium, direct imaging of gaseous material is possible. The gases are produced in a premagnetized form (hyperpolarized), with a magnetization much greater than that achievable by conventional means (i.e. placing the sample in a B_0 field, or so-called Boltzmann or thermal magnetization). The hyperpolarization is produced by 'spin exchange' or 'metastability exchange' using rubidium vapour as a spin transferring medium. Both xenon and helium are safe to use in humans, the former being soluble in blood, the latter not absorbed in the lungs and with properties well known from deep sea diving. Helium produces more signal but is restricted to studies of the air-spaces. With xenon various forms of physiological and functional imaging are possible.

15.8.1 Xenon and helium

[129]Xe has nonzero nuclear spin and is suitable for imaging with a Larmor frequency of 17.5 MHz at 1.5 T (compared with 63 MHz for hydrogen). It accounts for 26% of naturally occurring xenon. At high concentrations it acts as an anaesthetic and is soluble in blood with a high affiliation to lipids.

[3]He is a rarely occurring form of the inert gas helium ([4]He is the natural form – and is the stuff we put in cryogenic magnets!). Its resonant frequency at 1.5 T is 48 MHz. It will therefore give a higher MR signal than xenon and can attain higher levels of polarization. It is not taken up by the lungs and is therefore restricted to morphological studies of the airways, bronchi and alveolar structures. Figure 15.18 shows [3]He lung images.

15.8.2 Imaging considerations

One of the limitations of hyperpolarized gases is that the application of RF pulses for imaging progressively destroys the magnetization. Low flip angle techniques must therefore be used, as after each pulse the reduction in longitudinal magnetization is not recoverable. Rewound gradient echo sequences offer some advantages over spoiled gradient echo, as the transverse magnetization can be used for longer in the steady state. EPI with its single RF excitation and speed is also attractive despite its inherent resolution limitations. EPI also offers the prospect of dynamic ventilation studies, as do spiral imaging techniques.

In whole-blood [129]Xe has a T_1 of around 13 s, which reduces to about 4 s in venous blood because of the influence of paramagnetic deoxyhaemoglobin. This raises the possibility of using Xe-MRI to measure blood oxygenation in vivo. Detection of xenon in organs, such as the brain, is possible using MR spectroscopy. Dissolved xenon in blood has a chemical shift of 196 ppm from the main gaseous phase peak. When imaging the brain, it is necessary to protect the xenon

Production of hyperpolarization

The method of spin exchange is achieved by the initial excitation of rubidium vapour by optical 'pumping' by diode laser. This is similar to NMR excitation but acts on the electrons of the rubidium rather than the nucleus. Following electronic polarization, the nuclear spins of the xenon or helium are excited by collisions with the rubidium atoms. This process is lengthy, of the order of several hours, but polarization levels of 5–25% are achievable. In the case of xenon the gas is cooled to liquid nitrogen temperature (77 K), which freezes the gas so that it can then be transported as xenon ice. In this form the T_1 of the polarization is about 3 h. In the case of helium the gas is transferred in gaseous form in a special nonpermeable 'Tedlar' bag. Small 'holding' magnets are required to maintain the polarization.

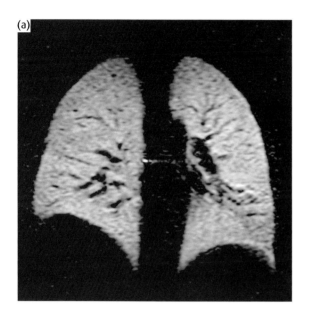
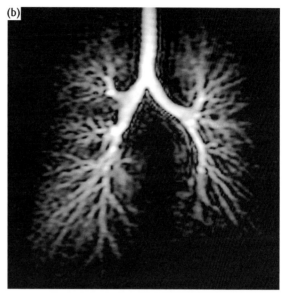

Figure 15.18 Hyperpolarized helium imaging. (a) Static, coronal, multi-slice lung image obtained during breath-hold of 1 litre of hyperpolarized ^{3}He gas with a GRE pulse sequence and 18° flip angle. (b) Dynamic, steady-state coronal lung projection image obtained during the inhalation of 1 litre of hyperpolarized gas using a fast GRE pulse sequence and 16° flip angle. Images courtesy of Mitchell Albert, PhD, Department of Radiology, Brigham and Women's Hospital and Harvard Medical School, Boston, MA.

gas in the lungs from unwanted RF excitation, which will destroy the hyperpolarization, by using an 'RF blanket'. In order to prolong the MR lifetime of xenon, various inert 'buffer' gases such as sulphur hexafluoride may be added. In the lungs ^{3}He has a T$_1$ of about half a minute.

Because the gas comes 'premagnetized' the strength of the B$_0$ field does not affect magnetization. The signal strength detected will be proportional to the Larmor frequency. However, we have already seen that electrical noise induced from the patient is generally proportional to the RF frequency. This means that hyperpolarized gas imaging should be broadly independent of magnet strength. Successful imaging has been carried out at field strengths as low as 0.01 T.

15.8.3 Applications

At the time of writing hyperpolarized gas imaging remains firmly in the research domain. However, possible clinical applications include ventilation studies prior to lung reduction surgery, the monitoring of lung transplants, and assessment of disease state in cystic fibrosis and asthma. Dynamic ventilation studies may be useful in studying emphysema and smoking-related pathology. The development of sophisticated gas-delivery systems could permit the quantitative study of intrapulmonary partial oxygen pressure and pulmonary perfusion. The study of perfusion phenomena in other organs, notably the brain, may be aided by the development of intravenous xenon delivery. Xenon imaging may be useful in identifying white matter disease and cerebrovascular disease. Diffusion-weighted imaging offers the possibility of studying alveolar morphology. The high diffusion coefficient of the hyperpolarized gases means that the ADC will be predominantly determined by the alveolar structure. The possibility of using lower strength magnets offers an intriguing future of hyperpolarized gas MRI alongside current nuclear medicine techniques.

Protons have the major advantage of increased SNR over any other nucleus, and so in those parts of the body where it can be measured it provides better information than other spectroscopic techniques. ^{13}C, ^{23}Na and ^{19}F are so far only used in research studies, and it may seem that they are of limited interest to workers in a clinical setting. However, if an important clinical indication is combined with efforts to maximize SNR and technical developments, they may become more common in routine MR.

See also:

- Slice-selective RF pulses: section 7.4
- 3D phase encoding: section 7.8

FURTHER READING

Abragam A (1983) *The Principles of Nuclear Magnetism.* Oxford: Clarendon Press (ISBN: 019852014X), Chapters I, II & III.

Danielsen EB and Ross B (1998) *Magnetic Resonance Spectroscopy Diagnosis of Neurological Diseases.* New York: Marcel Dekker (ISBN: 0824702387).

Hahn EL (1950) Spin echoes. *Phys Rev* **80**(4): 580–94.

Kauczor H-U (ed) (2000) Special Issue: hyperpolarized gases in MRI. *NMR Biomed* **13**(4): 173–264.

Salibi N and Brown MA (1998) *Clinical MR Spectroscopy First Principles.* New York: Wiley-Liss (ISBN: 047118280).

Van Hecke P and Van Huffel S (eds) (2001) Special Issue: NMR Spectroscopy Quantitation. *NMR in Biomedicine* **14**(4): 223–83.

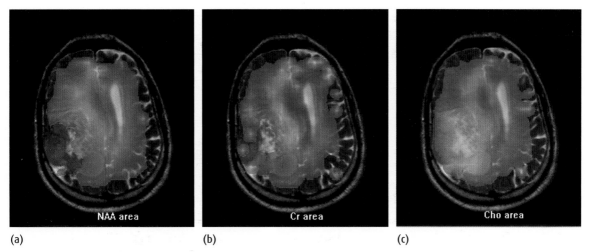

(a)   (b)   (c)

Figure 15.15 CSI metabolite maps from a patient with a brain tumour. (a) NAA, (b) Cr, (c) Cho.

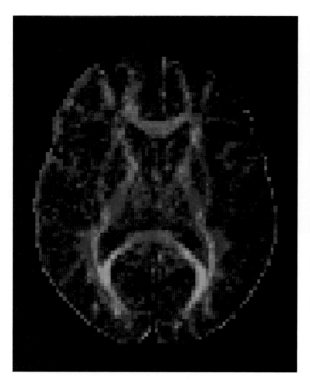

Figure 16.9 (e) Colour fractional anisotropy map. Hue represents direction (red = left-right, blue = foot-head, green = anterior-posterior) and intensity represents FA value. Courtesy of Philips Medical Systems.

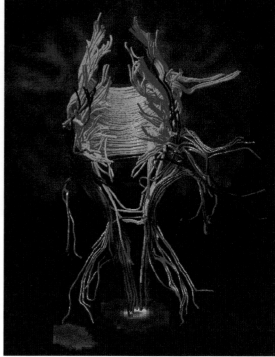

Figure 16.10 Tractography: the green tracts were launched from seed points placed at the centre of the body of the corpus callosum. The red tracts were obtained by defining seed points in the cerebral peduncles. The data were acquired using seven low b-values and 64 high b-values with a 40 mT m⁻¹ gradient system. Image courtesy of Dr. D. Jones, University of Leicester and Institute of Psychiatry, London, UK.

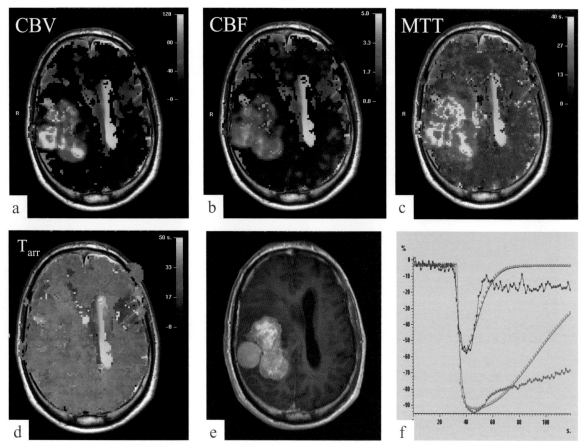

Figure 16.13 Perfusion parameter maps from DSC-MRI in a patient with a glioma. (a) CBV, (b) CBF, (c) MTT, (d) time of arrival (t_{arr}), (e) matching post-Gd T_1-weighted image, (f) time-intensity curves for normal brain (blue) and tumour (red). Note how the fitted gamma-variate curve deviates from the real data, due to rapid leakage of Gd into the tumour.

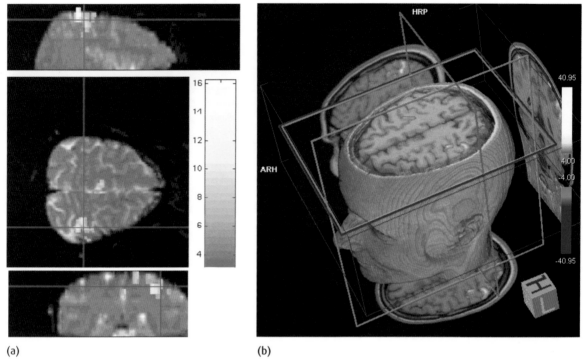

(a)   (b)

Figure 16.21 fMRI results: (a) motor (finger tapping) activation map output from Statistical Parametric Mapping (SPM) (the Wellcome Department of Cognitive Neurology, London) superimposed on raw EPI images in three orthogonal planes. (b) BOLD activation maps overlaid on a 3D surface rendering of the cerebral cortex in response to painful stimulation of the hand. The colour schemes indicate the degree of statistical significance of the signal changes: the colour scale is a 'hot body spectrum', where red is coolest, then yellow through to white. The signal changes due to the BOLD effect are only small percentages of the MR signal. The numbers are related to z-score values.

To BOLDly go: new frontiers

16.1 Introduction

We turn now to some of the more recent developments in MRI, to areas at the cutting edge between research and clinical practice. With the current pace of development, it is likely that some of these techniques will move swiftly forward; however, in this chapter we aim to explore the underlying principles.

The techniques we are exploring are all related to what is sometimes termed 'micro-contrast' mechanisms. This term is unfortunate because basic T_1 and T_2 relaxation depend upon the microscopic (at molecular level) interactions of spins. Nevertheless these new techniques give specific information about aspects of tissue not readily available through conventional contrast mechanisms. These are:

- Diffusion-weighted imaging, which relates to the mobility of water molecules, particularly when mobility is restricted to specific orientations, as in white matter tracts. Diffusion-weighted imaging is the method of choice for the imaging of acute stroke.
- Perfusion-weighted imaging relates to the delivery of blood to tissues, in terms of relative or absolute concentrations, or in terms of rates of delivery or mean transit times. Perfusion-weighted imaging can use exogenous contrast (i.e. a bolus of contrast agent) or endogenous contrast, by the 'spin labelling' of arterial blood.
- BOLD (**B**lood **O**xygenation **L**evel **D**ependent) imaging, sometimes called fMRI (functional MRI – note the small 'f'), is used to investigate regional brain activation, in lay terms, to observe the brain thinking. The BOLD effect uses the level of blood oxygenation to generate contrast.

Echo planar imaging (EPI) is the method of choice for diffusion, perfusion and BOLD imaging. The compromise for speed in EPI is extreme sensitivity to susceptibility-induced image distortion, low resolution and higher artefact levels.

16.2 EPI acquisition methods

We met EPI briefly in chapter 12. When using EPI what immediately strikes you is that it sounds very different from other sequences, giving a single very loud, moderately high pitched beep. Within this beep the whole of one slice is acquired, the sound being generated by a rapidly oscillating read gradient. EPI can be single or multi-shot, spin or gradient echo based. The acquisition is said to be blipped or unblipped depending on how the phase-encode gradient is applied.

EPI contrast can be amazing. In single-shot EPI, TR is effectively infinite. Thus one can obtain very highly T_2- or $T_2{}^*$-weighted contrast with no T_1 contribution at all.

Gradient-echo EPI is $T_2{}^*$-weighted and spin-echo EPI is T_2 weighted. T_1 weighting can be obtained by the addition of an inversion prepulse. In single-shot EPI, image slices are acquired sequentially, a whole slice at a time from a single RF excitation, usually at modest spatial resolution.

16.2.1 Blipped versus nonblipped single-shot EPI

In nonblipped EPI (figure 16.1) a constant phase-encode gradient is applied continuously during the oscillating readout gradient. Data are also sampled

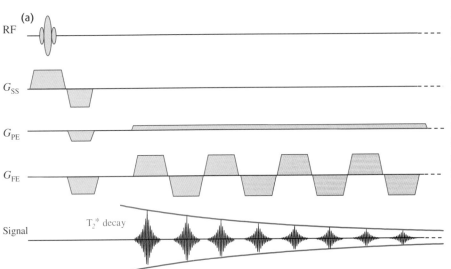

(a)

RF

G_{SS}

G_{PE}

G_{FE}

Signal

T_2^* decay

Figure 16.1 Constant phase-encode echo planar imaging (EPI). (a) Gradient-echo sequence – first 8 of typically 64 or 128 readout gradient lobes shown. The dotted lines indicate continuance of the sequence. (b) k-space path acquired following a single RF excitation.

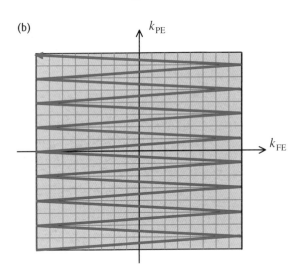

(b)

k_{PE}

k_{FE}

continuously throughout, with large bipolar read gradients creating a train of echoes. This results in an irregular zig-zag path through k-space (figure 16.1(b)) acquired from one RF excitation, with the phase encode continuously accruing over all k_{PE}. Prior to reconstruction, 'regularization' of the raw data to a rectilinear grid of points by mathematical interpolation is required.

In blipped EPI (figure 16.2(a)) a small phase-encoding gradient 'blip' is placed at each readout gradient reversal. This blip is of constant size and adds

further phase encoding to the previous blips. This results in a regular path through k-space (figure 16.2(b)), which makes reconstruction easier and quicker.

In both forms of EPI, large read gradient amplitudes are required so that the appropriate values of k_{FE} can be sampled quickly, and the whole set of k_{PE} collected within a single free induction decay (FID). This limits single-shot EPI acquisitions to the order of 100 ms resulting in a typical resolution of 64×64 or 128×128. The time limitation imposed by the duration of the FID means that in EPI data are usually acquired during the gradient ramp-up times. In so-called resonant systems (see 'Gradient considerations') the readout gradient lobes are sinusoidal. Two sampling strategies can be used: either sampling equally spaced in time, in which case interpolation within k-space is required, or sampling at equal k-space increments, in which case additional prescan calibration and specialist analogue-to-digital converter (ADC) hardware may be required. These are illustrated in figure 16.3.

As for other segmented sequences (e.g. Rapid Acquisition with Relaxation Enhancement, or RARE) an effective echo time, where the centre of k-space is acquired, applies. Because the phase encoding is accrued monotonically, line-by-line, TE is generally of moderate length (e.g. 30–60 ms). The options for manipulating TE are limited, although partial fourier techniques (see section 7.7) may help to reduce TE to an extent. Changing the matrix will also affect TE.

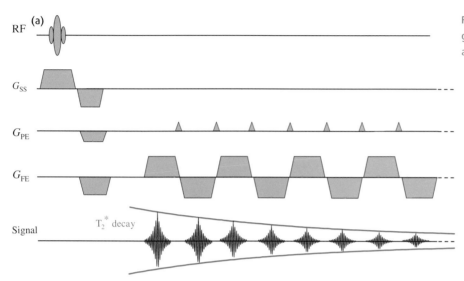

Figure 16.2 (a) Blipped gradient-echo EPI sequence and (b) k-space path.

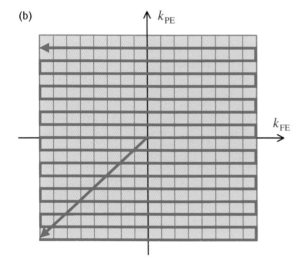

Gradient considerations

The ultimate speed of EPI is limited by the speed of gradient switching. Often specialist gradient hardware is employed to enable very fast switching times. A compromise in this instance is the use of resonant gradient systems that produce sinusoidal type waveforms. The limiting parameter is the gradient slew rate in $mT\,m^{-1}\,ms^{-1}$. Figures in excess of $100\,mT\,m^{-1}$ ms^{-1} are found in high-performance gradient systems. Limits on how large this can be are physiologically determined by the onset of peripheral nerve stimulation. The new techniques of SMASH and SENSE (chapter 17) offer ways around this limitation.

16.2.2 EPI artefacts

EPI is notorious for a high level of artefact. The classic EPI artefact, is the N/2 (or 'Nyquist') ghost (figure 16.4(a)). This is a phase ghost of the sort encountered in section 6.3 but displaced by exactly one-half the field of view. This arises because of imperfections in the rephasing-dephasing cycle of the rapidly switching bipolar frequency-encode gradient. In practice a ghost level of a small percentage is almost always present.

The other artefacts are consequences of bandwidth. Each frequency-encode lobe is sampled rapidly with a very high gradient amplitude resulting in a very large signal bandwidth. The phase encode is sampled 64 or 128 times over the whole gradient-echo train. This rather slow sampling rate means that the signal bandwidth in the phase-encode direction may be as little as 10 Hz per pixel. This has major consequences.

First, chemically shifted signals from fat will be displaced by many pixels, a significant fraction of the entire field of view *in the phase-encode direction* (figure

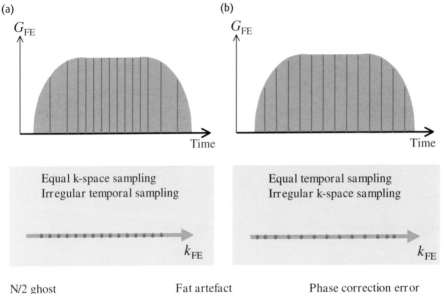

(a)

G_{FE}

Time

Equal k-space sampling
Irregular temporal sampling

k_{FE}

(b)

G_{FE}

Time

Equal temporal sampling
Irregular k-space sampling

k_{FE}

Figure 16.3 Two sampling strategies for k_{FE} in EPI during the rise and fall periods of a resonant catch-and-hold gradient. (a) Irregular temporal sampling, (b) regular temporal sampling.

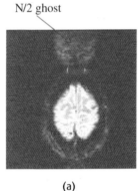

N/2 ghost

(a)

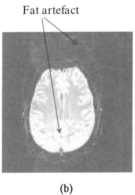

Fat artefact

(b)

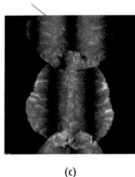

Phase correction error

(c)

Figure 16.4 EPI artefacts: (a) N/2 ghost also in the PE direction, (b) chemical shift: scalp fat is displaced in the PE direction (vertical) by a significant fraction of the field of view, (c) phase correction ("three brains") error.

16.4(b)). For this reason effective fat suppression is mandatory in EPI.

Second, small magnetic field differences (of the order of 1 ppm) will result in much greater spatial distortion. In particular air–tissue boundaries will result in large image distortions. Additionally signal drop-out may occur for locally shortened T_2^*. The orientation of tissue–air boundaries within the magnet can dramatically influence the extent and nature of these effects. Regions of brain close to the nasal sinuses, auditory meatus, frontal and temporal lobes are particularly affected (figure 16.5).

In a further artefact (we call it the 'three brains artefact') a combination of ghosting and banding occurs

because of cumulative phase differences between odd and even echoes over the echo train caused by eddy currents from the rapidly switched readout gradient (figure 16.4(c)). Clever techniques such as reference scans and variable timing of data acquisition are employed to reduce this (see 'Exorcism!').

16.2.3 Multi-shot EPI

Multi-shot EPI works a bit like RARE, in that it is a segmented k-space acquisition scheme. Typically the whole of k-space will be divided into two, four or eight segments, each of which is acquired by separate EPI trains. The advantages are that susceptibility effects can

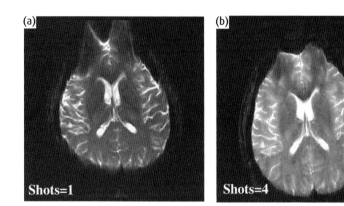
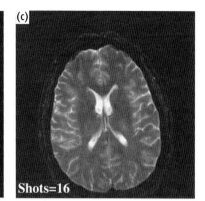

Figure 16.5 (a) Spatial distortion in single-shot EPI and improvements for multi-shot EPI: (b) 4 shots, (c) 16 shots.

Exorcism!

The origin of the N/2 ghost is a slight mis-positioning of every alternate refocusing of the FID, resulting from gradient imperfections (figure 16.6), which result in a mis-registration of alternate lines of k-space. Phase correction can be derived from a reference scan which is identical to a full scan but without phase encoding. From the 1D FT of these data lines, phase correction filters can be produced which will then be applied to every line of image data. Phase correction is also used in RARE imaging techniques. Additionally the position of the sampling points (the ADC raster) may be shifted to ensure the echoes are all centred. This requires a substantial prescan calibration procedure. To reduce artefacts, shimming using the gradients is required before an EPI acquisition. Even so, N/2 ghosts are almost always a small percentage of the main image signal.

be reduced as the PE bandwidth is effectively higher than for an equivalent single shot (figure 16.5) and that less gradient power is required. Scan time is obviously increased and there is a need for a finite TR as in conventional scanning. Multiple slice interleaving is possible, thereby helping to keep overall acquisition times short. The acquisition of 20 slices in 30 s, for example, is quite reasonable; however, the snapshot ability to freeze physiological motion is compromised.

16.2.4 Spiral EPI

One of the problems of single-shot EPI is that relatively short echo times are difficult to achieve. In spiral imaging the k-space trajectory takes the form of a spiral. This has the advantage that the low values of k-space are acquired first, and thus the effective echo time is short. Both single shot and multi shot spiral acquisitions are considered in section 17.7.4.

16.3 Diffusion imaging

The sensitivity of MR signals to random molecular motions, self-diffusion, has been known since the original pioneering work of Hahn, Carr and Purcell over half a century ago. More recently diffusion-weighted MRI (DW-MRI) has established itself as an important method in the assessment and diagnosis of acute stroke, revealing dramatic signal differences within an hour of the onset.

16.3.1 Pulsed gradient spin echo

The most commonly applied method for producing diffusion-weighted contrast is the **P**ulsed **G**radient **S**pin Echo (PGSE) method, sometimes called Stejskal and Tanner after its inventors. It consists of a 90°–180° spin-echo pair of RF pulses with large and equal gradients placed on either side of the 180° pulse (figure 16.7). By manipulating the strength of this gradient (G) and the

(a)

Sequence

G_{FE}

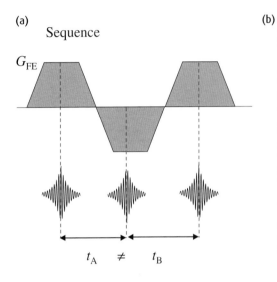

$t_A \quad \neq \quad t_B$

(b)

k-space

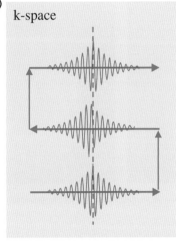

Figure 16.6 (a) Timing errors where the misplacement of the echo centre results in successive inter-echo timing t_A and t_B not being equal, and (b) consequence for k_{FE}, resulting in N/2 ghosting.

timing elements δ ('little delta'), the pulse width, and Δ ('big delta'), the leading edge separation or centre-to-centre spacing, we can control the degree of weighting or b-factor.

DW contrast behaves rather like inverse T_2 weighting, in that watery tissues that have very mobile molecules give lower signal intensity whilst more solid and static tissues give a stronger signal. The signal strength is described by the equation

$$S(b) = S(0)\exp(-bD)$$

where $S(b)$ is the signal for a particular b-value (see 'To b or not to b') and D is the self-diffusion constant of the tissue. In MRI we talk rather of an apparent diffusion coefficient (ADC) (see 'The diffusion coefficient – apparently'). This can be calculated from two or more images with different b-values and can be displayed as an ADC map.

The PGSE gradient scheme works a bit like the velocity-encoding gradients used in MR angiography. Indeed bulk flow will have its phase changed according to its velocity, but the phase angle will be many times 2π. With self-diffusion the molecules are moving about randomly, changing direction many times without actually getting anywhere. This is illustrated in figure 16.8. DW imaging works because all the spins accrue random and unique phase changes as they move about within the gradient. This results in a net loss of signal

To b or not to b

In the PGSE sequence the value of b is given by

$$b = \gamma^2 G^2 \delta^2 \left(\Delta - \frac{\delta}{3} \right)$$

and is determined by the gradient amplitude G and duration δ and trailing-to-leading edge separation $(\Delta - \delta)$. b has units of s mm^{-2}. Values of up to 1000 s mm^{-2} are required to obtain good contrast. Large gradient amplitudes (of up to 30 mT m^{-1}) are highly advantageous because their use means that the timing parameters can be minimized, thus avoiding very long TE values. Even so a DW acquisition will also have some T_2 weighting.

The quantity $(\Delta - \delta/3)$ is known as the diffusion time τ and is related to molecular motion through the Einstein equation

$$\langle r^2 \rangle = 6D\tau$$

where $\langle r^2 \rangle$ is the mean square displacement of a collection (or ensemble) of molecules.

within each voxel, provided sufficient DW is applied. Restricted diffusion applies where physical barriers, e.g. cell walls, prevent or limit this motion. A high value of D (the self-diffusion constant of the tissue) or ADC implies high motion and therefore low signal in DW-MRI. The corresponding ADC map will be bright.

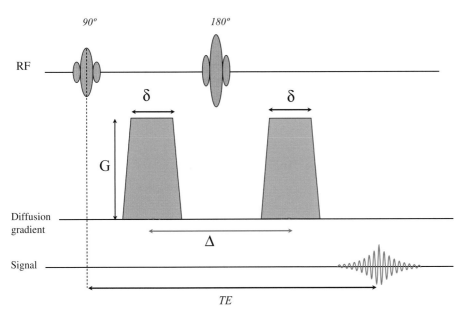

Figure 16.7 Basic pulsed
gradient spin echo (PGSE)
sequence for diffusion
weighting. For imaging this
precedes a spin-echo EPI
acquisition. δ denotes the
pulse width and Δ the
centre-to-centre spacing.
G is the magnitude of the
diffusion-weighting
gradient.

Table 16.1 Typical apparent diffusion coefficient (ADC) values for human brain tissues

	ADC ($\times 10^{-3}$ mm^2 s^{-1})	Relative signal (at $b=1000$)
CSF	2.94	0.05
Grey matter	0.76	0.47
White matter	0.45	0.63
White matter parallel to fibres	0.95	0.39

The diffusion coefficient D is measured in units of mm^2 s^{-1}. At room temperature pure water has a value of D approximately 2.2×10^{-3} mm^2 s^{-1}. With a b of 1000, the water signal will be reduced to 11% of its unweighted value. Typical tissue values are given in table 16.1.

16.3.2 Anisotropy

Pure water is said to have isotropic diffusion properties, meaning that the molecules are equally likely to wander off in any direction. So the diffusion gradients can be applied in any physical direction and the effect on the MR signal should be the same. In many

The diffusion coefficient – apparently

In practice what we measure in PGSE is related to the actual diffusion coefficient but may contain contributions from other movement sources. Microcirculation in pseudo-random capillary systems is one such source of incoherent-intravoxel motion. Bulk flow and motion will also seriously degrade the measurements and lead to image artefacts. Additionally the imaging gradients can contribute to the diffusion weighting, although with large diffusion gradients this effect is normally minimal. Because of this we usually refer to the apparent diffusion coefficient or ADC, which can be calculated from

$$\text{ADC image} = \frac{-1}{b}\ln\left(\frac{\text{DW image}}{\text{T}_2\text{w image}}\right)$$

for cases where an equal TE applies to both weighted and unweighted images. Alternatively a range of b-values can be applied and a 'least-squares' fit can be performed. This should give a more accurate value of ADC.

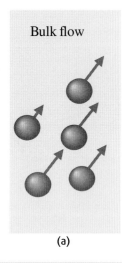

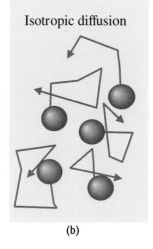

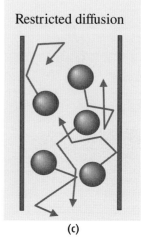

Figure 16.8 Three types of molecular motion (indicated by arrows) which may occur in tissue in (a) bulk flow, (b) isotropic diffusion where molecular motion is random and (c) restricted diffusion where random motion is constrained by physical barriers, e.g. by cell membranes.

Bulk flow (a)   Isotropic diffusion (b)   Restricted diffusion (c)

Diffusion tensor imaging (DTI)

For anisotropic tissues, the physical orientation of the tissue (e.g. fibre direction) in conjunction with the applied gradient direction will determine the signal intensity. If these two directions are the same, there is no problem, but usually this is not true. In this most general case the diffusion properties are described mathematically by a tensor. A tensor is a matrix of values. The diffusion tensor has nine such values, each corresponding to a gradient orientation and a cell orientation. The diffusion tensor is

$$DT = \begin{bmatrix} D_{xx} & D_{xy} & D_{xz} \\ D_{yx} & D_{yy} & D_{yz} \\ D_{zx} & D_{zy} & D_{zz} \end{bmatrix}$$

The first subscript (x, y, z) refers to the 'natural' orientation of the cells or tissue, and the second refers to the gradient orientation. The so-called orthogonal elements D_{xx} and D_{yy} and D_{zz} correspond to the simple three direction measurements found in commercial scanners. To make a full measurement of ADC in an anisotropic tissue all these components plus a $b = 0$ unweighted image is required. In practice there is a degree of redundancy (because D_{xy} is the same as D_{yx}, etc.) and only seven measurements are required, six tensor components and an unweighted $(b = 0)$ image.

Once the tensor terms have been found, the diffusivity can be described by three eigenvalues that describe the axes of an ellipsoid, which may be thought of as the 'diffusion space' of the protons. The display of such complex information is fairly difficult but a promising method is that of tractography, where the principal direction or eigenvector is traced in three dimensions. The resultant images display a striking resemblance to actual bundles of fibre tracts (figure 16.10, see colour section). Such methodology offers promise in determining connectivity between different parts of the brain.

From the diffusion tensor a so-called scalar invariant known as the trace diffusion constant can be computed as

$$Trace(D) = D_{xx} + D_{yy} + D_{zz}$$

from which an average ADC is obtained, equal to

$$\frac{1}{3} Trace(D).$$

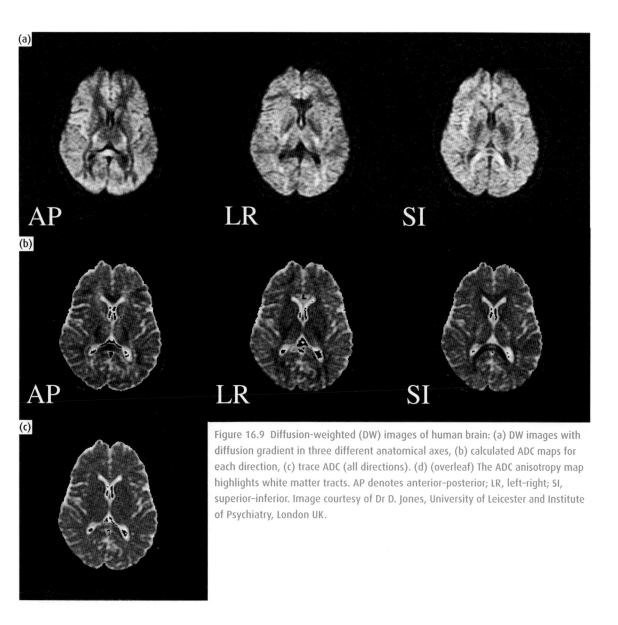

Figure 16.9 Diffusion-weighted (DW) images of human brain: (a) DW images with diffusion gradient in three different anatomical axes, (b) calculated ADC maps for each direction, (c) trace ADC (all directions). (d) (overleaf) The ADC anisotropy map highlights white matter tracts. AP denotes anterior–posterior; LR, left–right; SI, superior–inferior. Image courtesy of Dr D. Jones, University of Leicester and Institute of Psychiatry, London UK.

biological tissues (and especially white matter tracts) diffusion is restricted by the presence of cell membranes and there may be a preferential direction, e.g. along nerve fibres.

This type of diffusion behaviour is called anisotropic. The measurement of the degree of diffusion anisotropy can yield useful biological information on the tissue's microstructure, e.g. degree of myelination. To measure

anisotropy it is necessary to apply diffusion weighting on different axes, commonly the three principal axes of the scanner. The effect of this on a normal brain is shown in figure 16.9 as raw diffusion-weighted images and ADC maps. Colour maps (figure 16.9(e), colour section) for fractional anisotropy provide a way of displaying two types of information simultaneously: the hue represents the principal direction of the anisotropy

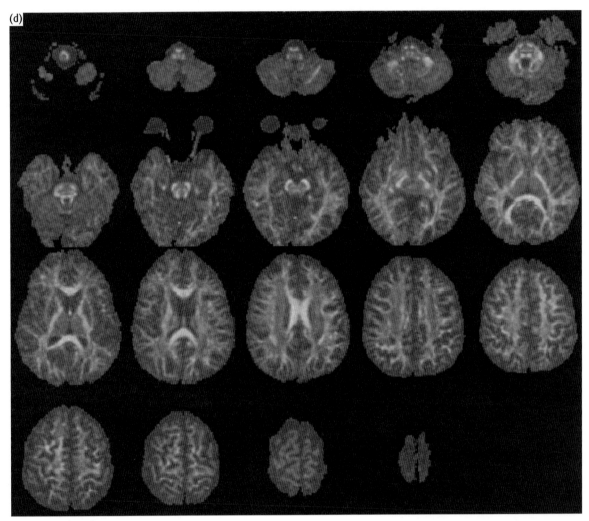

(d)

Figure 16.9 (*cont.*)

and brightness represents how strongly anisotropic the diffusion is within that voxel.

16.3.3 Diffusion sequences

Spin-echo EPI is the sequence of choice for DW imaging. Its very rapid acquisition time means that very little motion-induced artefact is encountered. The PGSE portion is appended to the front of the sequence as a preparation phase. Often sequences will be arranged to provide multiple images with a range of dif-

fusion directions and *b*-values, and sometimes the scanner software will calculate an ADC map. Because of the need to have a reasonable diffusion time in the PGSE preparation, the TE value is normally quite high, typically greater than 100 ms.

Conventional sequences such as spin echo can also be used for DW imaging. However, their long scan times render the images very sensitive to bulk motion. One way to address this is to apply corrections through the use of navigator echoes. Other fast sequences can be used for DW imaging, including turbo-FLASH, RARE

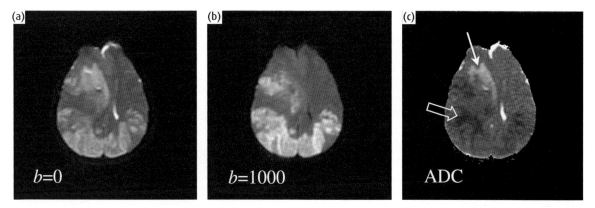

Figure 16.11 DW imaging of a stroke patient: (a) EPI image with b = 0, (b) b = 1000, (c) calculated ADC map. Notice that the ADC is depressed in areas where the DW image is bright. Also notice the signal elevation in the b = 0 image. This is caused by increased T_2 rather than by diffusion changes. Acute infarcts have reduced ADC (open arrow) while chronic infarcts have elevated ADC (arrow).

and time-reversed GE (see Chapter 12). These all have their inherent problems and to date none has rivalled spin-echo EPI.

16.3.4 Clinical applications

The major clinical application of DW imaging is in the investigation of ischaemic stroke, particularly in distinguishing between the acute ischaemia and chronic infarction (figure 16.11). Ischaemic stroke, arising from thrombotic or embolic occlusion of a cerebral artery, leads to cell swelling or cytotoxic oedema which results in a depressed ADC. Acute stroke thus displays hyperintense (bright) on DW imaging. These changes are apparent in under an hour on DW imaging (compared with over 6 h on CT or 12 h on T_2-weighted MRI). ADC maps are preferable to the raw DW images in order to rule out so-called T_2 shine-through. The ADC continues to reduce with a minimum between 1 and 4 days, thereafter it recovers over 5–10 days, and finally remains elevated compared with the nonischaemic value. DW imaging can act as a valuable guide to prognosis and management. It can also help to distinguish between acute stroke and other conditions with acute neurological deficits such as transient ischaemic attacks and atypical migraine, which show no abnormality in DW imaging. Another important application is in neonatal

ischaemia, particularly for detecting acute and subacute infarction in unmyelinated white matter. Other developing roles for DW imaging include differentiating solid tumours from cystic ones, and for trauma, haemorrhage and infections.

16.4 Perfusion imaging

Perfusion is a term that has different meanings to different professionals. Biotechnologists use it to mean the process of keeping tissues alive in a solution containing all the vital nutrients. In MRI it has a much more specific meaning, and refers to the capillary blood supply to a tissue, measured in ml min^{-1} g^{-1}. In the brain this is usually called the cerebral blood flow (CBF) or simply f. Two other measures are commonly used in perfusion MRI, the cerebral blood volume (CBV) and mean transit time (MTT). Often these terms are prefixed with 'r' (rCBF, rCBV and rMTT) meaning 'relative', since it is difficult to quantify them absolutely and it is usually preferable to find a ratio between the ipsi- and contralateral sides.

Two MRI techniques for imaging perfusion have been developed in the last few years, both using a contrast agent to distinguish perfused tissue from unperfused, primarily for neurological applications. (See chapter 14 for cardiac perfusion.) The quicker method is to image the required slices rapidly and repeatedly during the first pass of a gadolinium bolus, sometimes referred to as 'dynamic susceptibility contrast MRI' (DSC-MRI). The other technique tags protons in the arterial blood supply with a magnetic 'label', then images the required slices with and without the labelling. Although a slower technique with poor signal-to-noise ratio (SNR), it is completely noninvasive and can be repeated as often as required (without having to wait for excretion of the gadolinium). It is known as 'arterial spin labelling' or 'arterial spin tagging', and there are several variations on this basic theme (which produce another rash of acronyms!). We will start by considering DSC-MRI, which to date has been more popular in clinical applications.

16.4.1 Dynamic susceptibility contrast MRI

In DSC-MRI a volume of tissue, usually only a few slices, is imaged repeatedly using an EPI sequence. After a few images have been collected as a baseline, a bolus of gadolinium is injected as fast as possible. During the first pass through the intracranial circulation the gadolinium remains in the vasculature, causing a reduction of T_2 and T_2^*, which is seen as a dramatic drop in signal intensity on T_2-weighted or T_2^*-weighted images (figure 16.12). The second pass may also be detected as a slight drop in intensity, before the signal returns to baseline. The whole imaging sequence takes no more than 2–3 min.

Originally gradient-echo EPI sequences were used for DSC-MRI since they are most sensitive to changes in T_2^*. However, it is now more usual to use spin-echo EPI and measure changes in T_2, which has been shown to be due only to the microcirculation, excluding the confounding signals from larger arteries and veins. A TE of 35–60 ms is used to detect the T_2 changes, with a TR of no more than 1500 ms in order to maintain reasonable temporal resolution. This rather short TR usually restricts the volume coverage even on a system with high-power gradients, since only a few slices may be acquired in such a TR. The exception is on Philips scanners with a whole-head perfusion sequence called PRESTO, which uses a time-reversed gradient-echo

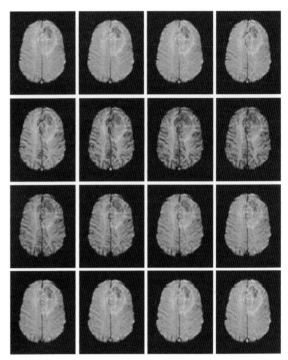

Figure 16.12 Sixteen images from a DSC-MRI examination of a low-grade glioma as the bolus of gadolinium passes through the vasculature. Time runs from left to right then down the rows, temporal resolution 1.2 s. As the bolus of gadolinium passes through the vasculature the signal intensities drop because of reductions in T_2^*.

sequence to produce a Hahn echo collected by an EPI acquisition. There should be at least five images (time points) in the baseline section for analysis purposes; since a bolus injection in the antecubital vein typically takes 8–10 s to reach the brain, the injection should be started soon after the start of the imaging sequence. Many groups regard a power injector as essential, as an injection rate of 3–5 ml s^{-1} is necessary to achieve a good bolus. (Contrast this with the requirements for contrast-enhanced MRA, where the timing of the injection is more critical relative to the image acquisition and the bolus shape should be rather longer.) If the injection is performed by hand, large gauge IV tubing with a minimum of connections and a mechanism for rapidly switching to saline flush should be used. It is also possible to make rapid hand injection easier by

Advanced processing and quantification

The starting point for perfusion quantification, or for generating parametric maps, is to find the Gd concentration as a function of time for each voxel, $C_{tissue}(t)$. This can be done by assuming an inverse linear relationship between the T_2 of the tissue and $C_{tissue}(t)$:

$$C_{tissue}(t) \propto \frac{1}{\Delta T_2} = -\frac{1}{TE} \cdot \ln\left[\frac{S_{tissue}(t)}{S_{tissue}(0)}\right]$$

where $S_{tissue}(t)$ is the tissue signal intensity at time t and $S_{tissue}(0)$ is the initial baseline signal intensity. From the concentration-time curve (figure 16.14) we can measure some simple parameters such as the time of arrival (t_{arr}), time to peak (t_p) and maximum concentration C_p. Maps of these parameters are particularly useful in stroke studies, where a delayed t_{arr} is an indication of collateral blood supply. However they are sensitive to differences in the bolus injection, which is a good reason for using a power injector in perfusion studies.

For more accurate quantification, we use indicator dilution theory (see Further reading for some useful references). This is a well-known model which describes how an indicator (gadolinium) is distributed (diluted) in the blood supply following an instantaneous bolus injection. In the ideal case of an intact blood-brain barrier, the concentration-time curve has a gamma-variate shape:

$$C_{ideal}(t) = C_p \cdot \left(\frac{e}{rs}\right)^r \cdot (t - t_{arr})^r \cdot \exp\left(-\frac{(t - t_{arr})}{s}\right)$$

where e is exp(1), $e \approx 2.718$. r and s are related to the rate of increase and rate of decrease respectively. Of course the bolus is certainly not ideal, and the tissue concentration curve is modified by the shape of the input concentration curve, known as the arterial input function, $AIF(t)$. Mathematically this is a convolution,

$$C_{tissue}(t) = C_{ideal}(t) \otimes AIF(t)$$

which means that if we measure the AIF, typically in a cerebral artery, we can find the ideal concentration-time curve by deconvolution. To do this, we divide the Fourier transform of $C_{tissue}(t)$ by the Fourier transform of $AIF(t)$ and take the inverse Fourier transform of the result:

$$C_{ideal}(t) = FT^{-1}\left\{\frac{FT(C_{tissue}(t))}{FT(AIF(t))}\right\}$$

It is usual to fit a gamma-variate curve to the measured $C_{ideal}(t)$, using $r = s = $ full-width-half-maximum as starting values for the fitting (figure 16.15). The fitted curve $C_{fit}(t)$ can then be integrated to provide the cerebral blood volume CBV, mean transit time MTT, and cerebral blood flow CBF:

$$CBV = \frac{\kappa}{\rho} \int C_{fit}(t)\,dt$$

$$MTT = \frac{\int t \cdot C_{fit}(t)\,dt}{\int C_{fit}(t)\,dt}$$

$$CBF = \frac{CBV}{MTT}$$

where ρ is the density of brain tissue and κ is a constant that accounts for the difference in haematocrit between large and small vessels.

There are many problems associated with quantification of perfusion from Gd bolus studies, not least being the requirement for good SNR for both the deconvolution and the fitting process. However with care it is possible to achieve reliable results.

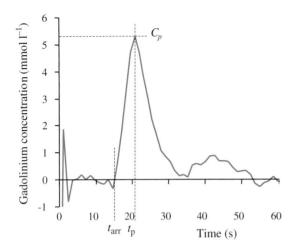

Figure 16.14 Concentration–time curve for white matter, showing the definition of various summary parameters. C_p denotes peak height; t_{arr} bolus time arrival and t_p time to peak.

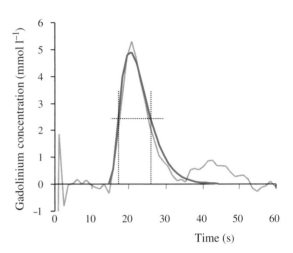

Figure 16.15 Gamma-variate fitting to the concentration–time curve. Starting points for the fitting parameters are found from the peak height and the times of the two half-heights.

warming the gadolinium to body temperature which reduces the viscosity by a factor of two. Repeated imaging of the volume should continue for a total of 2–3 min, subject to the limitations of the scanner.

Analysis of all these images in the clinical setting is best done with proprietary software on a workstation, although for quantitative results or research work it may be better to use home-written software which can be well controlled. Most software produces pixel-by-pixel maps of the required parameters and often colour scales are used for display (figure 16.13, see colour section), giving a similar 'look' to nuclear medicine or PET scans. At a simple level, so-called summary parameters can be measured directly from the signal intensity curves; for example, the area under the curve (or 'negative enhancement integral'), the bolus arrival time (t_{arr}) and the time to peak (t_p), and the peak height (C_p). These are roughly related to rCBV, rMTT and rCBF respectively, but have the disadvantage that they depend strongly on the shape of the bolus.

Full analysis for quantification uses deconvolution of the shape of the injected bolus, known as the arterial input function (AIF). This can be measured in the middle cerebral artery or any other easily identifiable vessel, but caution should be exercised in patients

with stroke who may not have a normal arterial supply. Good SNR is essential for the deconvolution to work successfully and it is common to use spatial filtering (smoothing) to reduce the noise level in the images.

16.4.2 Arterial spin labelling

Arterial **S**pin **L**abelling (ASL) imaging is based on magnetically labelling protons in the arterial blood supply, usually with an inversion pulse. When images are then acquired from slices in the brain, there will be a very small signal loss compared with unlabelled images. This is because there is an inflow enhancement even in the capillaries. The label decays in only 4–5 s due to T_1 relaxation of the blood protons, so EPI is used for the image acquisition. There are several different ASL techniques, differing mainly in the way they apply the labelling and control pulses. We will only describe one, **F**low-sensitive **A**lternating **I**nversion **R**ecovery (FAIR), in order to illustrate the principles. You should check out the references at the end of this chapter for the other ASL techniques.

In the FAIR labelled images, an inversion pulse is applied to the whole brain before a single-slice EPI

Nonselective inversion

Image slice

Slice-selective inversion

Image slice

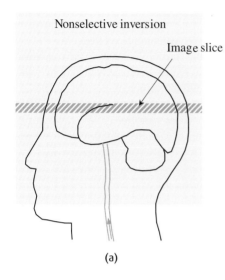

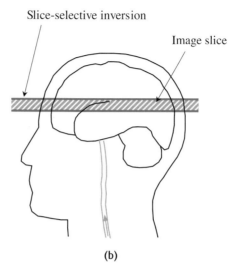

(a)

(b)

Figure 16.16 Schematic diagram for FAIR: (a) the labelled image is produced by applying a nonselective inversion pulse to the whole head while (b) the control image is produced with a slice-selective inversion pulse slightly wider than the image slice thickness.

image is acquired (figure 16.16). For the control experiment the inversion pulse is applied only to the imaged slice. In the labelled image, inverted protons in the arterial supply are carried into the capillary bed of the imaged slice and exchange with protons in the tissues. Depending on the time delay between inversion and imaging, the signal intensity of protons in perfused tissue is reduced. In the control experiment, arterial blood protons are unlabelled and the image will have a slightly higher SNR overall. Large bipolar crusher gradients (effectively diffusion weighting) are added to the pulse sequence to remove the signal in larger blood vessels, so one of the advantages of ASL over DSC-MRI is that it only measures capillary perfusion.

ASL suffers from several problems so currently it is mainly used in research centres. Chief among these problems is the very low SNR of the signal difference between the labelled and control images, even if the labelling efficiency is nearly 100% (which in practice is impossible to achieve). Many signal averages are necessary to overcome this, which extends the imaging time. A delay between labelling and imaging is necessary to allow time for the labelled protons to reach the imaged slice, but this very delay reduces the magnitude of the label. Another disadvantage is that only CBF maps are produced (figure 16.17), not CBV or MTT, and the latter in particular has been found to be very useful in stroke.

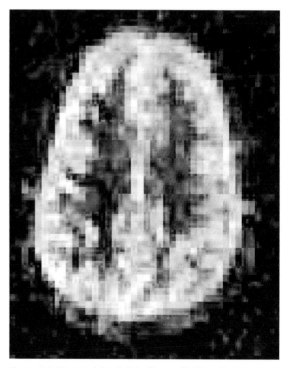

Figure 16.17 Arterial spin labelling perfusion map in a normal subject, showing higher perfusion as bright signal intensity. Grey matter has 2–3 times more blood flow per unit volume than white matter, in agreement with positron emission tomography (PET) studies.

ASL analysis

The difference in signal intensity can be shown to be related to M_0, T_1 and perfusion of the tissue. The theory for ASL is not derived from the indicator dilution theory, since the tracer (labelled water) is freely diffusible whereas gadolinium is merely transported by the blood. Instead the theory is derived from the Bloch equations using a two-compartment exchange model for water in the blood and tissues. For the FAIR technique

$$\Delta M = 2M_0 \frac{f}{\lambda} \left[\frac{\exp(-\text{TI} \cdot R_{1a}) - \exp(-\text{TI} \cdot R_1)}{R_1 - R_{1a}} \right]$$

where f is tissue perfusion, TI is the inversion time, R_1 is the relaxation rate $(1/T_1)$ of the tissue and R_{1a} is the relaxation rate of arterial blood. λ is a constant called the blood–brain water partition coefficient, which is usually assumed to be 0.9 (i.e. 90% of water is in the brain tissues and only 10% in the intracranial blood vessels). Although literature values for M_0 and T_1 could be used in theory, in practice it is usual to acquire images at a series of TIs, and to calculate M_0 and T_1 maps from the control images. With the M_0 and T_1 maps the signal differences can be fitted to the above equation to produce a perfusion map (figure 16.17).

However, it does have the advantage that ASL is sensitive to brain activation (in fact the sequence was first developed to measure activity – an alternative to the BOLD mechanism described in the next section) and it seems likely that in the future this will be a significant application of the techniques.

16.5 Brain activation mapping using the BOLD effect

In recent years the term functional MRI or fMRI (note the small 'f') has become synonymous with brain activation imaging using the BOLD effect. This is in some ways related to ASL perfusion imaging, except that intrinsic T_2^* contrast rather than T_1 contrast is utilized. In BOLD fMRI we 'see the brain thinking'.

16.5.1 The BOLD effect

The BOLD (**B**lood **O**xygenation **L**evel **D**ependent) effect was observed at the start of the 1990s in animal-based experiments. It was known that oxyhaemoglobin is diamagnetic (i.e. essentially nonmagnetic) and that deoxyhaemoglobin is paramagnetic. This means that deoxygenated blood has a shorter T_2^* and hence lower MR signal than fully oxygenated blood. That the opposite was observed in visual cortex during sensory stimulation was initially surprising – the MR signal increasing or 'lighting up' at times when oxygen consumption was heightened due to neuronal activity as in figure 16.18. The scientific consensus is now that the increased consumption of oxygen by neurones during activation is accompanied by a disproportionate

Brain or vein

In fMRI we detect blood oxygenation changes in the draining veins, i.e. downstream from the actual activation site (figure 16.18). The difference in magnetic susceptibility between fully oxygenated and deoxygenated blood is about 9.5×10^{-7}. However fully oxygenated blood has a magnetic susceptibility χ similar to that of the extra-vascular space in grey matter and so differences in oxygenation will affect the local field homogeneity and therefore change T_2^*.

The BOLD effect during activation is illustrated in figure 16.18 where following neuronal activity, although there is a greater number of de-oxygenated red blood cells, the increase in fresh oxygenated blood delivery results in a reduction of the concentration of de-oxyhaemoglobin and therefore T_2^* increases as does the MR signal.

MR perfusion can also detect neuronal activation by its sensitivity to the blood flow changes in the capillaries. It is thought that perfusion fMRI may pinpoint the actual activation site more directly than BOLD fMRI, although the sensitivity of BOLD is higher. The localised blood flow changes in activation can also be detected using non-EPI sequences such as spoiled gradient echo, although the high sensitivity to flow may result in vessels on the cortical surface being mistaken for activation.

Rest

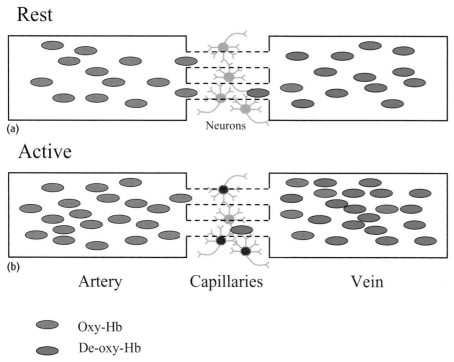

Active

Oxy-Hb

De-oxy-Hb

Figure 16.18 The origin of the BOLD effect. In activation (below) the over-provision of fully oxygenated blood leads to a reduction in de-oxy-Hb and an increase in local T_2^* in the draining veins compared with the rest condition (above).

increase in the supply of fully oxygenated blood, so that downstream from the site of activation the concentration of deoxyhaemoglobin decreases and so T_2^* is elevated and the MR signal increases. Gradient-echo EPI, with its strong T_2^* weighting, is the sequence of choice for many fMRI examinations.

16.5.2 fMRI acquisitions

To say that the 'brain lights up' during activation is a bit of an exaggeration as the actual signal intensity changes are no more than a few percent. In fMRI we detect these by modulating the oxygenation level at the site of brain activity and look for correlated signal changes. Rapid scanning, usually with EPI, is carried out continuously whilst the subject performs various mental tasks (known as the paradigm). These are commonly arranged in a block design with periods of activity interspersed with periods of contrasting activity or rest. The periods of activity might involve motor tasks, stimulus presentation or cognitive activity (e.g. generating words, doing mental arithmetic, etc.). A block length or 'epoch' will

typically be about 30 s with perhaps three or four complete cycles of the two contrasting tasks. This is shown in figure 16.19 for a simple on-off visual stimulus and in the box 'A typical clinical fMRI protocol'.

Block design paradigms are robust and simple to arrange. However, for some mental tasks it may be difficult to generate extended periods of activation to form an epoch. Some brain events, e.g. hallucinations resulting from psychosis, may be of a transient and unpredictable nature. One solution to this is to use so-called event-related (ER) fMRI. In ER-fMRI scanning is carried out continuously at a higher image acquisition rate (e.g. once per second) and we simply wait until the event occurs and look for corresponding changes in the MR signal that resemble the haemodynamic response of activation (see box 'Haemodynamic delay and convolution').

Having acquired the time series of scans, there is much post processing required. This is normally done off-line on an independent computer. Finally an image is produced that represents the statistical significance of signal changes correlated with the paradigm.

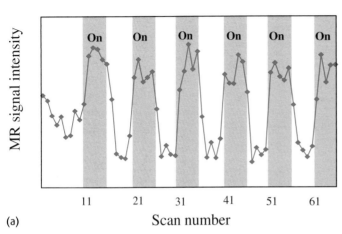

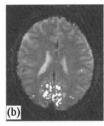

(b)

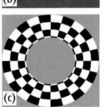

(c)

(a)   Scan number

Figure 16.19 (a) fMRI BOLD signal changes and (b) area of activation in the visual cortex resulting from (c) a visual (reversing chequerboard) paradigm. The first scans are used to establish equilibrium and are discarded from the analysis. A haemodynamic delay is apparent between the paradigm changes and the signal response.

A typical clinical fMRI protocol

Scout scan	Three orthogonal views.
EPI scan 1	Twenty transverse slices parallel to the anterior commissure–posterior commissure (AC–PC) line, 5 mm slice thickness, 1 mm slice gap, inplane resolution 64×64 or 128×128, 220 mm field of view, 35–50 volume acquisitions, interscan interval ('TR') 3–6 s. Alternating epochs of activity and rest of 30 s duration each. Scan time 5 min. Paradigm – left hand finger motion versus rest.
EPI scan 2	Parameters as above. Scan time 5 min. Paradigm – right hand finger motion versus rest.
3D structural scan	MP-RAGE $256 \times 256 \times 128$. Scan time 8 min

Total examination time approximately 20 min plus patient handling time.

16.5.3 fMRI processing

The common steps of fMRI processing are illustrated in figure 16.20. First the images are re-aligned or coregis-

Data meltdown

A typical fMRI scan may involve 24 slices of the brain, acquired with in-plane resolution of 128×128. We may collect 100 volumes in a single run, performing several runs on each subject. By the time we have done all the processing the data volume will have been at least trebled or quadrupled.

$$\text{Total raw data} = 24 \times 128 \times 128 \times 100$$

$$= 39\,321\,600 \text{ voxels}$$

$$= 80 \text{ MB}$$

and this represents 5 min scanning only. Generating several gigabytes (1 GB = 1000 MB) in one day is not hard.

tered with themselves. This is necessary because even the smallest shift in the position of a voxel can generate significant signal changes. Stimulus-correlated motion would result in false-positive 'activations' unless removed in this way. Normally the first few volumes will be discarded to ensure that the magnetization is in a steady state, usually required for the realignment algorithm to be accurate. Postacquisition re-alignment is required even if prospective slice positioning using navigator echoes has been used for the acquisition.

A second step is to spatially normalize the images to a standard brain space, often to the Talairach Brain

Atlas. This aids the neurological interpretation of the resultant activation maps and it also allows data to be averaged over groups of subjects. For individual patients with structural brain abnormalities or tumours this step is omitted.

The third step is to smooth the data. This helps to boost the SNR but has to be applied carefully to avoid excessive loss of spatial resolution. A fourth step may be to de-trend or normalize the data according to an overall or global mean or to apply a high-pass temporal filter. This step is designed to remove any bias resulting from scanner drift, for example, over the acquisition.

Next statistics are calculated. Various levels of sophistication are involved here but the simplest is to subtract the rest images from the active images and look for significant increases in signal, characterized by the Z-score defined as

$$Z = \frac{\text{mean signal difference}}{\text{standard deviation}}$$

In practice Z needs to be greater than 3 for any degree of confidence in the results. Z-scores are related to p-values commonly quoted with regard to the normal distribution (T-test). The resulting brain activation map is made by displaying only those voxels that have the appropriate statistical parameter (e.g. Z-score, p-value) greater than a given statistical threshold. Sometimes spatial extent thresholding is carried out to exclude isolated voxels or small groups and only show clusters of activation. Sophisticated analyses can be applied to obtain better inferences of the statistical significance of clusters of activated voxels. A number of statistical approaches other than T-tests are possible, including correlation, Fourier, wavelet and independent component analyses. Software packages are available through the academic domain as well as those supplied by MR manufacturers. It is common for an fMRI statistics program to model the haemodynamic effect either by introducing a fixed or variable time delay, or by a more complex convolution of the paradigm waveform over the time series with a notional haemodynamic response curve.

Finally the resultant statistical maps are combined with underlying anatomical information. It should be recognized that there may not be full geometric correspondence between the EPI BOLD images and the anatomical images (unless a similar EPI protocol is used for both). This is due to the inherent image quality limitations of EPI.

16.5.4 Interpreting fMRI: 'blobology'

What are we looking at in a functional MR image? fMRI brain activation maps are normally presented as coloured 'blobs' superimposed on a grey-scale anatomical background image, or as a colour overlay on a 3D surface-rendered image of cortical grey matter as in figure 16.21 (see colour section).

Haemodynamic delay and convolution

One of the complexities of BOLD imaging is that the effect we are detecting lags behind the actual firing of the neurones by as much as 6 s. This is known as the haemodynamic delay and can be allowed for in the data analysis. Similarly the effect will outlast the neural activation to a similar degree. This makes the temporal resolution of fMRI rather limited. There is also a considerable undershoot post-activation. The effects of the delay and undershoot can be seen in the actual data of figure 16.19 and schematically in figure 16.20.

Mathematically the combination of haemodynamic delay with the stimulus waveform, a boxcar or series of impulses, can be described by a convolution process. By deconvolution of the actual response the haemodynamic response function (HRF) may be obtained. In the case of an impulse stimulus (because of the mathematical properties of the delta-function) the MR signal intensity changes can directly yield the HRF although correction for the exact timing of the slices with respect to the stimulus timing is required.

One further feature of the HRF is an initial MR signal dip, thought to be due to the initial oxygen consumption increase, before the increase in blood delivery which causes the BOLD signal kicks in. This dip is usually too rapid to be observed with standard EPI sequences.

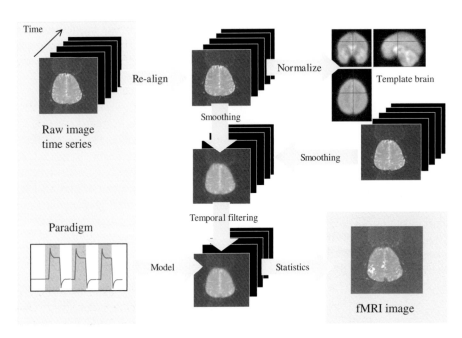

Figure 16.20 fMRI processing from the input of a time series of EPI data and a paradigm. The final image is a superposition of a statistical map on a raw image.

It is important to understand that the coloured blobs do not themselves signify brain activation, but represent areas of statistically different MR signals. The intensity of the colour represents the degree of statistical confidence that a voxel value or a group of voxels has changed according to the 'paradigm'. Actual signal changes may only be a small percentage or less. For this and other reasons the clinical interpretation of individual fMRI examinations is fraught with difficulty. BOLD signals can go down as well as up, and this so-called deactivation may be artefactual, due to inhibitory brain processes, or simply the result of the subject's mental processes, e.g. shifts in attention.

16.5.5 Clinical fMRI

Clinical fMRI can be used for patient selection and presurgical planning for epilepsy surgery or resection of brain tumours, or in the clinical evaluation of brain plasticity following injury. It can help with decision-making for patients with low-grade astrocytomas and arterio-venous malformations (AVMs) who have slight neurological impairments. It may be used in repeat studies for patients with slow growing tumours or congenital lesions. Most clinical examinations are of the motor cortex for hand, foot and facial movement control (figure 16.21(a), colour section). One specialized but promising application is in the determination of the hemispheric dominance of language, as an alternative to the invasive Wada test.

Typically in clinical fMRI the question is, 'if we operate, how close will the surgeons have to go to particular key functional areas of the brain?' Getting a definitive answer to this is difficult for a number of reasons. Patients may have some brain abnormality, AVM, tumour, etc., which makes spatial normalization to a standard brain atlas impossible. They may have impaired ability to cooperate, e.g. patients with an impaired motor function, and may find it harder to keep still when exercising their affected side. There is much scope for error and misinterpretation arising from false-positive and false-negative responses. Presurgical fMRI findings can be confirmed at the time of operation by direct electrical stimulation in the open skull situation. Further research will determine the role for fMRI in psychiatric illness.

16.5.6 Paradigm shift

fMRI is extremely difficult to do well. Very good subject cooperation is required, even a small degree of patient head movement is intolerable, and there are lots of data

T_2^* wars: the field strength question

As the BOLD effect is related to MR susceptibility, it should increase with field strength. Add to this the increase in SNR with B_0 and we would therefore expect the sensitivity of BOLD experiments to increase dramatically with the field strength. Reports in the literature suggest an increase in BOLD contrast of 30-40% for simple sensory-motor activations for 3 T compared with 1.5 T. However the overall picture is not clear as T_2^* is reduced at higher field strengths (T_2^* depends upon the field inhomogeneity in absolute units, i.e. microtesla). Moreover, in areas of particular neurological significance, e.g. the frontal or temporal lobes, the distortion and signal drop-out due to susceptibility differences may be excessive. Improving upon this is a particular focus of high-B_0 MRI research.

and much complicated analysis; but, more fundamentally, the paradigm itself may be flawed. Except for simple sensorimotor fMRI, it is quite hard to be certain that the subject is actually performing the task properly. Overt speech generally causes excessive head motion. Moreover, for subtle cognitive effects, the paradigm has to be psychologically effective, easily transferable to the inside of a scanner and capable of generating detectable BOLD responses. The scanner environment, with its excessive noise and claustrophobia-inducing space, presents a major limitation. Special stimulus delivery systems are required for the presentation of visual and audible stimuli. Despite these technical difficulties fMRI opens up new avenues of research into cognitive neuroscience, psychiatric illness and neuropathology that are not possible with positron emission tomography (PET) due to its limited availability and the radiation dose involved.

See also:
- Section 9.3, box 'High slew rates'.
- Section 10.3 Gradient effects.

FURTHER READING

Buxton RB (2002) *An Introduction to Functional Magnetic Resonance Imaging* (Book and CD-ROM Pack). Cambridge: Cambridge University Press (ISBN: 0521002745)

Calamante F, Thomas DL, Pell GS, Wiersma J and Turner R (1999) Measuring cerebral blood flow using magnetic resonance imaging techniques. *J Cereb Blood Flow Metab* **19**: 701–35.

Mansfield P (1984) Real time echo planar imaging by NMR. *Br Med Bull* **40**: 187–90.

Moonen CTW and Bandettini PA (Eds) (2000) *Functional MRI*. Berlin: Springer-Verlag (ISBN: 354067215X)

Schmitt R, Stehling MK and Turner R (1998) *Echo-Planar Imaging: Theory, Technique and Application*. Berlin: Springer-Verlag (ISBN: 3540631941)

Talairach J and Tournoux P (1988) *Co-planar Stereotaxic Atlas of the Human Brain*. New York: Thieme. (ISBN: 3137117011)

The Parallel Universe: parallel imaging and novel acquisition techniques

17.1 Introduction

We saw in chapter 11 that rapidly switched fields can lead to peripheral nerve stimulation. As figure 17.1 shows, in order to halve the scan time, the gradient slew rate must be quadrupled. Whilst producing higher and higher gradient slew rates is merely a matter for improved engineering, there comes a point when PNS becomes inevitable and thus the ultimate speed limit of MRI is physiologically determined. This imposes an apparently non-negotiable limit on the acquisition techniques we have encountered so far in this book. So does that mean fast imaging development has ground to a standstill? Surprisingly not, as even this fundamental limitation can be overcome, (or rather, circumvented) by using parallel imaging and reconstruction techniques together with phased array technology for even faster scanning. It needs to be stressed here that parallel imaging methods are not sequences, but entirely new ways of acquiring and reconstructing images. The two classic formulations of parallel imaging are SMASH and SENSE, working in k-space and image space respectively. This chapter will explain the various types of parallel imaging and other novel reconstruction and acquisition techniques, how they work, what advantages they provide and the image quality trade-offs involved.

In this chapter we will see that parallel imaging
- makes MR acquisitions faster by a factor known as the reduction factor R,
- can be applied to any existing MR sequence, including EPI,
- is enabled by phased array technology and may be performed in k-space or in image space,

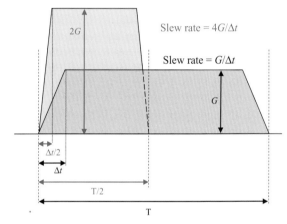

Figure 17.1 In order to halve the acquisition time whilst maintaining the same resolution and field of view, the gradient strength must be doubled and the gradient slew rate quadrupled.

- reduces the number of phase-encode steps you need to actually acquire an image,
- involves an image quality trade-off.
Additionally
- non-Cartesian acquisition methods can offer some advantages such as very short echo times, self-navigation and increased SNR.
- You will also learn lots of lovely new acronyms!

17.2 Groundwork

To understand parallel imaging we need to revisit two concepts considered earlier in the book, namely: array

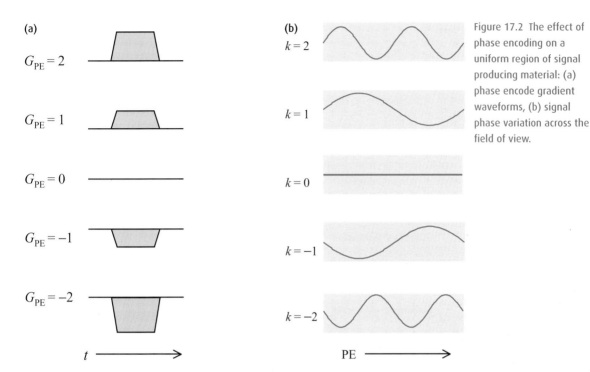

(a)

$G_{PE} = 2$

$G_{PE} = 1$

$G_{PE} = 0$

$G_{PE} = -1$

$G_{PE} = -2$

t ⟶

(b)

$k = 2$

$k = 1$

$k = 0$

$k = -1$

$k = -2$

PE ⟶

Figure 17.2 The effect of phase encoding on a uniform region of signal producing material: (a) phase encode gradient waveforms, (b) signal phase variation across the field of view.

coils (chapter 9) and phase encoding (chapter 7). If you are confident you understand both these you can skip forward to section 17.2.3.

17.2.1 Simple conceptual explanation of k-space and phase encoding

Phase encoding was explained in detail in chapter 7. For the present purpose we need to see that each phase-encode gradient step adds a further 2π of phase change across the image field of view (figure 17.2). Alternatively we can say that each line of k-space is separated by 2π/FOV. Each phase encoding step sensitises the MR acquisition to specific patterns of signal distribution, or in other words, picks out a particular spatial frequency of the image. The steps of phase encoding and signal acquisition need to be repeated until k-space is filled, prior to Fourier transformation to generate the final image. If we double the separation between the lines of k-space by skipping lines of k-space we halve the image field of view and if the imaged object exceeds this, aliasing or foldover will occur.

17.2.2 Basic principles of phased arrays

The conventional use of phased array coils is to achieve superior SNR. Each array element is sensitive to a smaller volume of tissue than an equivalent larger coil. Inductively coupled noise, which usually dominates the noise formation process, has a theoretical strong dependence on the volume of tissue to which the coil is sensitive. The smaller array elements thus 'see' less noise than larger coils (figure 17.3). Each array element has a separate receiver channel, with up to 8 channels being common. Additionally arrays benefit from the combination of uncorrelated noise sources offering the same sort of advantage that quadrature coils have over linear coils (see section 9.4.3). Separate reconstructions are carried out for each array element with the final image being a combination of these. The increased SNR can be used to achieve higher resolution, shorter scan times, greater anatomical coverage or a combination of all three. Many clinical applications would be impossible without array coils. In parallel imaging we are going to trade part of the superior SNR to give us shorter acquisition times.

17.2.3 Coil sensitivity profiles

In the conventional use of phased arrays, the images produced from each element are combined to form the resultant image. The spatial variations inherent to the individual coil responses, or the coil sensitivities, have been combined. This is illustrated in figure 17.4 where individual sensitivity profiles are shown for two coils. The determination of array element sensitivity profiles or maps and the linear combination of signals from array elements are both crucial aspects of parallel imaging.

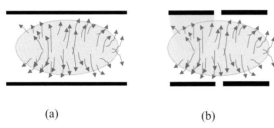

(a)   (b)

Figure 17.3 The inductive noise-reduction principle of phased array coils. (a) A larger single coil "sees" more noise from the greater volume of tissue it surrounds. (b) Smaller coil elements are less sensitive to inductive noise whilst adequate signal coverage is achieved by combining images from the separate elements.

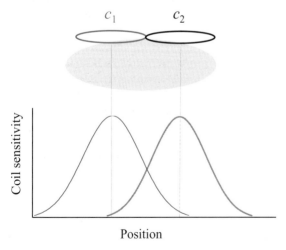

Figure 17.4 Coil sensitivity profiles: two loop surface coils.

17.3 Making SENSE: parallel imaging in image space

In parallel imaging we are going to speed up scanning by acquiring fewer lines of k-space and using our knowledge of the array coils used to unravel the aliased images or to generate the missing lines of k-space. The former technique employs parallel imaging reconstruction in image space, the latter in k-space. In both methods the scan time is reduced by a reduction factor R:

$$\text{Scan time}_{2D} = \frac{\text{NSA} \times \text{TR} \times N_{PE}}{R \times \text{ETL}}$$

where N_{PE} is the full (unreduced) PE matrix size and ETL the echo train length or turbo-factor (where appropriate) for 2D scans. For 3D scans

$$\text{Scan time}_{3D} = \frac{\text{NSA} \times \text{TR} \times N_{PE} \times N_{SS}}{R_{PE} \times R_{SS} \times \text{ETL}}$$

where R_{PE} and R_{SS} are reduction factors for each phase-encode direction.

17.3.1 SENSE

SENSE (**SENS**itivity **E**ncoding) was the first parallel imaging technique to be realised commercially (by Philips). ASSET on General Electric scanners and SPEEDER (Toshiba) are broadly similar. In SENSE a reduced k-space is acquired by using fewer phase-encode gradient steps in conjunction with phased array coil acquisition.

SENSE reconstruction works post-Fourier transformation on the images. In a conventional acquisition if we omit every second phase-encode step we will halve the scan time, but will get an aliased image. In parts of the image aliased signal is superimposed upon unaliased signal. However the position in the resultant image of the aliased signal contribution is entirely predictable from a knowledge of the field of view. What is unknown is the intensity of the aliased component. The trick in SENSE is to apply knowledge of the sensitivities of the coil elements to calculate the aliased signal component at each point.

An example with a reduction factor of 2 and two coil elements is shown in figure 17.5 where the point P in the aliased image can be seen to be composed of signal

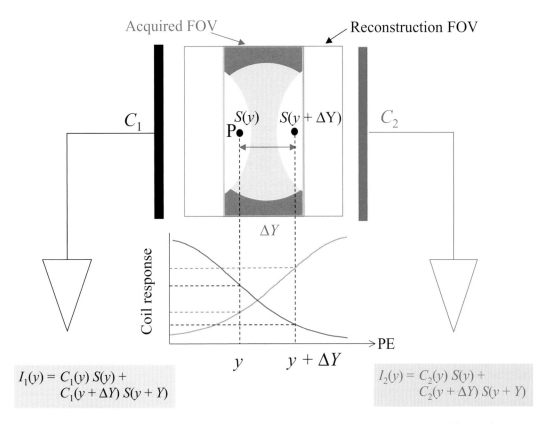

$$I_1(y) = C_1(y)\, S(y) + C_1(y + \Delta Y)\, S(y + Y)$$

$$I_2(y) = C_2(y)\, S(y) + C_2(y + \Delta Y)\, S(y + Y)$$

Figure 17.5 Image reconstruction in SENSE. Prior knowledge of the coil sensitivity profiles permits the unfolding of the image.

originating from two different locations: $S(y)$ from the true location y and $S(y + \Delta Y)$ from the aliased position. Provided we know the coil sensitivities we can calculate the true and the displaced signal components. Having computed the aliased signal component $S(y + \Delta Y)$, it can be reassigned to its proper location.

Figure 17.6 illustrates the acquisition and reconstruction with clinical images. Firstly sensitivity maps are generated for each coil element from a short, low resolution calibration scan, then an aliased image is reconstructed for each element before being fed into the SENSE reconstructor to produce the final image. The principle can be applied for a higher reduction factor R as shown in the box 'Making SENSE with maths'. For SENSE to work at all, there must be a coil sensitivity variation along the phase-encode direction. For array coils with appropriate geometry and in 3DFT acquisitions

SENSE can be applied in both phase-encode directions, thereby increasing the overall reduction factor.

Another feature of SENSE is that the reduction factor can be any value between 1 and the number of coil elements. It is not restricted to integer values. In prescribing a SENSE scan the operator chooses the reconstructed FOV. This must encompass all the signal-producing material otherwise serious artefacts will occur (figure 17.7). In other words SENSE cannot tolerate any inherent aliasing. The calibration procedure is explained further in the box 'To autocalibrate or not'.

17.3.2 mSENSE

Modified SENSE (mSENSE) is a version of SENSE which does not require a separate calibration scan. Instead additional lines are acquired at the centre of k-space

Making SENSE with maths

In the 2 coil example of figure 17.5, the signal at point y is made up of the correct signal for this position and one aliased signal. We can write

$$I_1(y) = C_1(y)S(y) + C_1(y + \Delta Y)S(y + \Delta Y)$$

$$I_2(y) = C_2(y)S(y) + C_2(y + \Delta Y)S(y + \Delta Y)$$

where I_1 and I_2 are the image intensities measured for each coil which have sensitivities C_1 and C_2. Hence we have two simultaneous equations and two unknowns which can be solved exactly by algebra. The aliasing distance ΔY is

$$\Delta Y = \frac{\text{FOV}_{\text{rec}}}{R}$$

where FOV_{rec} is the reconstruction field of view for PE and R is the SENSE reduction factor. With higher R, we may have two or more aliased signals at point y as well as the correct signal, and we can write

$$I_1(y) = C_1(y)S(y) + C_1(y + \Delta Y)S(y + \Delta Y) + \cdots + C_1(y + n_A\Delta Y)S(y + n_A\Delta Y)$$

$$I_2(y) = C_2(y)S(y) + C_2(y + \Delta Y)S(y + \Delta Y) + \cdots + C_1(y + n_A\Delta Y)S(y + n_A\Delta Y)$$

where n_A is the number of aliased signals which is spatially variant and depends on the size of the object being imaged. If the object exactly fills the reconstructed FOV, then $n_A = R$ at all points; in all other cases $n_A \leq R$. We can formalise this in terms of image intensities $I_j(x,y)$ for each of j coil elements:

$$I_j(x, y) = \sum_{n=0}^{n_A} C_j(x, y + n\Delta Y)S(x, y + n\Delta Y)$$

If there are L coil elements, we can write L simultaneous equations as above, most conveniently represented in a matrix equation as

$$\begin{bmatrix} I_1(x, y) \\ I_2(x, y) \\ \vdots \\ I_L(x, y) \end{bmatrix} = \begin{bmatrix} C_1(x, y) & C_1(x, y + \triangle Y) & \cdots & C_1(x, y + x_A\triangle Y) \\ C_2(x, y) & C_2(x, y + \triangle Y) & \cdots & C_2(x, y + x_A\triangle Y) \\ \vdots & \vdots & \ddots & \vdots \\ C_L(x, y) & C_L(x, y + \triangle Y) & \cdots & C_L(x, y + x_A\triangle Y) \end{bmatrix} \begin{bmatrix} S(x, y) \\ S(x, y + \triangle Y) \\ \vdots \\ S(x, y + n_A\triangle Y) \end{bmatrix}$$

which is more economically expressed as

$$\mathbf{I = CS}$$

and the solution arises from inverting the $L \times n_A$ element matrix $\mathbf{C}$ to obtain the true image signal $S(x,y)$ for every pixel. This is always possible if there are at least as many coil elements as the maximum number of aliased signals and if the coil sensitivities are sufficiently unique. Notice that since $R > n_A$ for the majority of images, it is possible for R to be greater than the number of elements in the coil. Pre-scan calibration data, or as in the case of mSENSE, reference lines are required to obtain the coil sensitivities.

during the diagnostic scan (figure 17.8). These central lines are extracted for each coil element and used on their own to reconstruct low resolution, unaliased, images from each coil element which may then be used to provide sensitivity maps. A SENSE reconstruction algorithm can then be used to unfold the images from the sparse k-space data (the blue arrows in figure 17.8). The full time saving by the reduction factor R is not achieved because of the additional lines required for calibration.

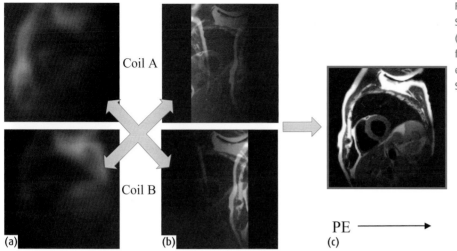

Coil A

Coil B

(a)

(b)

PE

(c)

Figure 17.6 Example of SENSE reconstruction steps: (a) reference scans, (b) folded images from each element, (c) reconstructed SENSE image.

17.4 SMASH hits: parallel imaging in k-space

Historically SMASH (**Si**Multaneous **A**cquisition of **S**patial **H**armonics) was the first parallel imaging technique. The term spatial harmonics refers to the spatial frequencies: SMASH works in k-space. It uses combinations of array coil element sensitivities to create virtual phase encoding. In principle it can be applied to any sequence. Just like SENSE it reduces the number of phase-encode gradient steps you need giving a scan time reduction by factor R.

17.4.1 SMASH

Looking back at figure 17.2 we see the signal distributions in the phase-encode direction for various values of k. The principle of SMASH is simply to generate a similar pseudo k-space phase encoding by using the spatial response of the RF reception. In practice this means using arrays of coils and combining the various elements to obtain the required sinusoidal variations in response across space.

Figure 17.9 shows how two simple linear coils could be combined to produce either a uniform response by adding the signals together, or a nonuniform response which resembles a sinusoidal variation by subtraction of the coil sensitivities. In other words by the appropri-

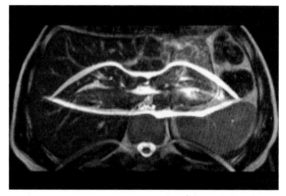

Figure 17.7 SENSE reconstruction "hot lips" artefact resulting from attempting to use SENSE when the unfolded field of view does not contain all of the anatomical region of interest.

ate combination of signals from different coil elements we can obtain a spatial signal distribution which can be made to match either zero spatial frequency (uniform response, $k = 0$) or the lowest nonzero spatial frequency ($k = 1$). In practice weighted combinations of the coil sensitivities are used. Figure 17.10 shows the coil weights necessary to produce $k = 0$ and $k = 2$ spatial harmonics for a notional 8 element array coil. Further details are given in the box 'More about spatial harmonics'.

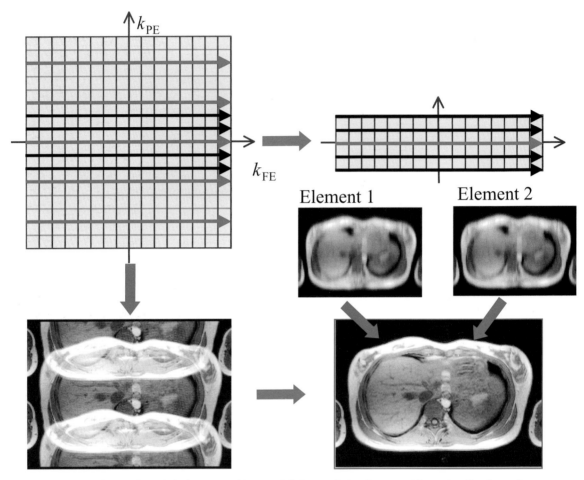

Figure 17.8 Modified SENSE (mSENSE). The centre of k-space is fully sampled and extracted for each coil to form a low resolution image which can be used as a sensitivity map in a SENSE reconstruction. Images courtesy of Siemens Medical Solutions.

This use of RF reception properties to achieve spatial encoding opens the intriguing prospect of an MR acquisition without the use of *any* phase-encode gradients. The RF engineering required to produce a sufficiently complex phased array coil is just too demanding at the moment – the coil would need at least 128 elements spread out along the phase-encode direction! Consequently in SMASH, a combination of phase encoding with gradients, and virtual phase encoding (with array coils) is applied. This is illustrated in figure 17.11 showing the phase change over the FOV for the $k = 2$ PE gradient from the uniform coil combination ($\Delta k = 0$). By combining the coils differently a modified response ($\Delta k = 1$) is obtained and when added to the effect of the gradient produces a line of virtual phase encoding with $k = 3$. Figure 17.12 shows combinations of gradient and array coil phase encoding to generate six lines of k-space from only three actual acquisitions. In this example then, we can halve the number of phase-encode gradient steps required, and therefore halve the number of excitations required and halve the scan time. The reduction factor R is therefore equal to 2.

To Auto-calibrate or not

In the calibration method used by SENSE low resolution images are acquired from each array element and also from the body coil. The array element images are divided by the body coil image (to remove sensitivity variations due to anatomy rather than coil response). Then various image processing steps (thresholding, filtering, extrapolation, smoothing) are performed to produce the sensitivity map for each coil. Note that due to the thresholding step, the background noise is suppressed in SENSE images.

The calibration scan takes about 20 seconds and once acquired can be used on all subsequent parallel image acquisitions provided the geometry or the patient's position does not change. ASSET (GE) and SPEEDER (Toshiba) also require calibration scans. ASSET does not require the body coil division step.

In mSENSE and GRAPPA (see section 17.4.3) the calibration data is inherent to the main scan acquisition. No body coil image is required and there is no image division. This means that the background noise is not suppressed. Having the calibration (ACS) lines integral to the acquisition also means that there will be no misregistration problem if the patient moves between scans. However, the scan time will be increased by the number of ACS lines used, thus the full reduction factor will not be realised. In GRAPPA, the ACS lines may also be included in the reconstruction, giving a slight increase in SNR.

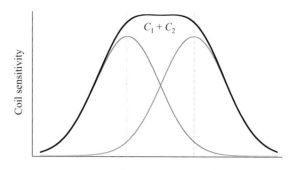

(a)

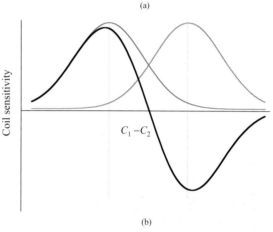

(b)

Figure 17.9 Coil sensitivity profile combinations for two loop surface coils, (a) coil combination (addition) to achieve uniform spatial response, (b) coil combination (subtraction) to produce, non-uniform spatial response.

The acquisition in k-space is illustrated in figure 17.13(a) where we see that k-space is filled completely using a sparser set of phase-encode gradient steps (represented by the blue arrows) and the synthesising of virtual phase-encode lines (the dotted lines) from the combinations of the coils.

17.4.2 Auto-calibrating SMASH

The constraints of coil design make true SMASH very hard to realise on a clinical scanner. In order to make SMASH techniques more applicable to real phased array coils a change of strategy was needed. Instead of making coils to give a 'spatial frequency-type' signal response, why not accept whatever spatial sensitivity response the coils actually give and then work out how to combine their signals to get the desired lines of k-space? The first technique to do this was Auto-SMASH. The principle is shown in figure 17.13(b) where a reduced k-space is acquired by skipping lines (e.g. every third line to give a reduction factor $R = 3$). However we also acquire additional 'auto-calibrating signal' (ACS) lines near the centre of k-space. The scanner then computes from the signals acquired from the array coil elements the nearest linear combination of these signals to match the actual acquired ACS line. The coefficients calculated can then be applied throughout the remainder of k-space to fill in

(a)

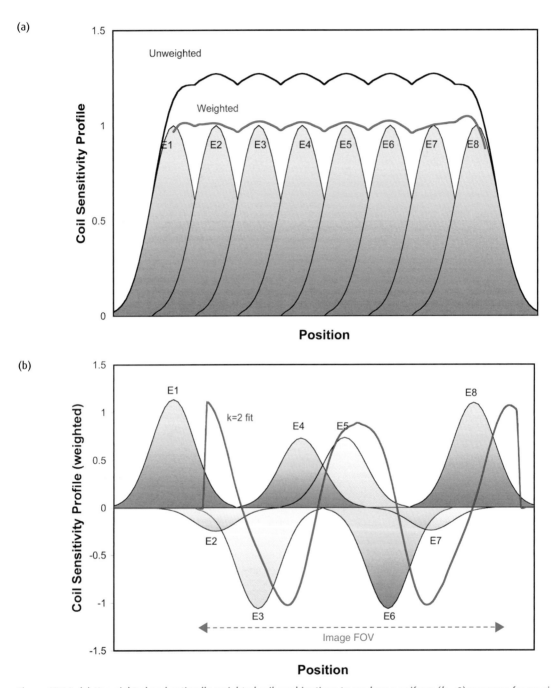

Figure 17.10 (a) Unweighted and optimally weighted coil combinations to produce a uniform ($k = 0$) response for an eight element array coil. (b) Weighted coil sensitivity functions to produce the second harmonic ($k = 2$). Grey areas represent the coil sensitivity profiles multiplied by their respective weights.

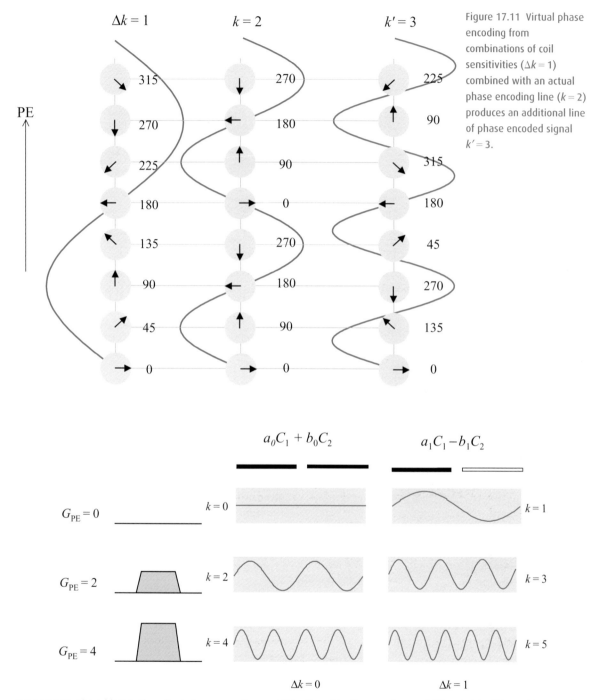

Figure 17.11 Virtual phase encoding from combinations of coil sensitivities ($\Delta k = 1$) combined with an actual phase encoding line ($k = 2$) produces an additional line of phase encoded signal $k' = 3$.

Figure 17.12 The addition of gradient phase-encoding and RF coil combinations produces additional virtual lines of k-space. In this example 2 lines of k-space can be acquired per gradient, the original with $\Delta k = 0$ and one additional with $\Delta k = 1$.

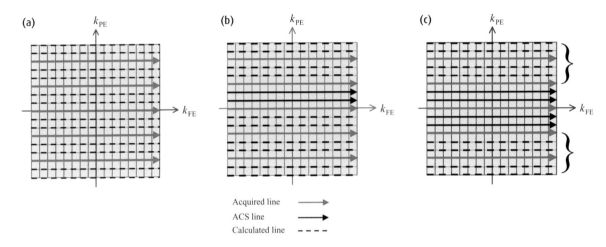

Figure 17.13 k-space scheme for (a) SMASH, (b) Auto-SMASH with 2 ACS lines and (c) VD-Auto-SMASH where an outer reduction factor (ORF) applies away from the centre of k-space. In each example $R = 3$. Arrowed lines are acquired with gradients, the interspersed (non-arrowed) lines are computed from combinations of the coil element signals. The fully filled k-space is Fourier transformed to generate the image.

More about spatial harmonics

The purpose of phase encoding is to produce a linearly varying phase change to the MR signal along the phase-encode axis, as illustrated in the clockface diagram in figure 17.11. In order to generate the rotational nature of phase encoding, we need to add sine and cosine functions (see appendices A2 and A5). Mathematically this is:

$$\exp(i\,2\pi y k_{PE}) = \cos(2\pi y k_{PE}) + i\sin(2\pi y k_{PE})$$

remembering that k-space uses complex maths. The first harmonics are shown in figure 17.14 for the example of an 8 element coil, along with the $\Delta k = 1$ combination. The figure shows both the calculated harmonics and the ideal ones.

Figure 17.14 also shows the higher harmonic, $\Delta k = 3$, for the same eight element coil, showing that significant deviations exist between the ideal and the fitted harmonics. Errors in the generation of the coefficients will result in image artefacts (see also figure 17.23).

the unacquired lines, before standard reconstruction by Fourier transformation. In practice a minimum of R-1 ACS lines are required.

Variable density Auto-SMASH (VD-Auto-SMASH) extends the above principle, but adds additional ACS lines, illustrated in figure 17.13(c). This makes it more robust from artefacts and reconstruction errors. The centre of k-space is more highly sampled and we can talk of an inner and an outer reduction factor. The scan time compared with Auto-SMASH will be longer because of the additional ACS lines. As in Auto-SMASH, a composite k-space (i.e. just one for all the array elements) is acquired and estimated.

17.4.3 GRAPPA

GRAPPA (GeneRalized Autocalibrating Partially Parallel Acquisitions) is a further extension of the Auto-SMASH principle. GRAPPA is illustrated in figure 17.15. It deploys multiple ACS lines and uses data from every coil for the fitting of the appropriate weights for each ACS line. A separate sub-k-space is filled for each array element, which is then reconstructed, giving an image for each element. These separate images are then combined by the usual 'sum-of-squares' algorithm used in

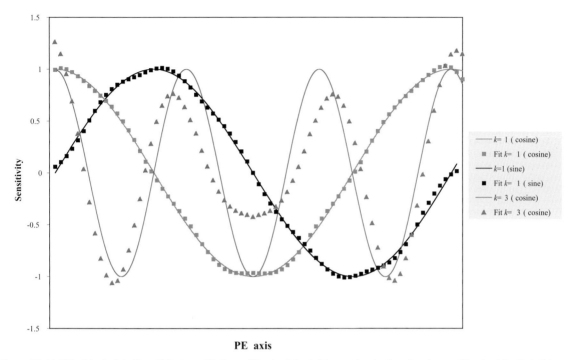

Figure 17.14 Fitted (calculated) and ideal sensitivity profiles for $\Delta k = 1$ (sine and cosine) and cosine profiles for $\Delta k = 3$. Solid lines show the ideal response, points show the weighted fits for an 8-element array.

conventional array coil reconstructions. GRAPPA has been implemented commercially in Siemens scanners where the reduction factor is known as the iPAT factor and parallel imaging (both mSENSE and GRAPPA) goes under the generic name iPAT (where PAT stands for **P**arallel **A**cquisition **T**echnique and the 'i' stands for 'integrated' - but we suspect is really just to appear trendy.)

17.5 k-t BLAST (or as we prefer to call her, Katie Blast)

This technique is very new and not yet available on any clinical systems, but it is very promising for dynamic techniques such as cardiac imaging and dynamic contrast enhancement. k-t BLAST (**B**road-use **L**inear **A**cquisition **S**peed-up **T**echnique) takes advantage of the fact that most of the image does not change at all during these acquisitions. For example in a typical short-axis cine of the heart, the chest wall, lungs, spine and muscles do not vary (much) from one frame to another. Once we have the first frame, these voxels do not need to be re-sampled during the rest of the cine. The remaining voxels can therefore be sampled quicker and provide better temporal and/or spatial resolution.

Figure 17.16 illustrates the principle for a single line through the cardiac frame. If we take the Fourier transform of this line through time, we find ourselves in x-f space, which shows the spectrum of motional frequencies. In the middle are all the voxels which do not change through the frames of the cine acquisition: out to the edges are the faster moving voxels which represent the ventricle walls and moving blood. It is obvious that most of this space is empty!

In normal imaging, every point in k-space is sampled at each of t time-points. By skipping some of the k-space points for some of the time-points, k-t space is undersampled. In x-f space, the periodic nature of the signal means that they are folded in. Reconstruction of

SMASH and k-space methods

As usual in MRI, those of a mathematical nature get it easy as the whole thing can be reduced to one equation:

$$S(k_x, k_y) = \iint \rho(x, y) \cdot C(x, y) \cdot \exp\left(\frac{-t}{T_2^*}\right) \cdot \exp(i2\pi x k_{FE}) \cdot \exp(i2\pi y k_{PE}) \cdot dxdy$$

This is similar to the equation for 2DFT given way back in chapter 7, but with one additional term: $C(x,y)$ which represents the coil sensitivities. For an array of coils with sensitivities $C_j(x,y)$

$$S(k_x, k_y) = \iint \rho(x, y) \cdot \left[\sum_j n_j C_j(x, y)\right] \cdot \exp\left(\frac{-t}{T_2^*}\right) \cdot \exp(i2\pi x k_{FE}) \cdot \exp(i2\pi y k_{PE}) \cdot dxdy$$

$$= \sum_j n_j \cdot S_j(k_{FE}, k_{PE})$$

where n_j are weighting factors for a superposition of coil and signal sensitivities. By judicious choice of weights we can obtain the combinations

$$\sum_j n_j C_j(x, y) = 1 \quad \text{or} \quad \sum_j n'_j C_j(x, y) = \exp(i2\pi \cdot y \Delta k_{PE})$$

where Δk is a step in spatial frequency.

Using the first of these yields the standard 2DFT equation for a uniform coil. Using the second gives

$$S' = \int \rho(x, y) \cdot \exp\left(\frac{-t}{T_2^*}\right) \cdot \exp(i2\pi x k_{FE}) \cdot \exp(i2\pi y [k_{PE} + \Delta k_{PE}]) \cdot dxdy$$

$$= S(k_{FE}, k_{PE} + \Delta k_{PE})$$

which is the acquired line of k-space offset by Δk. With the appropriate linear combination of coil signals we can therefore acquire purely gradient-phase-encoded signals or we can calculate additional virtual lines of k-space without having to acquire them.

In SMASH the sensitivities are computed from a calibration scan. In Auto-SMASH and GRAPPA additional auto-calibration signal (ACS) lines are acquired and the coil weights calculated from a fit of the ACS data with the known (acquired) neighbouring line or lines:

$$S(k_{FE}, k'_{PE}) = \sum_j n_j S_j(k_{FE}, k_{PE})$$

thus the coefficients n_j can be calculated to give a particular k-space offset.

these signals will give foldover in real space and under-sampling of the temporal frames, just like real-space signals are folded in during parallel imaging. To unfold the signal intensities, k-t BLAST uses a set of training data, usually a low-resolution cine with relatively few frames (figure 17.17). The training data gives an estimation of the signal distribution in x-f space. Combining the training data with the undersampled dynamic data allows the reconstructor to produce the final cine images.

k-t SENSE is k-t BLAST plus sensitivity encoding. By using the coil sensitivities of a multi-element receive coil, k-t space is undersampled even more, allowing speed-up factors up to 8. The reduced scan time can be traded for more slices (better coverage), higher spatial resolution, better temporal resolution, or a

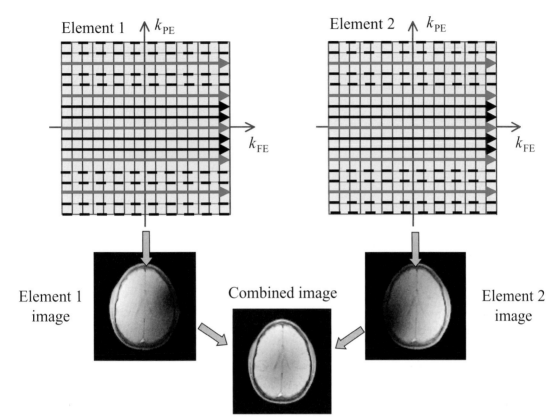

Figure 17.15 GRAPPA acquisition and reconstruction with $R = 2$. A separate k-space for each coil element is generated using multiple ACS lines and signal combinations from all the coil elements. Each element's k-space is Fourier transformed to generate images from each element which are then combined as in conventional phased array reconstruction.

combination of all three. For example, velocity mapping through the aorta can be achieved in a 10 s breath-hold instead of a 3 min scan time, or 6 slices may be acquired instead of only one in the same 3 min scan time.

In dynamic contrast enhanced imaging, the anatomy is not changing position but certain voxels will show higher intensity during the injection of gadolinium. In this situation one could acquire a training data set using a small test bolus, but it is preferable to acquire small bits of training data throughout the main bolus injection. k-t BLAST has great potential for applications in dynamic liver imaging, where we need to acquire a large number of slices at a temporal resolution of at least one frame per second.

17.6 Clinical benefits of parallel imaging

The benefits to parallel imaging can be summed up by the 'five Fs': namely **f**aster, **f**urther, **f**iner, (more) **f**aithful and **f**ainter (meaning quieter).

Figure 17.18 illustrates how shorter scan times can be achieved with very little discernable loss of image quality. Faster scanning also means shorter breath-holds as shown in figure 17.19 with the potential for reduced respiratory motion artefact or the second F: further, or more slices per breath-hold. The reduction in the number of phase-encode steps acquired means that higher matrices, and hence better resolution, finer images, may be acquired within a reasonable scan time. Thus a 1024 matrix image using $R = 2$ can be acquired in

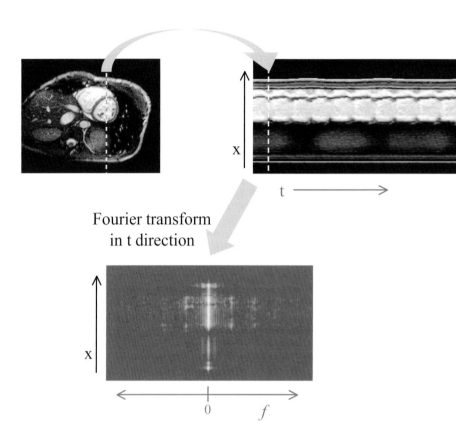

Figure 17.16 In a cine
cardiac scan, most of the
voxels do not change
between frames. By Fourier
transforming a line of
pixels in the time direction,
we can see the frequency
distribution of voxel
'motion' (actually it is
signal intensity which is
changing).

Fourier transform
in t direction

the same time as a convention 512 matrix image (figure 17.20).

Parallel imaging may be used to advantage in echo planar acquisitions (EPI) to reduce the effect of susceptibility artefacts (figure 17.21) and to reduce T_2 blurring in single shot fast spin echo or HASTE images (figure 17.22). In addition to reducing the echo train length, it also can enable a shortening of TE. For high field systems, the susceptibility distortions in EPI can be particularly bad. Parallel imaging helps reduce this. Also, particularly for EPI, parallel imaging can help to reduce the acoustic noise.

Parallel imaging and high field systems

There is an additional 'F' that we didn't consider earlier which is particularly relevant to high field MR systems: fry. We don't want to overheat our patients! As the SAR increases with the square of field strength (or frequency) high field systems (e.g. 3 T and above) are potentially limited by the permissible SAR. Of course these limits prevent us from frying our patients, but they do result in a need to length TR, or reduce the number of slices or the echo train length (as seen in section 10.2.2). Parallel imaging helps by reducing the number of RF excitations required to form an image, and indeed, without it, even the simplest head scan can prove problematical at 3 T.

17.7 Image quality in parallel imaging

We saw in chapter 5 that the image SNR was dependent upon the number of phase-encode lines acquired. This

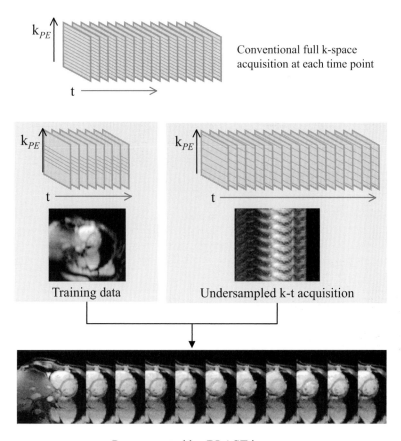

Conventional full k-space acquisition at each time point

Training data

Undersampled k-t acquisition

Reconstructed k-t BLAST images

Figure 17.17 A conventional cine scan acquires the whole of k-space at every time point. In k-t BLAST, a set of training data is acquired with low spatial and temporal resolution. This is followed by a rapid acquisition which undersamples in both k-space and time in a well defined pattern. The training data can then be used to unwrap the aliased signals

is also true in parallel imaging. So if we use a reduction factor R, then the SNR will be reduced theoretically by at least $\sqrt{R}$. In practice it may also be reduced by a geometric efficiency factor g which is dependent upon the geometrical arrangement of the array elements and their sensitivities.

If too high a reduction factor is used then artefacts may also appear in the image. These are shown for mSENSE and GRAPPA in figure 17.23. Artefacts also appear if too few ACS lines are used in the auto-calibrating techniques. Typical parallel imaging artefacts are increased noise in the centre of the image (or wherever the coil sensitivities are weakest), and residual foldover ghosts particularly if there is a very strong signal (like fat on T_1-weighted images).

SNR and SENSE

The SNR in SENSE can be expressed as

$$SNR_{SENSE} = \frac{SNR_{full}}{g\sqrt{R}}$$

where g is a geometry factor which is always greater than or equal to 1. An additional feature of SNR in SENSE is that the noise is not uniformly distributed access the image as in conventional acquisitions. This can be seen in 17.24 for different R with the level of noise and artefact increasing with R.

The SNR in mSENSE and GRAPPA does not have such a simple relationship with R, as ACS lines can be used in the reconstruction to boost the SNR. Like SENSE, the noise varies spatially across the image in SMASH-type techniques.

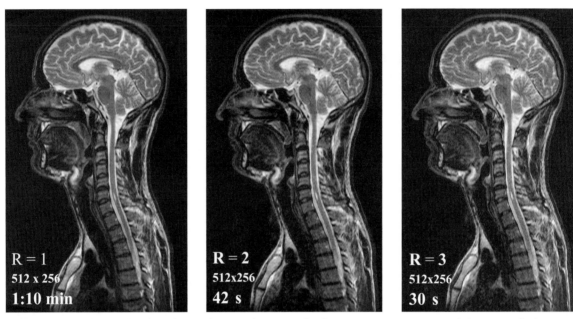

Figure 17.18 Use of parallel imaging (GRAPPA) to speed up T_2 weighted FSE scans. Images courtesy of Siemens Medical Solutions.

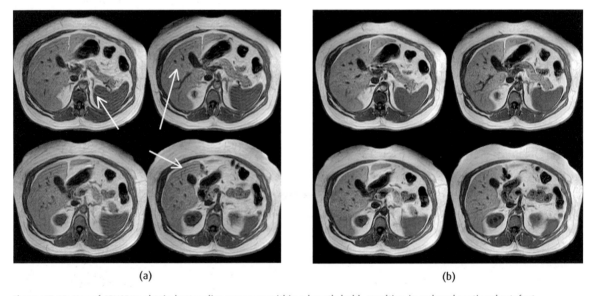

(a)   (b)

Figure 17.19 Use of SENSE to obtain better slice coverage within a breath-hold, resulting in reduced motional artefact (arrowed), (a) without SENSE: 22 s breath hold (25 slices), (b) with SENSE: 13 s. Images courtesy of Philips Medical Systems.

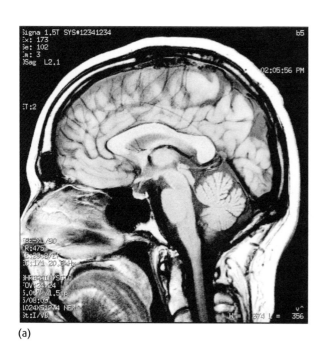

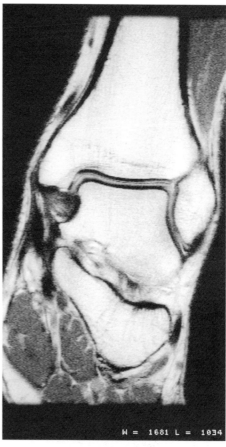

(a)

(b)

Figure 17.20 Use of parallel imaging (ASSET) to reduce acquisition time for a 1024 matrix acquisitions. Images courtesy of GE Healthcare.

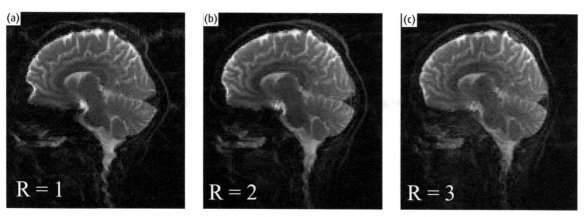

Figure 17.21 Parallel imaging reduces T_2^* distortion in EPI, by shortening the echo train length (increasing the PE bandwidth): (a) Conventional, (b) $R = 2$, (c) $R = 3$. Images courtesy of Siemens Medical Solutions.

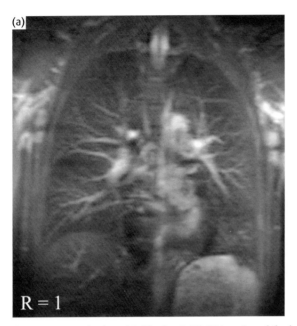
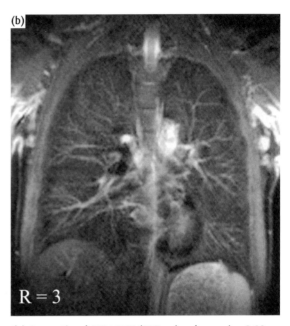

Figure 17.22 Reduction of T_2 blurring in HASTE imaging of the lungs. (a) Conventional 128×256 (207 ms), echo spacing 2.88 ms, (b) 256×256 (149 ms), effective echo spacing 0.96 ms. Images courtesy of Siemens Medical Solutions.

Parallel EPI

Figure 17.25 shows a reduced k-space trajectory for EPI and the related gradient scheme with and without reduction. The shorter echo train results in a higher PE bandwidth and hence less susceptibility distortion artefacts and reduces the minimum TE. The single shot nature of EPI however has implications for the reference images and calibration procedure. For SENSE and similar techniques, a standard calibration is run prior to the EPI acquisition(s) as for other sequences. For GRAPPA, the autocalibration traversal of the centre of k-space takes place before the reduced acquisition. In a repeated series of acquisitions as required for fMRI, this results in one additional 'TR' period. Another odd thing about EPI-GRAPPA is that, because the ACS data is real data and can be used in the reconstruction, the SNR for a reduction factor of 2 is higher than without parallel imaging, even if TE is kept the same. For $R=3$ and above SNR and image quality is degraded as the fitting to the ACS lines becomes more approximate.

We have already noted that for a SENSE acquisition, the field of view must be sufficiently large to encompass all the signal producing regions. If it is not, then the images cannot be unfolded properly.

17.8 Non-Cartesian acquisition schemes

Projection reconstruction (PR) was the first MR k-space trajectory used by Lauterbur to produce the first MR image of two tubes of water. This method is similar to the reconstruction of computerised tomography (CT) images. In CT, projections of the object are acquired at a number of angles around the object. The images are then reconstructed by 'back-projecting' the individual projections. Since simple back projection results in blurred images the projection data is usually filtered before reconstruction. In the earliest MR scanners magnetic field inhomogeneity and gradient nonlinearities resulted in excessive image blurring (see figure 1.3) and PR was subsequently replaced by the 'spin-warp' (2DFT) technique which was much more forgiving (see chapter 7). However with technical improvements in

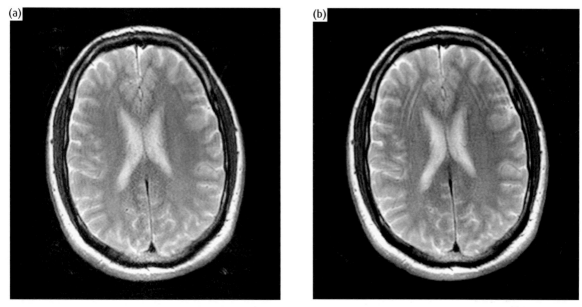

Figure 17.23 Parallel imaging artefacts at high reduction factor ($R = 3$) with 8 element head array coil: (a) GRAPPA (b) mSENSE.

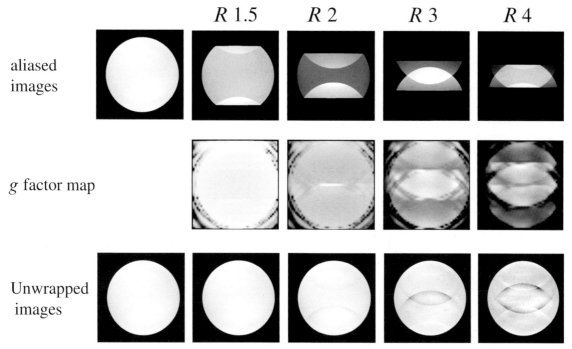

Figure 17.24 Image noise and reconstruction artefacts in SENSE at various reduction factors. Image courtesy of Philips Medical Systems.

scanner performance PR has been reborn with a new name: radial imaging.

17.8.1 2D radial imaging

In radial imaging we acquire a number of 2D projections through the object at different angles, ϕ. To

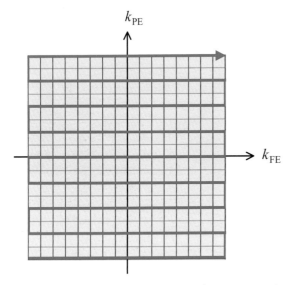

produce the radial projection pattern frequency encoding is applied simultaneously on two physical axes (e.g. x and y for transverse slices) with varying amplitudes to produce the rotational pattern. The pulse sequence simply involves slice selection and frequency encoding; there is no concept of a phase encoding direction. Figure 17.26(a) shows a 2D gradient echo radial sequence and twelve radial projections overlaid on a Cartesian k-space. In figure 17.26(b) the sequence is shown for the projection at $\phi = 45°$ i.e. the G_x and G_y gradients have the same amplitude. In radial imaging the data is no longer reconstructed using filtered back projection but is 'regridded' onto a conventional Cartesian (x,y) k-space and then reconstructed via direct Fourier transformation (see box 'Re: gridding').

17.8.2 3D radial imaging

The radial approach can also be extended into 3D by acquiring radial projections in 3D, i.e. spherical k-space coverage, this has sometimes been termed the Koosh ball trajectory due to its similarity with the child's toy and adult stress-buster! The proper name for this method is VIPR (**V**astly **U**ndersampled **I**sotropic

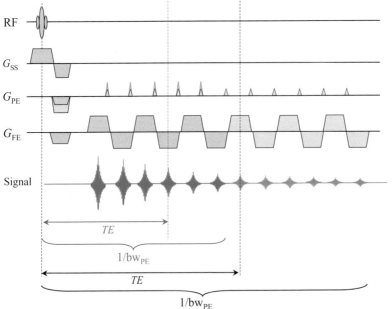

Figure 17.25 Parallel imaging and EPI: (a) k-space path of EPI with $R = 2$. (b) EPI sequence corresponding to k-space in (a) with (blue) and without (grey) a reduction factor of 2. The use of parallel imaging reduces TE and increases the PE bandwidth, resulting in less susceptibility distortion.

Projection **R**econstruction). A VIPR acquisition of 27 000 projections can result in a 3D volume with an isotropic resolution of $256 \times 256 \times 256$ being acquired every few seconds, ideal for dynamic 3D contrast enhanced MRA studies.

Re: Gridding

In conventional MRI raw data are acquired along a uniformly sampled rectilinear k-space trajectory and the image reconstructed by direct Fourier transformation. In radial and spiral imaging the k-space trajectories are nonuniform. Whilst any nonuniform data can be reconstructed using extensions of the standard discrete Fourier transform (DFT) algorithm the methods are generally far too slow to be clinically useable. Instead, in a process called 'regridding', the data is resampled or interpolated onto a uniform rectilinear grid prior to a standard FFT. Figure 17.27 shows the principle of gridding in a very simple way where each acquired data point contributes to the signal in four nearest neighbours on the Cartesian grid. An important part of gridding is that that the data also need to be corrected for the nonuniform sampling density, i.e. some sequences like radial and spiral imaging heavily oversample the centre of k-space. Each data acquisition point therefore needs to be multiplied by an appropriate 'weighting' factor to compensate for this effect, usually based on a Bessel function.

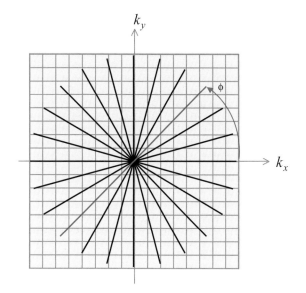

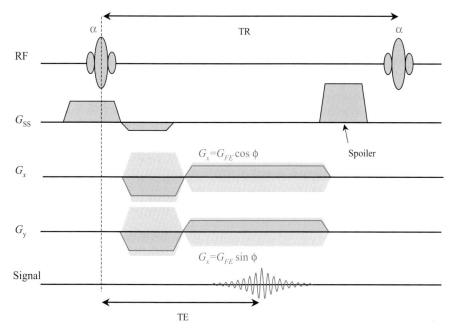

Figure 17.26 Radial scanning: (a) k-space for radial acquisition, the projection for $\phi = 45°$ shown in blue. Regridding to the underlying Cartesian k-space is required prior to reconstruction. (b) Pulse sequence for radial acquisition for $\phi = 45°$. There is no phase encoding and the amplitude of G_x and G_y vary to produce the radii, represented by the grey areas.

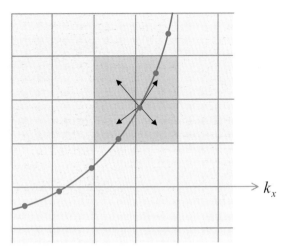

Figure 17.27 Regridding: each point affects four nearest neighbours. The blue line and points represent actual k-space trajectory and sampled points.

17.8.3 Applications of radial imaging: ultra short TE

Radial imaging has a number of advantages. Firstly because no phase encoding gradient is used the minimum TE for gradient echo based radial imaging can be made very short. Using nonselective or half-pulse excitation together with half-Fourier readout and ramped sampling TE can be as short as a few hundred microseconds. Furthermore if hardware changes are made to the system such that system delays and switching times are substantially reduced then echo times as short as $8\mu s$ can be achieved. This makes it possible to image previously unobservable tissues such as cortical bone, tendons, ligaments and menisci which have very short T_2 (figure 17.28). The term **Ultra-short TE** is used to describe these applications and it gives us another new acronym, UTE. The UTE images themselves are heavily PD weighted, so it is common to acquire a second echo at a later time (e.g. 4 ms) and subtract it from the UTE image. The subtracted image highlights the short T_2 tissues as bright structures against a darker background.

Secondly, because each radial projection passes through the centre of k-space the signals are effectively heavily averaged. This means that motion artefacts are

Sampling in radial imaging
The oversampling of the centre of k-space means that radial acquisitions take $\pi/2$ times longer than conventional Cartesian acquisitions for the same matrix. The scan time can be reduced by undersampling the radial data, i.e. decreasing the number of spokes. In conventional Cartesian imaging this results in image aliasing. In radial imaging it results in radially positioned streak artefacts (figure 17.29). In the same way as for undersampled Cartesian imaging, reducing the number of radial spokes does not compromise spatial resolution but reduces SNR and leads to increased streaking artefacts. However, with a high enough degree of undersampling the artefacts become a nearly uniform background haze instead of discrete streaks. With an appropriate trade-off between acquisition time and artefact then undersampled PR offers a means of rapidly acquiring high resolution images.

considerably reduced but at the expense of increased blurring.

17.8.4. PROPELLER

PROPELLER (**P**eriodically **R**otated **O**verlapping Parall**EL L**ines with **E**nhanced **R**econstruction) is a hybrid Cartesian/radial acquisition. PROPELLER acquires a number of parallel lines, each rotated about its centre through a series of angles in order to fully sample k-space (figure 17.30). The k-space path then resembles an aircraft propeller, the 'blades' being the rotating block of parallel lines. If each blade only comprised one line of raw data then the technique would be identical to a conventional radial acquisition.

The most common implementation of PROPELLER uses a fast spin echo (FSE) train to acquire each blade. Like radial imaging PROPELLER takes $\pi/2$ times longer than a conventional Cartesian FSE acquisition, e.g. in order to match a conventional acquisition with an N_{PE} of 480 lines, using a PROPELLER acquisition with an FSE ETL of 28, would require $(480 \div 28) \times \pi/2 \approx 27$ blades. The scan time would therefore be TR $\times 27$.

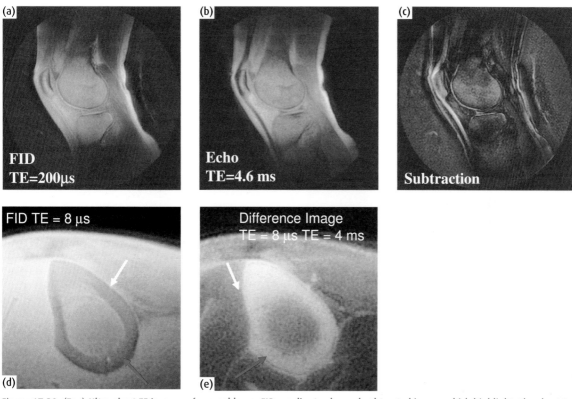

Figure 17.28 (Top) Ultra-short TE images of normal knee: FID, gradient echo and subtracted image which highlights the short T_2 components such as the femoro-patellar tendon. Images courtesy of Philips Medical Systems. (Bottom) Normal tibia: FID and subtracted image, showing high signal in cortical bone ($T_2 = 500$ μs, blue arrows) and periosteum ($T_2 = 5$-11 ms, white arrows). Images courtesy of Jean Brittain, GE Healthcare Technologies.

The advantage of using PROPELLER is that the centre of k-space is heavily oversampled reducing any artefacts due to patient motion. Furthermore, since each blade samples the centre of k-space any rotational or translational motion between blades during the PROPELLER reconstruction can be identified by any inconsistencies between each blade. Depending upon the similarity between blades data can either be corrected to account for the motion or individual blades may even be discarded. PROPELLER can therefore produce good quality images even in the presence of quite severe motion. Figure 17.31 shows two T_2-weighted FSE acquisitions in a normal volunteer who was asked to rotate their head from side to side during a conventional FSE acquisition and a PROPELLER acquisition.

PROPELLER can also been used with diffusion weighting. Although PROPELLER is significantly slower than EPI, the use of an FSE readout means that susceptibility issues are significantly reduced and that the overall image SNR is much higher. The issue of patient motion during the extended acquisition time is addressed by the inherent PROPELLER motion correction.

17.8.5 Spiral

In spiral imaging the k-space trajectory samples data along an Archimedean spiral (see box 'k-space spirograph'). Spiral acquisitions can achieve greater scan efficiency than conventional Cartesian acquisitions, i.e.

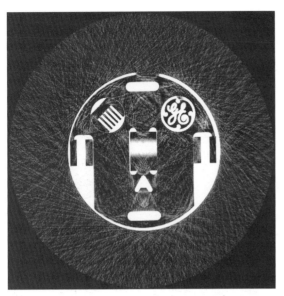

Figure 17.29 Radial artefacts: streak artefacts (very similar to CT) can be seen in the background.

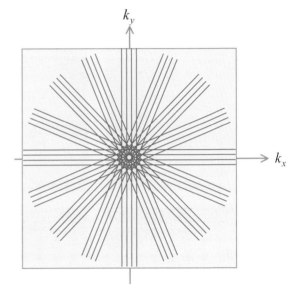

Figure 17.30 k-space trajectories for PROPELLER acquisition with 4 echoes per blade and 8 blades.

k-space spirograph

Spiral trajectories use an Archimedean spiral which is defined by

$$r = a\theta$$

where r is the radius, a is a constant and θ the angle. The k-space path for a simple constant spacing spiral is given by

$$k_x = \frac{N_{shot}}{2\pi \cdot \text{FOV}} \theta \sin\theta$$

$$k_y = \frac{N_{shot}}{2\pi \cdot \text{FOV}} \theta \cos\theta$$

where N_{shot} is the number of interleaved spirals or shots. The gradient waveforms necessary to produce a spiral k-space trajectory come from the derivative of k with respect to time:

$$G_x = \frac{N_{shot}}{\gamma \cdot \text{FOV}} \cdot \frac{d\theta}{dt} (\sin\theta + \theta\cos\theta)$$

$$G_y = \frac{N_{shot}}{\gamma \cdot \text{FOV}} \cdot \frac{d\theta}{dt} (\cos\theta - \theta\sin\theta)$$

These are shown in figure 17.32a. In practice slew rate constraints need to be considered and the rotation velocity $d\theta/dt$ may not be constant.

a spiral acquisition can cover a greater portion of k-space with each RF excitation. As the spiral readout starts at the centre of k-space spiral sequences can have very short echo times. Spiral acquisitions may be either single-shot or multi-shot. In a single-shot acquisition all of the k-space data is acquired following a single RF excitation. Figure 17.32 shows the k-space trajectory for a single shot acquisition and the in-plane gradient waveforms required to generate this trajectory. Like radial imaging there is no longer any concept of phase or frequency encoding and data is constantly acquired during the spiral readout.

For multi-shot acquisitions a number (N_{shot}) of spiral interleaves are performed, each shot being rotated by an angle of $\pm 2\pi/N_{shot}$ (figure 17.33). Figure 17.34 shows a phantom image acquired with a single shot spiral comprising 16384 complex data points, and a multi-shot with 16 interleaves each of 4096 data points.

Since spirals are a method of in-plane data readout then they can be combined with any other pulse sequences, for example spin echo. The spirals can also be acquired in a reverse fashion so that the centre of

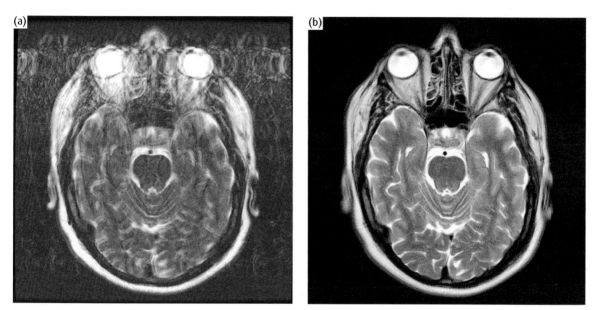

Figure 17.31 Effect of head motion on (a) convention FSE (scan time 2 min 41 s) and (b) PROPELLER (scan time 3 min 12 s).

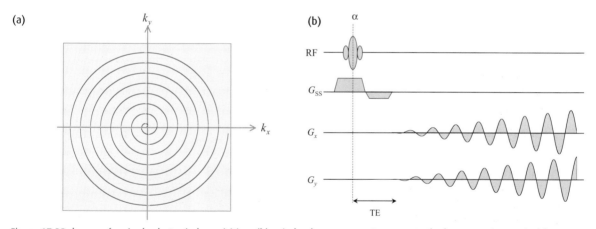

Figure 17.32 k-space for single shot spiral acquisition, (b) spiral pulse sequence to generate the k-space trajectory in (a).

k-space is acquired last. This is one way of acquiring a T_2^*-weighted spiral acquisition suitable for fMRI studies. Spirals can also be extended to 3D, the simplest method being to incorporate a conventional slice select phase encoding, the resultant data is often called a stack of spirals.

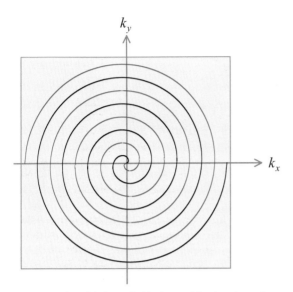

Figure 17.33 Multi-shot spiral k-space with 2 interleaved shots.

17.9. Epilogue: the final frontier

To quote the old human rights song, we've come a long, long way – both since the genesis of modern MRI and since the start of the book. We started with an allusion to rocket science. In this last section we delve into what may turn out to be science fiction, or mere star-gazing. What will tomorrow's MR scanner be like, and what will it do – or possibly, what won't it do? Expect the following:

- The use of interventional MRI will increase and expand, coupled with a proliferation of minimally invasive therapies, including gene therapies.
- Interventional MR systems may use high-temperature superconducting flat magnets (like fridge

Problems with spirals

The major problem with spiral acquisitions is the blurring due to off resonant spins. These frequency offsets can come from B_0 field inhomogeneity, local susceptibility effects and chemical shifts. In conventional Cartesian imaging these frequency offsets result in a simple shift in the frequency encoding direction, e.g. chemical shift artefact, whilst in spiral imaging, since the trajectory is changing simultaneously in both in-plane directions the effect is a 2D blurring (figure 34(c)). To reduce this blurring spiral imaging sequences are usually performed with a water-only excitation (spatial-spectral) excitation (Chapter 12). To correct for the effects due to B_0 inhomogeneity, it is usual for the system to rapidly acquire a field map to determine the frequency offset as a function of spatial location. This can easily be done during the prescan period by acquiring two single shot spiral images with slightly different TEs and constructing a phase map by complex subtraction. The calculated frequency shifts can then be incorporated into the spiral gridding algorithm to correct for the off-resonance spins.

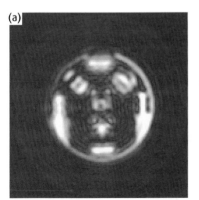
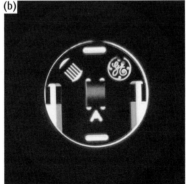
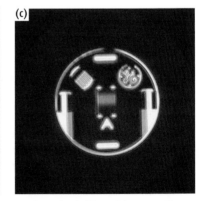

Figure 17.34 (a)Single shot spiral image (b) 16 shot interleaved spiral image (c) 16 shot interleaved spiral but with 50 Hz offset.

magnets) incorporated into the operating room couch.

- For screening we may see walk-through magnets.
- New extensions to parallel imaging will render EPI unnecessary except in some functional neurological examinations (i.e. just like the present!).
- Field strengths will of course keep increasing, and 3T will become the norm for state-of-the-art clinical scanning.
- There will be new 'intelligent' contrast agents for molecular-specific proton imaging.
- Finally spectroscopy will be deployed as a routine clinical application.

See also:

Section 7.7.2 Totally fazed: phase encoding

Section 9.4.6 Phased array coils

FURTHER READING

Bernstein MA, King KF and Zhou XJ (2004) *Handbook of MRI Pulse Sequences* Elsevier Academic Press (ISBN: 0120928612). Chs 13 and 17.

Griswold MA, Jakob PM, Heidemann RM, et al (2002). Generalized autocalibrating partially parallel acqusitions (GRAPPA). *Magn Reson Med* **47**: 1202–1210

Haacke EM, Brown RW, Thompson MR and Venkatesan R (1999) *Magnetic resonance imaging: Physical principles and sequence design* Wiley-Liss (ISBN: 0471351288). Chs 14 and 19.

Pruessmann KP, Weiger M, Scheidegger MB, Boesiger P (1999). SENSE: sensitivity encoding for fast MRI. *Magn Reson Med.* **42**: 952-962

Sodickson DK and Manning WJ (1997). Simultaneous acquisition of spatial harmonics (SMASH): Fast imaging with radiofrequency coil arrays. *Magn Reson Med* **38**: 591-603

Tsao J, Boesiger P and Pruessman KP (2003). k-t BLAST and k-t SENSE: Dynamic MRI with high frame rate exploiting spatiotemporal correlations. *Magn Reson Med* **50**: 1031–1042

Appendix: maths revision

Many people find maths challenging and are very happy to drop it after school. This appendix contains simple descriptions of the main mathematical concepts that will help you to understand MRI. These are:

- vectors;
- sine and cosine waves;
- exponentials;
- complex numbers;
- simple Fourier analysis.

A.1 Vectors

A vector quantity is one that has both magnitude and direction. For example, velocity describes the rate of movement in a particular direction (in comparison speed is a scalar quantity which just measures the rate of travel). Vectors are commonly depicted using arrows with the length denoting the magnitude. They can be added together by putting the arrows end-to-end and then joining the start and end points, creating the resultant vector. Alternatively a vector may be divided into components along the x, y and z axes in any frame of reference (figure A.1).

In equations vectors are either shown with little arrows over the top (like this $\vec{M}$) or in bold typeface (**M**). In this book we have used the bold notation, but only in equations where the vector directions are important. Components of vectors can be denoted by their magnitude and unit vectors **i**, **j** and **k** along the three directions. Vectors can be multiplied together using either the dot product (which has a scalar result) or the cross product (which has a vector result).

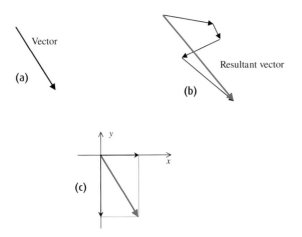

(a) Vector

(b) Resultant vector

(c) Component vectors along x and y

$\mathbf{A} = A_x\mathbf{i} + A_y\mathbf{j} + A_z\mathbf{k}$

$\mathbf{A}\cdot\mathbf{B} = AB\cos\theta = A_xB_x + A_yB_y + A_zB_z$

$\mathbf{A}\times\mathbf{B} = -\mathbf{B}\times\mathbf{A}$
$= (A_yB_z - A_zB_y)\mathbf{i} + (A_zB_x - A_xB_z)\mathbf{j} + (A_xB_y - A_yB_x)\mathbf{k}$
$= AB\sin\theta\mathbf{n}$

where θ is the angle between the two vectors, and $\mathbf{n}$ is a unit vector perpendicular to both $\mathbf{A}$ and $\mathbf{B}$.

Figure A.1 (a) A vector is shown as an arrow. (b) Several vectors can be joined together end-to-end to create the resultant vector. (c) A vector can be broken down into components along principal axes.

A.2 Sine and cosine waves

The simplest waves are pure sine or cosine waves, which have the same shape but are shifted with respect to each other (figure A.2(a)). They have three basic properties: the amplitude is the peak height (how large it is), the frequency, measured in hertz (Hz), describes how rapidly in time the magnitude of the wave is

(a)

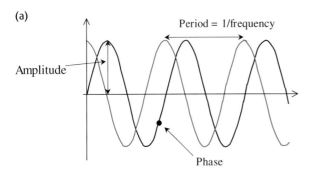

Period = 1/frequency

Amplitude

Phase

Sine wave

Cosine wave

Figure A.2 (a) A wave has amplitude, frequency and phase. A cosine wave differs from a sine wave by a phase angle of 90°. (b) A rotating unit vector creates two waves along the x and y axes.

(b)

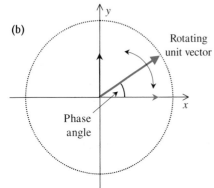

Rotating unit vector

Phase angle

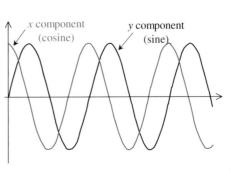

x component (cosine)

y component (sine)

changing, and the phase describes where we are within the cyclic variation.

A unit vector rotating around a circle produces sine and cosine components along the x and y axes (figure A.2(b)), and this gives us an easy way of thinking of phase, which is just the angle between the unit vector and the reference axis. Phase angles can vary from 0° to 360°, and angles larger than 360° just overlay themselves.

Angles around the circle can also be measured in radians, with the full 360° being equal to 2π rads. π (pronounced 'pie') is the ratio of the circumference of a circle to its diameter, and is approximately equal to 3.14. There are some important angles to know: $\pi/2$ is 90°, π is 180°, and in general $2n\pi$ is in line with 0°.

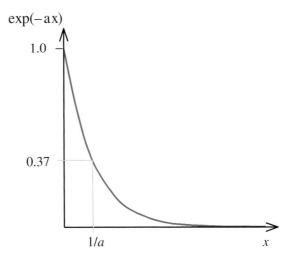

Figure A.3 Exponential decay describes spin-spin relaxation in MRI as well as radioactive decay.

A.3 Exponentials

Exponentials are rather difficult to explain but you really only need to know some important properties of these useful numbers. They are based on the number e which is approximately equal to 2.718. In equations exponentials may be denoted either as e^x or $\exp(x)$ – we have used the latter in this book – and x is known as the exponent. Exponentials are the inverse of natural logarithms (denoted ln), and in particular if $y = \exp(x)$ then $\ln(y) = x$.

Let's start with some general results for exponentials:

$$\exp(-x) = \frac{1}{\exp(x)}$$

$$\exp(x)\exp(y) = \exp(x+y)$$

$$\exp(0) = 1$$

$$\exp(\infty) = \infty$$

$$\exp(-\infty) = 0$$

In MRI we are particularly interested in exponential decays, $\exp(-x)$, which reduce down to zero (see figure A.3). This not only describes radioactive decay and the free induction decay in MRI, it also shows how the temperature of a cup of coffee drops – fast at first but getting slower and slower until it is stone cold. In contrast exponential growth, when the exponent is positive, just keeps getting bigger and bigger – like the world's population!

A.4 Complex numbers

Complex numbers have a real part and an imaginary part. The imaginary part is multiplied by i, the square root of –1, so a complex number can be written as

$$A = \mathrm{Re} + i\mathrm{Im}$$

The complex conjugate of A is defined by

$$A^* = \mathrm{Re} - i\mathrm{Im}$$

so when A is multiplied by its complex conjugate the result is a pure real number

$$A \cdot A^* = \mathrm{Re}^2 + \mathrm{Im}^2$$

You may see j used instead of i, particularly in engineering textbooks. Of course in real life it is impossible to find the square root of a negative number, so the imaginary parts don't really exist. However, complex numbers are useful for describing the rotational movement in MRI. We can define any point on the circle by a complex number

$$A = x + iy = \cos\theta + i\sin\theta$$

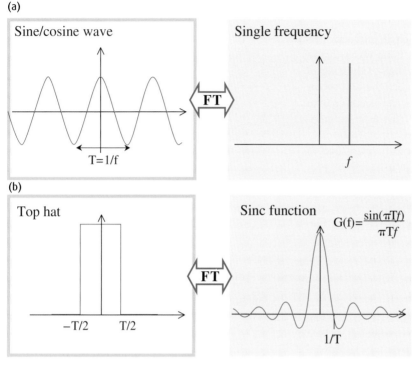

(a)

(b)

Figure A.4 Some important Fourier transform pairs. A simple sine wave with frequency f has a period T, and its Fourier transform is a spike function at frequency f. The FT of a top hat function with width 2T is a sinc function, with the first zero crossing points at 1/T. A Gaussian function transforms to another Gaussian, and finally an exponential decay transforms to a Lorentzian function.

We can use a complex exponent to define the rotational operator $\exp(i\theta)$, so that

$$\exp(i\theta) = \cos\theta + i\sin\theta$$

and if we use $\theta = \omega t/2\pi$, we can denote a rotating vector as $\exp(i\omega t/2\pi)$, which allows us to combine any number of rotational movements simply by adding their exponents.

A.5 Simple Fourier analysis

Fourier's theorem states that any complex waveform can be created from a sum of sine and cosine waves with appropriate frequencies and amplitudes. We write this as

$$s(x) = \frac{a_0}{2} + \sum_{n=1}^{\infty}(a_n\cos nx + b_n\sin nx) = \sum_{n=-\infty}^{\infty} a_n\exp(inx)$$

where a and b are the amplitudes and $i = \sqrt{-1}$. For MRI the most important feature of Fourier analysis is the *Fourier transform*, which is defined by the equations

$$S(k) = \int_{-\infty}^{\infty} s(x)\exp(-i2\pi kx)dx$$

$$s(x) = \int_{-\infty}^{\infty} S(k)\exp(i2\pi kx)dk$$

Although these integrals look nasty, you don't have to work them out, you just need to recognize them. $S(k)$ and $s(x)$ are functions of k and x respectively, called a Fourier transform pair, and k and x have an inverse relationship. Some important Fourier transform pairs are shown in figure A.4. In MRI, x is real space and k is spatial frequency. Another useful Fourier transform pair is time t and frequency f. A two-dimensional Fourier transformation involves integration over two directions and 3D FT is over all three:

$$S(k_x, k_y) = \iint_{x, y} s(x, y)\exp(-i2\pi k_x x)\exp(-i2\pi k_y y)dx\,dy$$

Figure A.4 (*cont.*)

(c)

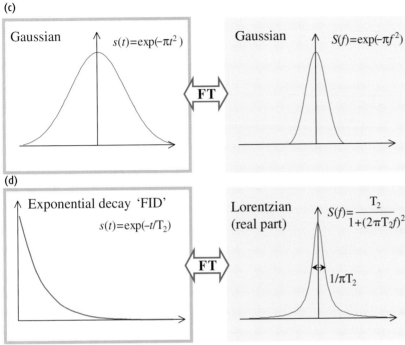

Gaussian $s(t)=\exp(-\pi t^2)$

FT

Gaussian $S(f)=\exp(-\pi f^2)$

(d)

Exponential decay 'FID'

$s(t)=\exp(-t/T_2)$

FT

Lorentzian (real part) $S(f)=\dfrac{T_2}{1+(2\pi T_2 f)^2}$

$1/\pi T_2$

$$S(k_x,k_y,k_z) = \iiint_{x,y,z} s(x,y,z)\exp(-i2\pi k_x x)\exp(-i2\pi k_y y)$$

$$\exp(-i2\pi k_z z)\mathrm{d}x\,\mathrm{d}y\,\mathrm{d}z$$

Planck's constant	h	6.63×10^{-34} J s
	$\hbar=\dfrac{h}{2\pi}$	1.05×10^{-34} J s
Proton gyromagnetic ratio	γ	2.68×10^{8} rad s^{-1} T^{-1}
	$\gamma=\dfrac{\gamma}{2\pi}$	42.57 MHz T^{-1}

A.6 Some useful constants

Boltzmann's constant k 1.38×10^{-23} J K^{-1}
Note this k is not related to k-space

Scanning completed at 12:55pm

The patient got off the table and JD removed the venflon.
JD informed the patient that the results of the scan would go back to her GP. She said she would like them to go to another Dr instead. I informed her that our policy was to send back to the referral source only and that her GP would forward them on to whoever necessary. She asked again about getting them referred not to her GP but to her consultant. I repeated what I had already said. She said she had a review appointment the following Tuesday night at Liverpool Spire and would they be available for her consultant to look at. I said that they most likely would.
JD assisted the patient off the scanner and down the steps.
8 mins after the end of scan time we started the next patient. 38 mins late for his appointed time.

PROBLEMS IDENTIFIED

Different protocols for msk radiologists
Protocolling radiologist not necessarily the reporting radiologist
Addressing patient demands

Index

Page numbers in *italics* refer to tables or figures only, page numbers in **bold** refer to boxes only.

2-D imaging *see* two-dimensional (2D) imaging
3-D imaging *see* three-dimensional (3D) imaging
absolute SNR (ASNR) **209**
ACR (American College of Radiology) standards **205–6, 217**
ADC (analogue-to-digital converter) **48, 49, 187**
ADC (apparent diffusion coefficient 330, *331*, **331**, 334–5
adiabatic pulses 96, **234**
air-cored resistive magnets 169
aliasing **50**, 130
Alzheimer's disease 308, *309*
American Association of Physicists in Medicine (AAPM) standards **205, 206**
American College of Radiology (ACR) standards **205–6, 217**
amplifiers
   gradient 174, 175
   pre-amplifiers 185–6
analogue images 47–51
analogue-to-digital converter (ADC) **48, 49, 187**
anatomy scans 32, *33*
angiography *see* magnetic resonance angiography (MRA)
anisotropy 331–4
apodization 316, *317*
apparent diffusion coefficient (ADC) 330, *331*, **331**, 334–5
array processor (AP) 188
arrhythmia rejection (AR) 288, **289**
artefacts 79
   cause determination *106*, 107
   chemical shift artefacts 89, *93*, 217–18, **316**
      practical exercise **95**
      severity **92**
   digital imaging artefacts 79

artefacts (*cont.*)
  echo planar imaging (EPI) 327–8
  equipment artefacts 103–5, **107**
    gradient nonlinearities 104
    halo artefact *104*, 105
    herring-bone artefact *104*, 105
    zipper artefact 103
  Fourier imaging 130–3
  inhomogeneity artefacts 79, **103**
  insufficient spoiling **243**, *244*
  metal artefacts 101–3
  motion artefacts 79–89
    cardiac motion *80*, 84–5, *86*, 282–3
    from flow 86–9
    peristaltic motion *80*, 85–6
    respiratory motion *80*, 81–3, **83**, 285, 293, *295*
  parallel imaging 361, *365*
  partial volume artefact 96–8
  phase cancellation artefact 90–1
  phase sampling artefacts 98–100
    Gibbs' artefact 99–100, **100**, *101*, 132
    phase wrap-around artefact 98–9, *100*, **100**
    ringing artefact 100, 132
  radial *370*
  susceptibility artefacts 13, 38, 101–3
arterial input function (AIF) 338
arterial spin labelling (ASL) 338–40
  analysis **340**
arterio-venous malformations (AVMs) 344
ASSET 348, **353**, *363*
astrocytoma *309*, 344
auto-calibrating signal (ACS) 353–6
Auto-SMASH 353–6
  variable density (VD-Auto-SMASH) 356

b-factor 330
B$_0$ *see* magnetic field
B$_1$ *see* radiofrequency (RF) coils, radiofrequency (RF)
    pulses
bandwidth *see* receive bandwidth
bandwidth reduction 77
binomial pulses 96, **234**
bio-effects of magnetic fields 16–17, 192–201
  gradient effects 194–7
    exposure standards 195–7
    noise 195
    stimulation effects 194–5
  occupational exposure *199*, **199**
  RF effects 192–3

exposure standards 193, *194*
    specific absorption ration (SAR) 16, 193
  static field effects 197–200
    exposure standards 198–200
    flow effects 198
    force fields 198
    occupational exposure **199**
birdcage coil 179, *180*, **182**
black-blood technique 288, **289**, *304*, 305
BLAST (broad-use linear acquisition speed-up technique)
    357–9, *361*
Bloch equations **158**
Bloch, F. **4**, **5**, *6*
Bloembergen, N. **5**, *6*
Bloembergen, Purcell and Pound (BPP) relaxation theory
    155
  body tissues 160
blood flow 44–5
  effects in conventional MRI 258–63
    phase shift effects 260–1
    time-of-flight (TOF) effects 259–60
  motion artefacts 86–9, 258–9
    avoidance 88–9, 261–3
    in-flow effects 86–8
    velocity-induced phase effects 88
  see also cardiac MRI
blood suppression preparation (BSP) 288, **289**, *290*, 305
BOLD (blood oxygenation level dependent) effect 340–5
  acquisitions 341
  clinical applications 344
  field strength and **345**
  haemodynamic delay **343**
  interpretation 343–4
  problems 344–5
  processing 342–3
Boltzmann distribution **140**
bolus chase MRA 27
BPP (Bloembergen, Purcell and Pound) relaxation theory
    155
  body tissues 160
brain imaging 19–20, *34*, *36*, *38*
  diffusion-weighted imaging *333–4*
  tumour *31*
  see also BOLD (blood oxygenation level dependent)
    effect
breast imaging 20, *21*
  cancer detection 20
  implant rupture detection 20
breath-hold cine imaging 296, *297*, *298*

broad-use linear acquisition speed-up technique (BLAST) 357–9, *361*
burns **17**

carbon spectroscopy 321
cardiac motion artefacts *80*, 84–5, *86*, 282–3
cardiac MRI 21, 282–305
  artefact challenges 282–5
  cardiac gating 84–5
    ECG gating *86*, 282–3
    peripheral pulse gating (PPG) 85, *86*, *284*, 285
    retrospective gating 290–1, *292*
  cine phase-contrast velocity mapping 298–300, *301*
  coronary artery imaging 304–5
  functional imaging 288–98
    fast prospective imaging 291–3, **294**
    fast retrospective imaging 294–6
    flow compensation 291
    functional analysis 296
    improving myocardial/blood contrast 296
    myocardial tagging 296–8
  morphological imaging 285–8
  myocardial perfusion imaging 300–3
  myocardial viability 303–4
carotid artery 26
Carr–Purcell sequence 149, *151*
Carr–Purcell–Meiboon–Gill (CPMG) sequence **149**, *152*
cerebral blood flow (CBF) 335
cerebral blood volume (CBV) 335
chemical shift artefacts 89, *93*, 217–18, **316**
  practical exercise 95
  severity 92
chemical shift imaging (CSI) 318–19, *320*
  technical difficulties 320
CHESS (chemical shift selective) pulse 94, 96, **309**
choline (Cho) 308
cine phase-contrast velocity mapping 298–300, *301*
circle of Willis 26, *45*
circularly polarized (CP) coils 180
circulation time 272, **274**, *275*
CISS (constructive interference in steady state) **248**
Clariscan(™) 281
clinical procedures
  brain 19–20
  breast 20, *21*
  cardiac 21
  carotid/intracerebral arteries 26
  hip 24, *25*
  knee 24, *26*
  liver 21–3
  pelvis 23–4
  renal arteries 27
  shoulder *23*, 24
  spine 20
  thoracic aorta 24–5
CNR *see* contrast-to-noise ratio (CNR)
coherence **239**, *241*, *245*, *249*
coils
  gradient coils 13–14, 173
  sensitivity profiles 348, *353*, *354–5*
  see also radiofrequency (RF) coils
cold sores **17**
complex numbers 377–8
complex subtraction 269, *271*
composite pulses *see* binomial pulses
computed tomography (CT) 2, 30, 47
computer system 14, 188
constructive interference in steady state (CISS) **248**
contrast 66, *70*
  definition **66**
  GE images **40**
  magnetization transfer contrast (MTC) *161*
  measurement 216
    contrast-detail detectability **216**, *217*
  normalized contrast behaviour *67–8*
  prediction **68**
  SE images **37**
contrast agents 19, 42–3, 162–6
  adverse reactions 16–17
  novel agents 279–81
  relaxivity **165**
  see also gadolinium; SPIO (super-paramagnetic iron oxide)
contrast-detail detectability **216**, *217*
contrast-enhanced (CE) MRA 271–7
  4D CE-MRA 277
  elliptic centric phase encoding **276**, *278*, *279*
  fat suppression 273, *275*
  novel contrast agents 279–81
  peripheral MRA 277–8
  ringing artefact 100
  timing 272–3, **274**, *275*
contrast-to-noise ratio (CNR) 66–9, *70*, 71
  definition **66**, 216
  effect on image quality 71–3, **74**
corduroy artefact *104*, 105
coronary artery imaging 304–5
cosine waves 376–7

coupling 185
creatine (Cr) 308
cross-talk 96–8
cryogens, hazards of 16
CT (computed tomography) 2, 30, 47

Damadian, R. 2, **4**
dementia 308
demodulation **187**
dephasing 112
depth-resolved spectroscopy (DRESS) 319–20
DESS (double echo steady state) **248**, *250, 251*
diamagnetic materials 39, **199**
diffusion imaging 329–34
    anisotropy 331–4
    brain 19–20
    clinical applications 335
    diffusion sequences 334–5
    pulsed gradient spin echo (PGSE) 329–31
diffusion tensor imaging (DTI) **332**
digital data 47
    versus analogue data 47–51
digital subtraction angiograms (DSA) 47
digital-to-analogue conversion 57
direct contrast MR venography 278, *280*
distortion 211
Dixon method 20, **93**
dobutamine **301**, 303
double echo steady state (DESS) **248**, *250, 251*
DRESS (depth-resolved spectroscopy) 319–20
driven equilibrium 229
DW-MRI *see* diffusion imaging
dynamic shimming **173**
dynamic susceptibility contrast MRI (DSC-MRI) 336–8

ECG gating *86*, 282–3
ECG-triggered gradient-echo imaging 288, *290, 293*
ECG-triggered spin-echo imaging 286, *289*
echo planar imaging (EPI) 4, **177**
    acquisition methods 325–9
        blipped versus nonblipped single-shot 326
        multi-shot 328–9
        spiral 329
    artefacts 327–8
    gradient considerations **327**
    gradient echo based (GE-EPI) 253–4, *255, 326, 327*
    parallel EPI **364**, *366*
    spin echo based (SE-EPI) 231–2, *233, 236*
echo time *see* TE (echo time)

echo train *see* fast spin echo (FSE)
echoes 144–8
    see also gradient echo (GE) sequences; spin echo (SE) sequences
eddy currents 174, **175**
edge response function (ERF) **213**
effective echo time *see* TE (echo time)
Einthoven's triangle 282, *283*
electromagnets 12, 169, **170**
electromotive force (EMF) **195**
elliptic centric phase encoding **276**, *278, 279*
EPI *see* echo planar imaging (EPI)
equipment *see* MR equipment
equipment artefacts *see* artefacts
Ernst, R. **5**, *6*
Ernst angle **243**
Eurospin Test System **205, 206**
event-related fMRI (ER-fMRI) 341
exponentials 377

FADE (fast acquisition dual echo) **248**
FAIR (flow-sensitive alternating inversion recovery) 338–9
Faraday cage 13
Faraday induction **195**, *196*
fast imaging with steady precession *see* FISP
fast spin echo (FSE) 35, 222–31, *236*
    3D FSE **231**
    cardiac imaging 286–8, *289*
    compromises 226–7
    driven equilibrium 229
    inversion recovery FSE 228–9
        interleaving 229, *230*
    single-shot 230–1
fat 89
    chemical shift artefacts 89, *93*, 217–18, **316**
    fat–water separation **93**
    phase cancellation artefact 90–1
    signal suppression 92–6, **234**, *235*
        binomial pulses 96
        CHESS 94, 96
        contrast-enhanced MRA 273, *275*
        fat sat 92–5
        measurement 217–18
        STIR 40–1, **42**, 92, 95
fat/water separation (Dixon technique) 20, **93**
ferromagnetic materials **39**
FFT *see* Fourier transforms (FT)
FID (free induction decay) 143–4, 236–8
    single-voxel spectra processing 316, *317*

field of view (FOV) 56
  matrix size and **70**
  optimization 75, 77
  rectangular 76, 133–5
  resolution relationship 127, **129**
field strength **13**, 168
  BOLD effect and **345**
  SNR and **13**, **208–9**
  strength–duration (SD) curve **197**
filtering 77–8
FISP (fast imaging with steady precession) 243–5
  cardiac imaging 296, *297*
  resonant offsets **246**
  true FISP 244–5, *247*
FLAIR (fluid attenuated inversion recovery) 41–2, 228–9
  brain imaging 19
flip angle _ 37–8
flow *see* blood flow
flow compensation 89, 261–2, 291
flow-sensitive alternating inversion recovery (FAIR) 338–9
fluoroscopy 2
fMRI *see* functional magnetic resonance imaging (fMRI)
focused ultrasound (FUS) 189
force fields **15**, 198
Fourier, Joseph 112
Fourier transforms (FT) 112–13, 378–9
  2-D FT imaging (2D FT) 3, 73, 113, **128**
    encoding for **128**
    image reconstruction 127
    resolution and field of view 127
  3-D FT imaging (3D FT) 113, 135–6
  consequences of Fourier imaging 129–33
    artefacts 130–3
    k-space 129–30
    T_2 blurring 130
  FT pairs 113, *114*, 378–9
  half Fourier 76, 133
free induction decay (FID) 143–4, 236–8
  single-voxel spectra processing 316, *317*
frequency encoding (FE) 123–5, 221
  axis selection **54**, *57*
  matrix 51–6
frequency-selective fat saturation (fat sat) 92–5, **95**
fringe field 15–16, 189, *190*
FSE *see* fast spin echo (FSE)
FT *see* Fourier transforms (FT)
full-width at half-maximum (FWHM) 96
functional magnetic resonance imaging (fMRI) 189, 340
  acquisitions 341

  clinical applications 344
  event-related (ER-fMRI) 341
  interpretation 343–4
  problems 344–5
  processing 342–3

gadobenate dimeglumine 280
gadolinium 19, 43, 162–3, *164*
  brain imaging 20
  carotid artery imaging 26
  direct contrast MR venography 278, *280*
  effect on T_2 **44**
  increased concentration 280
  increased relaxivity 280–1
  liver imaging 22–3
  see also contrast-enhanced (CE) MRA
Gadomer-17 280–1
gauss (G) **13**
GE sequences *see* gradient echo (GE) sequences
generalized autocalibrating partially parallel acquisitions (GRAPPA) **353**, 356–7, **359**, *362*
  SNR **361**
ghost artefacts 79, *218*
  evaluation 217
  Fourier imaging **132**, 133, *262*
  Nyquist (N/2) ghost 327, *328*, **329**, *330*
  respiratory **83**
  see also artefacts
ghost-to-signal ratio (GSR) 217
Gibb's artefact 99–100, **100**, *101*, 132, 247–8
glioma *34*, *43*, *309*
glutamate 308
glutamine 308
Golay coil configuration *174*, **174**
gradient echo (GE) sequences 32, 108–9, 144–6, 235–48
  3D GE sequences 246–8
  blood flow effect 86–8, 260
  contrast **40**, *68*
  family tree *222*
  PD-weighted images 40
  rewound 238, 243–5, **246**, *247*
  signal genesis 236–40
  signal strength calculation **69**
  spoiled 238, 240–3
  T_1-weighted images 32, 36–8
  T_2-weighted images 38–40
  terminology **237**
  time-reversed 245–6, **248**, *249*
  ultra-fast *see* ultra-fast GE sequences

gradient moment nulling 89, **90**, *91*, 261–2
gradient nonlinearities 104, 211
gradient pulses *see* pulse sequence
gradients 13–14, 110, 173–5
    amplifiers 174, 175
    dephasing **112**
    effects of *111*, **111**, *113*
    exposure standards 195–7
    linearity 174–5, *176*
    noise 195
    slew rates 174, **177**
    warping 175, *176*
GRAPPA (generalized autocalibrating partially parallel
    acquisitions) **353**, 356–7, **359**, *362*
    SNR **361**
GRASE (gradient and spin echo) **228**, 231–2, *236*
    k-space schemes **236**, *237*
GRASS (gradient recalled acquisition in the steady state)
    243
gridding **367**
gyromagnetic ratio 110, 138–139

Hadamard encoding 268
haemangioma *35*
haemodynamic delay in BOLD imaging **343**
Hahn echoes **238**, *239*, *240*, *241*
    amplitude **242**
half Fourier 76, 133
halo artefact *104*, 105
HASTE (half Fourier single shot TSE) 86, 231,
    364
hazards *see* safety
heart *33*
    see also cardiac MRI
helium, hyperpolarized 322, *323*
herring-bone artefact *104*, 105
high field systems **218**, **360**
hip imaging 24, *25*
history of medical imaging 2–4
homogeneity *see* magnetic field
hyoscine butylbromide 85–6
hyperbolic secant pulse **234**, *235*
hyperpolarized gases 322–4
    applications 323–4
    helium 322, *323*
    imaging considerations 322–3
    production **322**
    xenon 322
hypoperfusion 302

image artefacts *see* artefacts
image contrast *see* contrast
image display 57–8
image formation 108
    dephasing and rephasing 112
    Fourier imaging *see* Fourier transforms
    gradients 110
    image slice 113–17
        manipulation 116–17
        multiple slices 117, *119*
        oblique **117**
        rephasing 117
        selection of 113–16
    in-plane localization 117–27
        frequency encoding 123–5
        phase encoding 120–3
        spatial encoding 125–7
        spatial frequencies 117–20, *122*
    Larmor equation 109–10
    pulse sequence 108–9
    speeding up 133–5
        half Fourier 133
        rectangular field of view 133–5
        reduced matrix 133
image optimization 65–78
    basic parameters 65–9
        relationships between parameters 69–74
    contrast 74
    field of view 75
    scan time 75–6
image quality *see* quality assurance
image selective in vivo spectroscopy (ISIS) 319
image slices *see* image formation; slices
in-flow effect *see* time-of-flight (TOF) effect
inhomogeneity artefacts 79, **103**
Institute of Physics and Engineering in Medicine
    (IPEM) standards **205**
integrated parallel acquisition technique (iPAT) 357
inter echo spacing (IES) 224
internal auditory meatus (IAM) 96
international standards *see* standards
interventional MRI systems 189
intracerebral arteries 26
inversion recovery (IR) 40, *41*, **150**
    FSE 228–9
        interleaving 229, *230*
    normalized contrast behaviour *67*
    real-valued (true) IR 229, *230*
    signal strength calculation **69**

inversion time (TI) **150**
iPAT (integrated parallel acquisition technique) 357
iron oxide contrast agents *see* SPIO (super-paramagnetic iron oxide)
iron-cored electromagnets 169, **170**
ISIS (image selective in vivo spectroscopy) 319

J coupling 161–2

k-space 53, *54*, 129–30, **131**, 347
   cardiac imaging *294, 295, 297*
   contrast-enhanced MRA **276**, *278*
   GRASE **236**, *237*
   ordering schemes **252**, *253*
   PROPELLER *370*
   radial imaging *367*
   shutter 133
   signal and resolution information *55*
   SMASH 351–6, **358**
   spiral imaging **370**, *371*
   turbo-FLASH *252*
k-t BLAST (broad-use linear acquisition speed-up technique) 357–9, *361*
key-hole technique **253**, *255*
knee imaging 24, *26, 33, 36*
   meniscal tear *35*

lactate (Lac) 307
laminar flow 260–1
Larmor equation 109–10, 138
   derivation **138**, **139**
Lauterbur, P. 2–3, **5**, *6*
line spread function (LSF) **213**
   derivation *213*
linearity 211
   nonlinearities 104, 211
lipoma *34*
liver imaging 21–3, *33*
   tumour *44*
look-up table (LUT) 57–8
low-pass filter **51**

magnetic field
   field strength **13**, 168
      BOLD effect and **345**
      SNR and **13**, **208–9**
      strength–duration (SD) curve **197**
   fringe field 15–16, 189, *190*
   hazards 15–16

occupational exposure **199**
   shielding 172, 190
   see also bio-effects of magnetic fields
magnetic moment 139–41
   measurement of 141–4
magnetic resonance angiography (MRA) 21, 44–5, 63–4
   3D CE-MRA 25–7
   bolus chase MRA 27
   contrast-enhanced *see* contrast-enhanced (CE) MRA
   difficulties **45**
   peripheral 27, 277–8
   phase contrast 265–70, *271*
      2D 269–70, *272*
      3D 270, *273*
   time-of-flight MRA 263–5
      2D TOF 263–5
      3D TOF 265, **267**, *268*
magnetic resonance spectroscopy (MRS) 306–24
   basic chemistry 307–8
   carbon spectroscopy 321
   challenges **309**
   chemical shift imaging 318–19, *320*
      technical difficulties **320**
   dementia 308
   fluorine spectroscopy 321–2
   hyperpolarized gases 322–4
      applications 323–4
      helium 322, *323*
      imaging considerations 322–3
      xenon 322
   multiple sclerosis 310
   phosphorus spectroscopy 319–21
   quality assurance 218–19
   single-voxel spectroscopy 310–13
      PRESS 313, *314*, **315**, 319
      processing 316–18
      STEAM 310, *311*, **315**, 319
      voxel positioning 313, *315*
   stroke 308
   terminology **306**
   tumours 308–10
magnetization prepared rapid acquisition by gradient echo (MP-RAGE) 252–3, *254*
magnetization transfer (MT) 161, **162**, *163*, **266**, *267*
   MT contrast (MTC) *161*
magneto-hydrodynamic effect 198
magnets 167–72
   field strength **13**, 168
   homogeneity **13**, 168

magnets (*cont.*)
  quenches 12–13, 171
  shielding 172, 190
  shimming 171–2
  types of 12–13, 169–71
    electromagnets 12, 169, **170**
    permanent 12, 169, **170**
    resistive 12, 169, *170*
    superconducting *1*, 12–13, 169–71, **171**, *172*
Maki artefact 100
Mansfield, P. **5**, *6*
matrices 51–6
  reduced matrix 76, 133
  size, field of view and **70**
maximum intensity projection (MIP) 45, 64, 263, **264**
Maxwell pair *174*, **174**
MDE (myocardial delayed-enhancement) imaging 303–4
mean transit time (MTT) 335
medical imaging, history 2–4
metal artefacts 101–3
MIP *see* maximum intensity projection (MIP)
modified SENSE (mSENSE) 349–50, *352*
  artefacts 361, *365*
  SNR **361**
modulation transfer function (MTF) **213**
Moiré fringes **103**
motion artefacts *see* artefacts
MOTSA (multiple overlapping thin slab acquisitions) 26, **267**, *268*
MP-RAGE (magnetization prepared rapid acquisition by gradient echo) 252–3, *254*
MR cholangiopancreatography (MRCP) 22
MR equipment 167–91
  computer system 14, 188
  open systems 188–9
  siting and installation 189–91
    environment 190–1
    fringe field 15–16, 189, *190*
    RF shielding 190
  see also gradients; magnets; radiofrequency (RF) system
MR unit 11–15
  layout *12*
  patient's journey through 18–19
  safety *see* safety
  typical working week 27–9
MRA *see* magnetic resonance angiography (MRA)
MRCP *see* MR cholangiopancreatography (MRCP)
MRS *see* magnetic resonance spectroscopy (MRS)
MS 325 C 280

multi-shot EPI 328–9
multi-slice imaging 62–4
multiple overlapping thin slab acquisitions (MOTSA) 26, **267**, *268*
multiple sclerosis (MS) *42*, 310
multiple spin echo 223
myo-inositol (mI) 308
myocardial delayed-enhancement (MDE) imaging 303–4
myocardial perfusion 21, 300–3
myocardial perfusion reserve index (MPRI) 302
myocardial tagging 296–8
myocardial viability 303–4
myocardial/blood contrast 296

N-acetyl aspartate (NAA) 307
N/2 ghost 327, *328*, **329**, *330*
National Electrical Manufacturers Association (NEMA)
  image quality standards **205**, **206**
  SNR measurement method 205, **207**, 210
navigator echoes 83, *84*, **285**, *286*
noise 66, **69**
  acoustic, safety issues 16
  gradient 195
  measurement **209**
  see also contrast-to-noise ratio (CNR); signal-to-noise ratio (SNR)
noise figure (NF) **186**
nonlinearities 104, 211
nuclear magnetic resonance (NMR) 1, 2, 137–41
  classical mechanics explanation 137–8
  early history **4**
  quantum mechanics explanation 139–41
number of signal acquisitions (NSA), increasing 81
number of signal averages (NSA) 73
number of signal excitations (NEX) 73
Nyquist frequency **50**, *52*
Nyquist (N/2) ghost 327, *328*, **329**, *330*
Nyquist theorem 49

occupational exposure to magnetic fields *199*, **199**
open MRI systems 188–9
optic nerve *64*
optimization *see* image optimization
out-of-phase scanning (OOPS) 91
oversampling **51**, *52*, 99, *100*

parallel imaging 76, 185, 346–72
  artefacts 361, *365*
  clinical benefits of 359–60

coil sensitivity profiles 348, *353*, *354–5*
GRAPPA **353**, 356–7, **359**, **361**, *362*
high field systems and **360**
image quality 360–4
k-space 347
k-t BLAST 357–9, *361*
non-Cartesian acquisition schemes 364–71
  2D radial imaging 366
  3D radial imaging 366–7
  applications 368
  PROPELLER 368–9, *371*
  spiral imaging 369–71, *372*, **372**
parallel EPI **364**, *366*
phase encoding 347
phased arrays 347
SENSE 348–50, *351*, *362–3*
  calibration **353**
  maths **350**
  modified (mSENSE) 349–50, *352*, 361, *365*
SMASH 351–6, **358**
  auto-calibrating 353–6
paramagnetic materials **39**
partial volume effects **60**, *61*, 96–8
patient handling system 14–15
PD-weighted images 35, *36*, 40
  timing parameters **36**
pelvic imaging 23–4
perfusion imaging 335–40
  arterial spin labelling (ASL) 338–40
    analysis **340**
  dynamic susceptibility contrast MRI (DSC-MRI) 336–8
  quantification **337**
  see also myocardial perfusion
periodically rotated overlapping parallel lines with
    enhanced reconstruction (PROPELLER) 368–9, *371*
peripheral MRA 27, 277–8
peripheral nerve stimulation (PNS) 194
peripheral pulse gating (PPG) 85, *86*, *284*, 285
peristaltic motion artefacts *80*, 85–6
permanent magnets 12, 169, **170**
PGSE (pulsed gradient spin echo) 329–31
phantoms 20
  contrast-detail detectability *217*
  filling factors **207**
  geometric 211
    distortion measurement *212*
  MRS 218–19
  problems with **219**
  spectroscopy 307

phase cancellation artefact 90–1, *94*
phase contrast angiography 265–70, *271*
  2D 269–70, *272*
  3D 270, *273*
phase encoding (PE) 120–3, 221, 347, **356**
  axis selection **54**
  matrix 51–6
phase sampling artefacts 98–100
  Gibb's artefact 99–100, **100**, *101*, 132
  phase wrap-around artefact 98–9, *100*, **100**
  ringing artefact 100, 132
phased array coils 185, 347
  coil sensitivity profiles 348, *353*, *354–5*
phosphorus spectroscopy 319–21
photoplethysmograph 285
pixels 47, *48*, 56, 57–61
plug flow 260
point-resolved spectroscopy (PRESS) 219, 313, *314*, 319
  versus STEAM **315**
polarization 179–80
  linear 179–80, *184*
positron emission tomography (PET) 2
Pound, R. 5
pre-amplifiers 185–6
pre-scan 186–8
presaturation bands 261
PRESS (point-resolved spectroscopy) 219, 313, *314*,
  319
  versus STEAM **315**
PRESTO sequence 336
progressive saturation **267**, *268*
projection reconstruction (PR) 364–5
PROPELLER (periodically rotated overlapping parallel
    lines with enhanced reconstruction) 368–9, *371*
prostate cancer 23
proton density (PD) 31
  PD-weighted images 35, *36*, 40
protons 137
  behaviour in an external magnetic field 137–41
  energy states **140**
  exchange **160**
  spectroscopy 307
    challenges **309**
PSIF sequence 245
pulse programmer (PP) 188
pulse sequence 13, 31, 108–9
  conversion chart *256–7*
  family tree 221–2
  physiology of 221

pulse sequence (*cont.*)

   see also gradient echo (GE) sequences; radiofrequency

       (RF) pulses; spin echo (SE) sequences

pulse width modulated (PWM) voltage supplies **177**

pulsed gradient spin echo (PGSE) 329–31

Purcell, E **4**, **5**, *6*

quadrature coils 180

quadrature detection **187**

quality assurance (QA) 203

   fat suppression 217–18

   geometric parameters 211–16

      distortion 211

      linearity 211

      resolution 212–14

      slice parameters 214–16

   ghosting 217

   high-field systems **218**

   quality cycle 204

   relaxation parameters 216

   signal parameters 204–11

      SNR 204–10

      uniformity 210–11

   specialized programmes **218**

   standards **205–6**

   see also phantoms

quantum mechanics (QM) 137–8, 139–41, **144**

quenches 12–13, 171

radial imaging 366–8

   2D 366

   3D 366–7

   applications 368

   sampling **368**

radiofrequency (RF) coils 13, *14*, **181**, **185**

   arrays 13, 185, 347

   body coil 13

   circularly polarized (CP)/quadrature coils 180

   receiver coil 13, 181–3

   surface coils 183

   transmitter coil 13, 178–9

   uniformity 210–11

radiofrequency (RF) pulses 31, **32**, **233**

   adiabatic pulses 96, **234**

   binomial pulses 96, **234**

   effect of 142–3

   hyperbolic secant pulse **234**, *235*

   ramped excitation pulses **267**

   see also pulse sequence

radiofrequency (RF) system 175–88

   polarization 179–80

   pre-amplifier 185–6

   pre-scan 186–8

   receiver 186

   shields 185, 190

   transmitter 177–8

   see also radiofrequency (RF) coils

radiographer, week in the life of 27–9

radiology, history of 2

real functions **133**

receive bandwidth **51**, *52*

receiver 186

receiver coils 13, 181–3

rectangular field of view (RFOV) 76, 133–5

reduced matrix 76, 133

regridding 366, **367**, *368*

relaxation times 148–53

   BPP relaxation theory 155, 160

   measurement 161–2

      biological variability 161

      field strength/temperature dependence 161

      J coupling 161–2

      magnetization transfer 161

      multi-exponential behaviour 161

      sources of error 162

   mechanisms 153–60

   T_1 (spin–lattice) 31, 151–3, *155*, 156–9

   T_2 (spin–spin) 31, 149–51, *155*, *156*, 159–60

renal arteries 27, *45*

repetition time *see* TR (repetition time)

rephasing 112, *113*, 117

resistive magnets 12, 169, *170*

resolution 69, 212

   effect on image quality 71–3, *72*, **74**

   field of view relationship 127, **129**

   limits **214**

   measurement 212–14

   optimization 75

   scan time and 71

   signal-to-noise ratio and 69–71, **71**

resonance condition 138, 141

resonant offset averaging steady state (ROAST) **246**

resonant offsets **246**, *248*

respiratory gating 81–2

respiratory motion artefacts *80*, 81–3, **83**, 285

   avoidance 81–3, **83**

      breath-hold cine imaging 296, *297*, *298*

      cardiac imaging 285, 293, *295*, *297*, *298*

navigator echoes 83, *84*, **285**, *286*
  respiratory compensation 81–3
  respiratory gating 81–2
respiratory-ordered phase encoding (ROPE) *81*,
    82–3
retrospective gating 290–1, *292*
rewound gradient echo 238, 243–5, **246**, *247*
RF *see* radiofrequency (RF) pulses, radiofrequency (RF)
    system
rheobase values *197*
ringing artefact 100, 132
ROAST (resonant offset averaging steady state) **246**
ROPE (respiratory-ordered phase encoding) *81*,
    82–3
rotating frame of reference **141**, **143**

saddle coil 179, *180*
safety 15–18, 192–201
  acoustic noise protection 16
  burns **17**
  contrast agents 16–17
  cryogen contact 16
  magnetic field hazards 15–17
    fringe field 15–16, 189, *190*
  occupational exposure **199**
  standards **17**, 193
    gradient exposure 195–7
    RF exposure 193, *194*
    static field exposure 198–200
  see also bio-effects of magnetic fields
sampling frequency **49**, *50*
SAR *see* specific absorption rate (SAR)
saturation bands 88–9, **117**
scan time
  optimization 75–6
  resolution and 71
SE sequences *see* spin echo (SE) sequences
selective excitation 3, 113–16
SENSE (sensitivity encoding) 185, 277, 348–50, *351*,
    362–3
  artefacts *365*
  calibration **353**
  maths **350**
  modified (mSENSE) 349–50, *352*
    artefacts 361, *365*
  SNR **361**
shaded surface display 64
shielding 172, 190
shimming 171–2, **306**, **310**, 313

dynamic **173**
  effects of *315*
  fixed **173**
short TI inversion recovery *see* STIR
shoulder imaging *23*, 24
signal averaging 73
signal-to-noise ratio (SNR) 65, 66
  absolute (ASNR) **209**
  definition **66**
  effect of parameter changes *75*
  effect on image quality 71–4
  improving 77
  magnetic field strength and **13**, **208–9**
  measurement 204–10
    NEMA method 204–5
    signal-background method 204, *205*
  parallel imaging 360–1
  prediction of **74**
  resolution and 69–71, **71**
simultaneous acquisition of spatial harmonics (SMASH)
    185, 277, 351–6, **358**
  auto-calibration 353–6
sine waves 376–7
single photon emission computed tomography (SPECT) 2
single-shot FSE 86, 230–1
single-voxel spectroscopy *see* magnetic resonance
    spectroscopy (MRS)
slew rates **177**
slices
  excitation profile *98*, **98**
  gaps 62, *63*, **63**
  multiple 117, *119*
  oblique **117**
  optimization 76–7
  orientation *56*, 57, 116–17
  position 214, *215*
  profile *215*, **216**
  quality assurance 214–16
  selection 113–16
    maths **116**
  thickness 56, 77, 116–17, *118*, 214–16
SMASH (simultaneous acquisition of spatial harmonics)
    185, 277, 351–6, **358**
  auto-calibrating 353–6
SNR *see* signal-to-noise ratio (SNR)
solenoidal coil 179, *180*
SPAMM (spatial modulation of magnetization) 296
spatial encoding 125–7
spatial frequencies 117–20, *122*

specific absorption rate (SAR) 16, 193
  limits *194*
  maths **193**
  reducing 193, 227
SPECT (single photon emission computed tomography)
  2
spectra 307–8
spectral density function *159*, **159**
spectral inversion at lipid (SPECIAL) 95
spectral inversion recovery (SPIR) 95
SPEEDER 348, **353**
spin echo (SE) sequences 32, *34*, 146–7, 222–32, **223**
  blood flow effect 86–8, 259–60
  contrast 37, *67*
  echo planar imaging (SE-EPI) 231–2, *233*, *236*
  family tree *222*
  fast SE (FSE) *see* fast spin echo (FSE)
  multiple spin echo 223
  pulse sequence options *221*
  pulsed gradient spin echo (PGSE) 329–31
  runners on a track analogy 148
  signal strength calculation **69**
  T$_1$-weighted images 32, **33**
  T$_2$-weighted images 33
spin–lattice (T$_1$) relaxation time 31, 151–3, *155*
  field strength/temperature dependence 161
  measurement **150**
  mechanisms 153–4, 156–9
  see also relaxation times
spin–spin (T$_2$) relaxation time 31, 149–51, *155*,
    156
  measurement **149**
  mechanisms 153–5, 159–60
  see also relaxation times
spinal imaging 20
SPIO (super-paramagnetic iron oxide) 43, *44*, 163–6, **207**,
    281
  ultra-small particles (USPIO) 281
SPIR (spectral inversion recovery) 95
spiral imaging 369–71, *372*
  problems **372**
  spiral EPI 329
spoiled gradient echo 238, 240–3
spoiling 240–1, *243*, *244*
  artefacts from insufficient spoiling *243*, *244*
staircase effect 63, *64*
standards
  image quality **205–6**
  safety **17**, 193, *194*, 195–7, 198–200

STEAM (stimulated echo acquisition mode) 219, 310, *311*,
    319
  versus PRESS **315**
stimulated echoes 238, **239**, *241*, **311**, *312*
STIR (short TI inversion recovery) 40–1, 228
  breast imaging 20
  fat suppression 41, **42**, 92, 95
streak artefacts *370*
strength–duration (SD) curve **197**
stress, pharmacological **301**
stroke 308, *309*, *335*
sum-of-square technique 185
super-paramagnetic materials **39**
  see also SPIO (super-paramagnetic iron oxide)
superconducting magnets *1*, 12–13, 169–71, **171**, *172*
surface coils 183
surface rendering 64
susceptibility **102**
susceptibility artefacts **13**, 38, 101–3

T$_1$ spin–lattice relaxation time 31, 151–3, *155*
  field strength/temperature dependence 161
  measurement **150**
  mechanisms 153–4, 156–9
  reduction **273**, *274*
  see also relaxation times
T$_1$-weighted images 32, *33*, *34*, 39
  angiographic images 44–5
  GE images 32, 36–8
  sequence timing effect **33**
T$_2$ blurring 130
T$_2$ spin–spin relaxation time 31, 149–51, *155*, *156*
  measurement **149**
  mechanisms 153–5, 159–60
  see also relaxation times
T$_2$-weighted images 33, *35*, 39
  gadolinium effect **44**
  GE images 38–40
  sequence timing effect **35**
T$_2^*$ effective spin – spin relaxation time 32, 38, *39*, 40, 148,
    see also gradient echo (GE) sequences
TE (echo time) 31, *32*, *33*
  effective 226
  ultra short TE (UTE) 368, *369*
tesla (T) **13**
thoracic aorta 24–5
'three brains' artefact 328
three-dimensional (3D) imaging 61–4
  3D CE-MRA 25–7

3D Fourier transform imaging (3D FT) 113, 135–6, 236
3D FSE **231**
3D GE sequences 246–8
3D radial imaging 366–7
angiography
    phase contrast (3D PC) 270, 273
    time-of-flight (TOF) 265, **267**, *268*
versus 2D imaging 74, **135**
TI inversion time *see* inversion time (TI)
tilted optimized nonsaturating excitation (TONE) **267**
time resolved imaging of contrast kinetics (TRICKS) 277
time-of-flight (TOF) effect *44, 45*, 259–60
time-of-flight (TOF) MR angiography 263–5
2D TOF 263–5
3D TOF 265
    progressive saturation **267**, *268*
time-reversed gradient echo 245–6, **248**, *249*
tissues
    BPP relaxation theory 160
    classification of 30
    magnetic properties of **39**
    relaxation times *155*
TOF *see* time-of-flight (TOF)
TONE (tilted optimized nonsaturating excitation) **267**
TR (repetition time) 31, *32*, **33**, 153–5
transcranial magnetic stimulation (TMS) **195**
transmit coils 13, 178–9
transmitters 177–8, *179*
TRICKS (time resolved imaging of contrast kinetics) 277
true FISP 244–5, *247*
tumours 308–10
turbo gradient spin echo (TGSE) *see* GRASE
turbo spin echo (TSE) *see* fast spin echo (FSE)
turbo-FLASH (TFL) 249–52, *253*
two-dimensional (2D) imaging
    2D Fourier transform imaging (2D FT) 3, 73, 113
        encoding for **128**
        image reconstruction 127
        resolution and field of view 127
    2D radial imaging 366
    angiography

phase contrast (2D PC) 269–70, *272*
time-of-flight (TOF) 263–4
versus 3D imaging 74, **135**

ultra short TE (UTE) 368, *369*
ultra-fast GE sequences 248–54
    GE echo planar imaging (GE-EPI) 253–4, *255*
    MP-RAGE 252–3, *254*
    terminology **250**
    turbo-FLASH 249–52
ultrasound 2
uninterruptible power supplies (UPS) 191

variable density Auto-SMASH (VD-Auto-SMASH) 356
vastly undersampled isotropic projection reconstruction
    (VIPR) 366–7
vector cardiac gating (VCG) 283
vectors 375–6
velocity compensation 261–2, *263*
velocity encoding (venc) 266, **269**, *270, 272*
velocity mapping 298–300, *301*
viability imaging *see* MDE (myocardial delayed-
    enhancement) imaging
VIPR (vastly undersampled isotropic projection
    reconstruction) 366–7
volume rendering 64
voxel bleed **316**
voxels 47, 56, 58–60
    partial volume effect **60**, *61*
    positioning 313, *315*

water binding **159**
window level 58, *59*
window width 58, *59*

xenon, hyperpolarized 322

Z-score 343
zebra stripes **103**
zero-filling 133, **135**, *317*
zipper artefact 103